my brush with depression

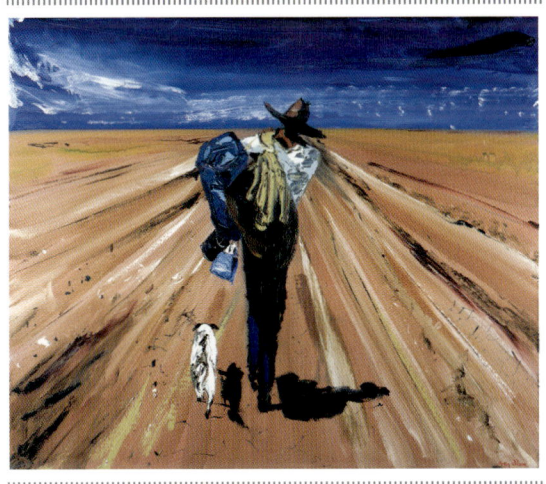

aaron cootes   greg wilson

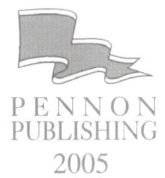

PENNON
PUBLISHING
2005

Greg and I would like to dedicate this book to the memory of those who have lost their fight with mental illness. To those that are still fighting, our thoughts are with you, please don't give up. With each new day comes hope.

I first met Greg Wilson four years ago, when I was invited to open his art gallery in the Hunter Valley, in New South Wales. As I wandered around looking at Greg's art, I realised the paintings and sculpture were about so much more than just art; this is because of the story and the dreams of the man behind the artwork. Greg Wilson's personal experience is nothing short of inspirational. Greg developed a mental illness after surviving a terrible motorcycle accident when he was twenty-four years of age. He turned to art to help himself survive. The extraordinary paintings and sculptures he created were just the beginning of an exciting and rewarding journey. Greg wasn't content to enjoy the spoils of his art career, instead he began using his talents to fight the stigma and fear surrounding mental illness.

This path has taken him around the world, where he has bravely shared his personal story, to ensure others don't feel alone in their suffering.

But Greg didn't embark on this journey by himself. His story is also about the bonds of love and friendship. Greg has been surrounded by an inspiring bunch of people, among them his partner Josie, and his best friend Aaron. These beautiful people have stood right beside Greg and helped him survive his rocky journey.

I feel incredibly proud to call this group of people my friends. And my life is so much richer now they're in it. And I'm sure that as readers, you will also feel richer for having shared in the story of Greg Wilson and his 'family'.

Jessica Rowe, March 2005

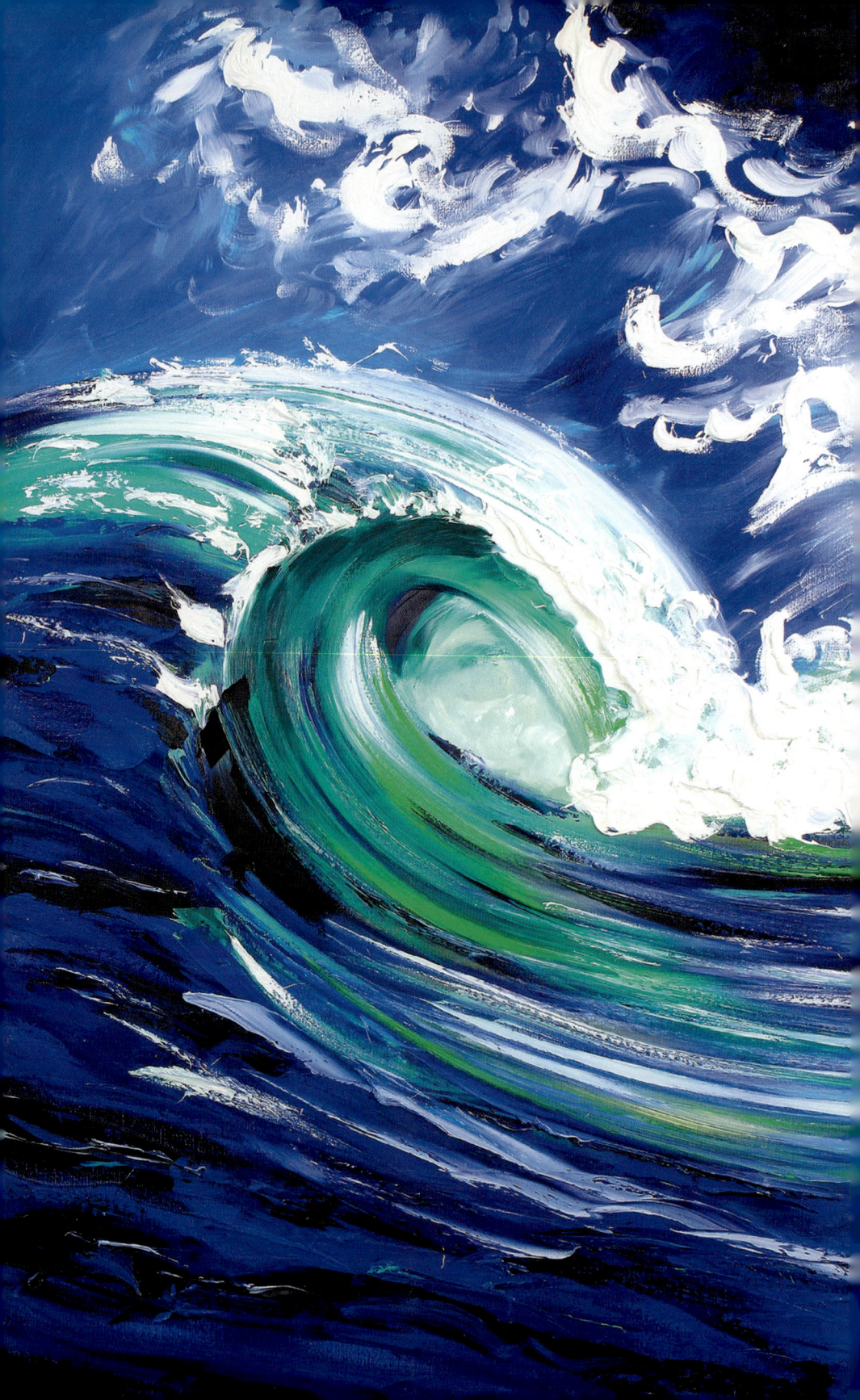

Greg and I would like to thank our inspiration, Josie and Joyce. Without your help this book would not exist. We love you both. Special thanks also to our dear friend Barbara Williams. Your selfless dedication and example, helping not only Greg but also those afflicted with depression, have been a shining light in the darkness.
I would like to dedicate this book to 'Me Darlin' grandmother who has left this world but whose loving memories remain.
Thanks also to: Andy and Kerrie Chrysillou, Bill and Trish Tilley, Michael and Soraya Salvatico, Robert and Simone Miletic, Don Champagne, John Tyrrell (our adopted brother), Kavita Payall, Jonathon Alder, Ken and Jenny Hipwell, Maria Biviano and Councillor John Clarence, mayor of Cessnock. Your understanding, your encouragement and your support have given Greg great assistance throughout his troubled journey. If the world had in it more people like all of you, what a wonderful place it would be.
Aaron would like to acknowledge his mentor, the immensely talented and influential writer, Ernest Hemingway, for the lasting impression his work has made on the world – his books and his legacy continue to be a source of inspiration for young authors.
Finally we would like to thank Bev Friend and Allan Cornwell from Pennon Publishing for taking a risk and for believing in our story.

Opposite
'Wave of Emotion' – Oil on linen 1525 x 1010 mm
At times the ocean can seem wild and threatening. The wave can make you feel fearful, yet the same wave can envelop you, roll you around, and then wash you to the shore – it becomes gentle – this is life – Greg Wilson.

Following pages
'Spring Bloom' – Oil on linen, 510 x 760 mm

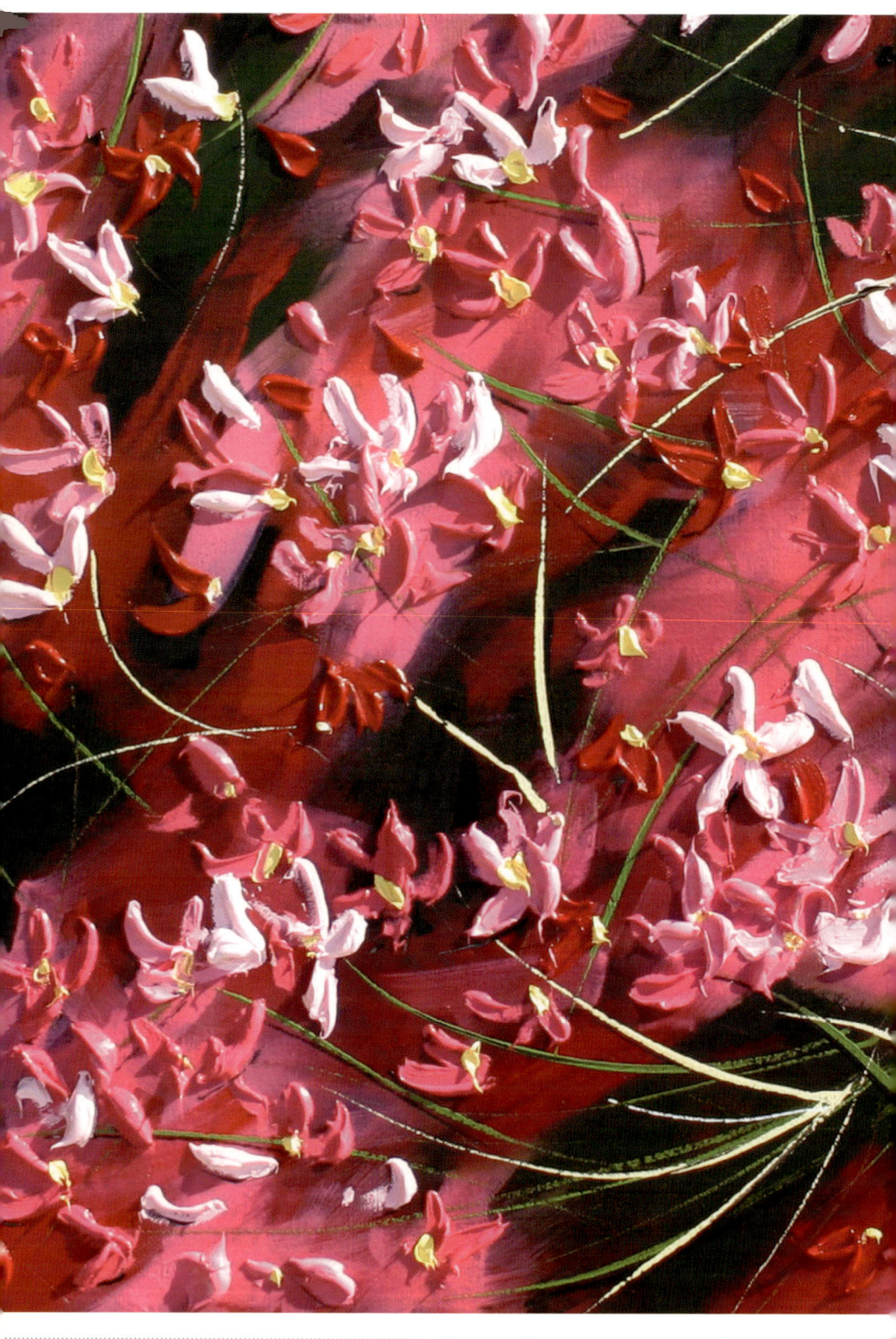

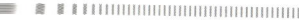

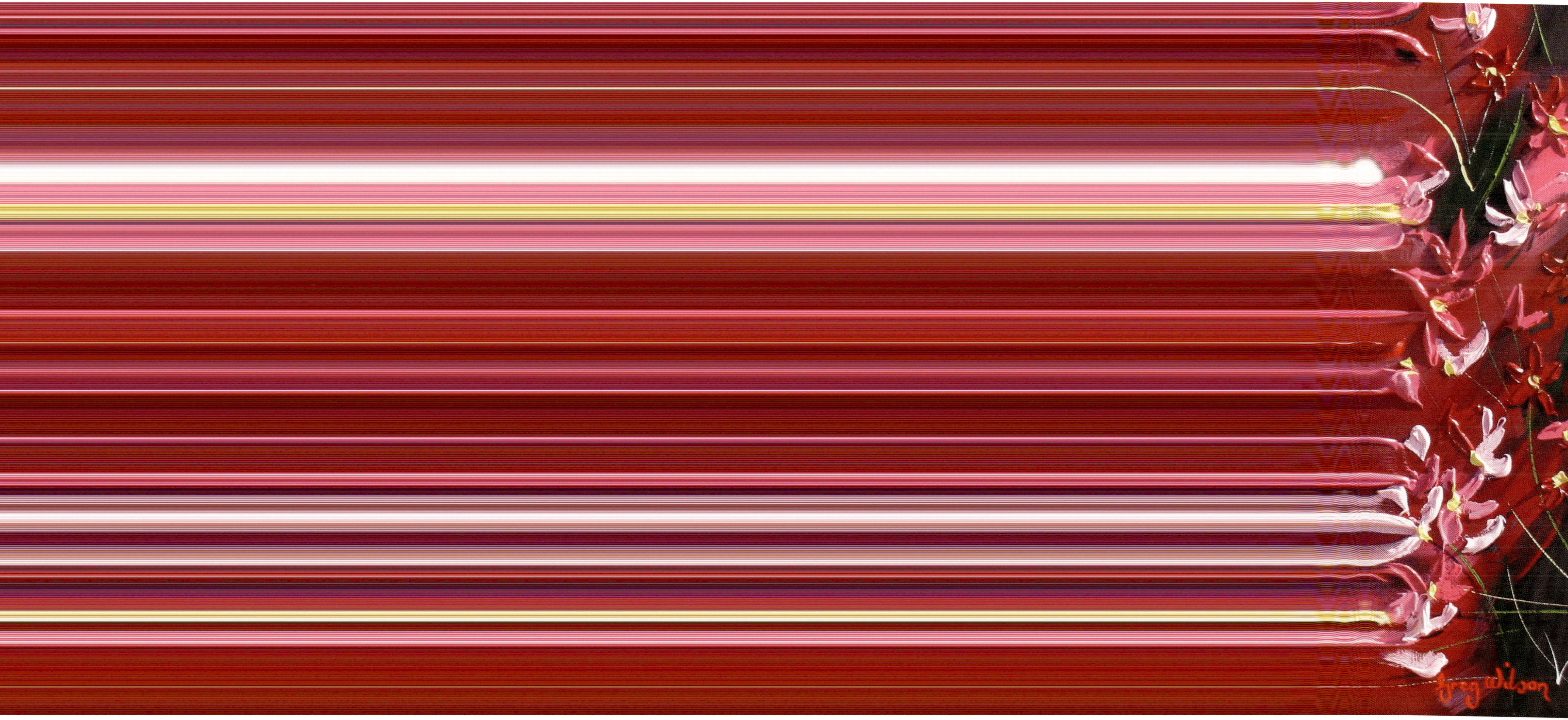

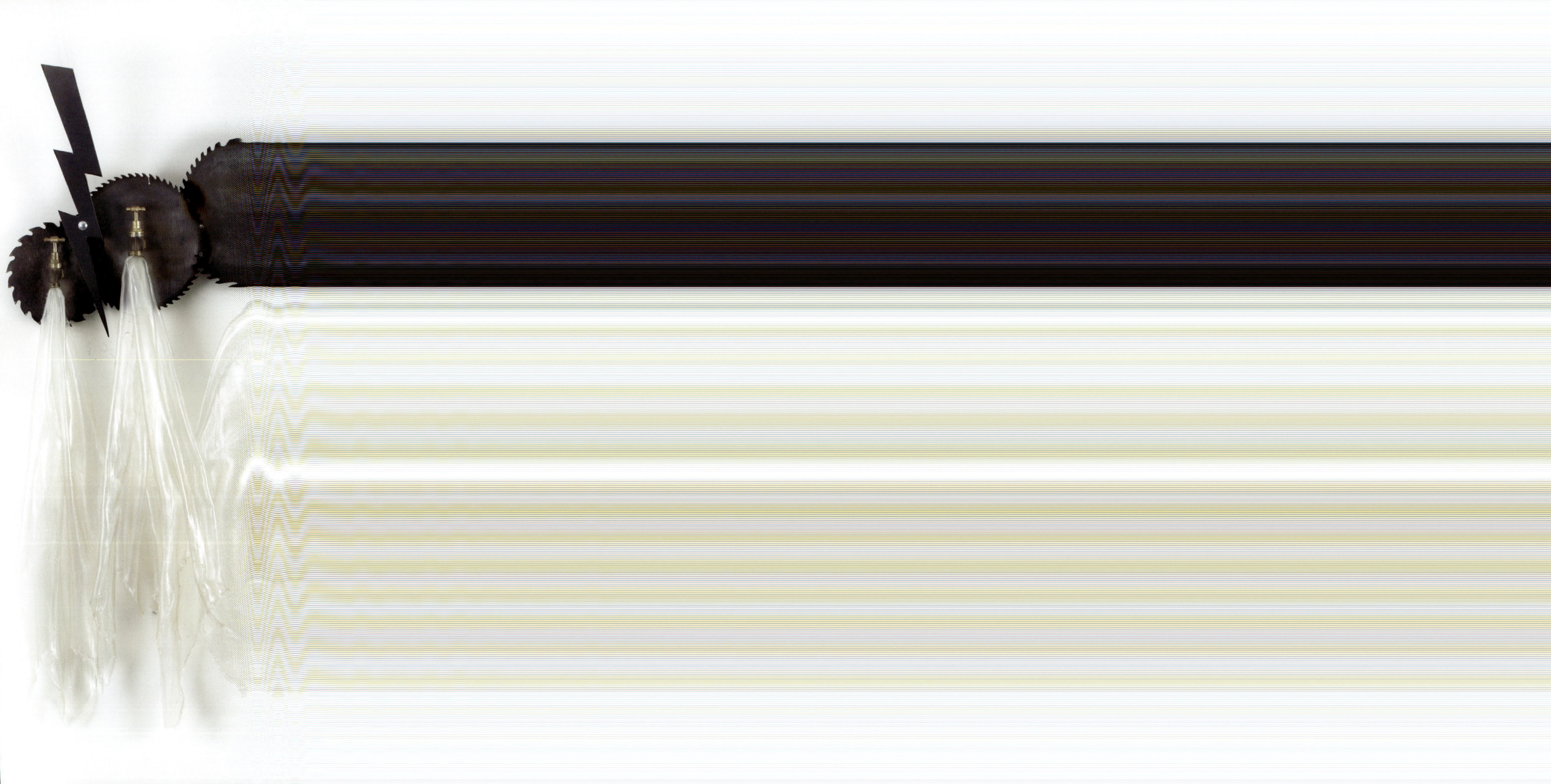

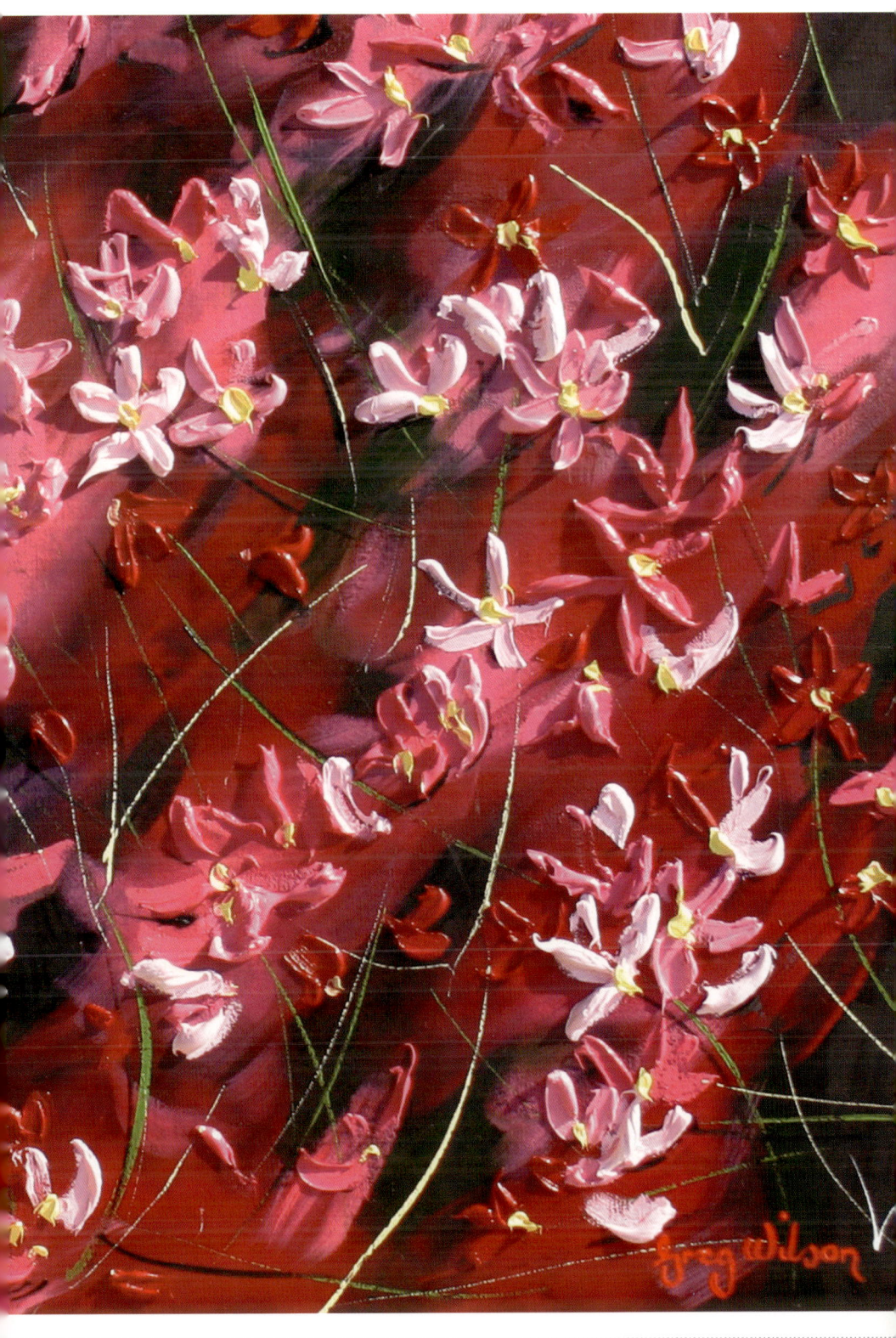

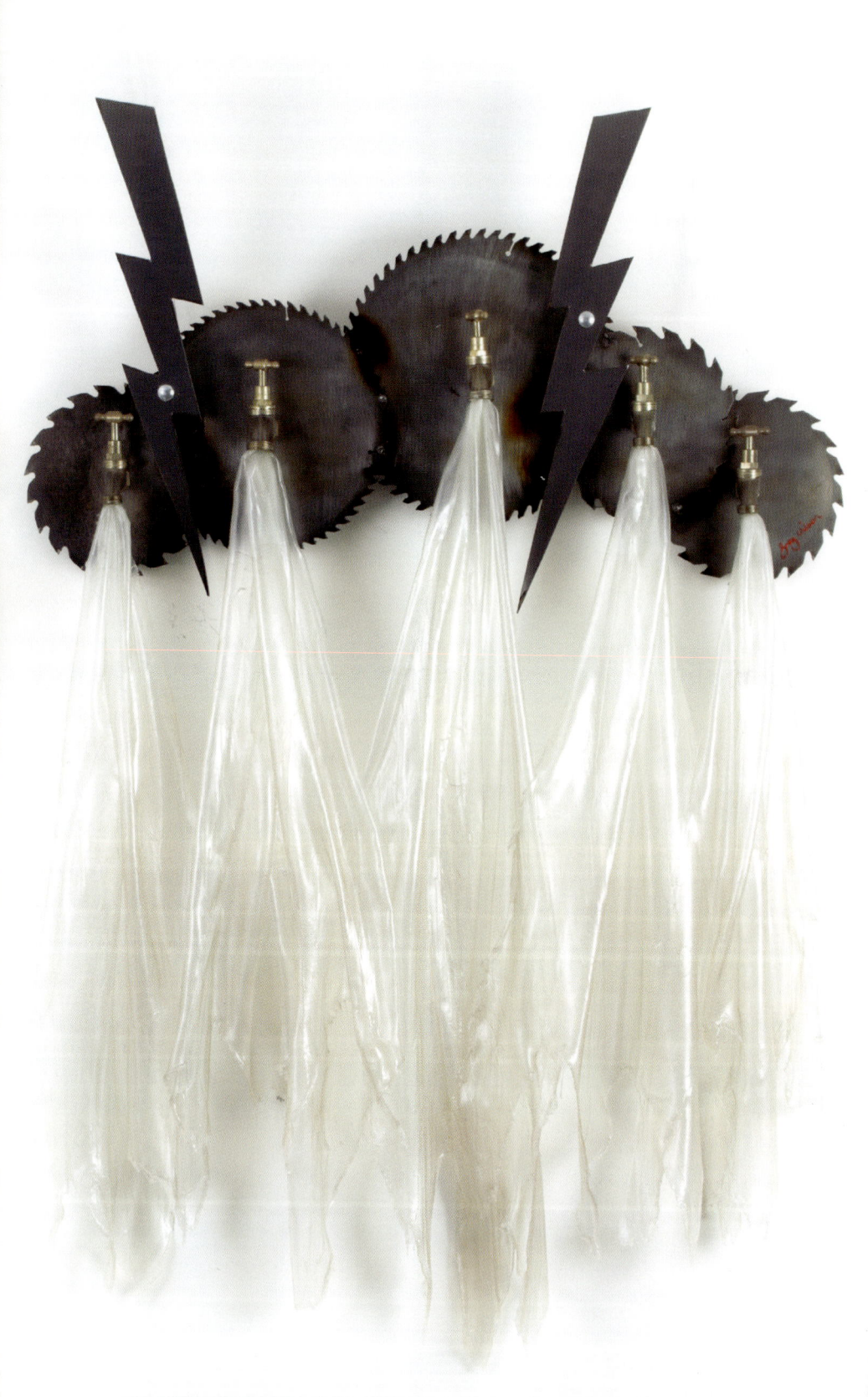

Greg and I would like to thank our inspiration, Josie and Joyce. Without your help this book would not exist. We love you both. Special thanks also to our dear friend Barbara Williams. Your selfless dedication and example, helping not only Greg but also those afflicted with depression, have been a shining light in the darkness.
I would like to dedicate this book to 'Me Darlin' grandmother who has left this world but whose loving memories remain.
Thanks also to: Andy and Kerrie Chrysillou, Bill and Trish Tilley, Michael and Soraya Salvatico, Robert and Simone Miletic, Don Champagne, John Tyrrell (our adopted brother), Kavita Payall, Jonathon Alder, Ken and Jenny Hipwell, Maria Biviano and Councillor John Clarence, mayor of Cessnock. Your understanding, your encouragement and your support have given Greg great assistance throughout his troubled journey. If the world had in it more people like all of you, what a wonderful place it would be.
Aaron would like to acknowledge his mentor, the immensely talented and influential writer, Ernest Hemingway, for the lasting impression his work has made on the world – his books and his legacy continue to be a source of inspiration for young authors.
Finally we would like to thank Bev Friend and Allan Cornwell from Pennon Publishing for taking a risk and for believing in our story.

Opposite
'Wave of Emotion' – Oil on linen 1525 x 1010 mm
At times the ocean can seem wild and threatening. The wave can make you feel fearful, yet the same wave can envelop you, roll you around, and then wash you to the shore – it becomes gentle – this is life – Greg Wilson.

Following pages
'Spring Bloom' – Oil on linen, 510 x 760 mm

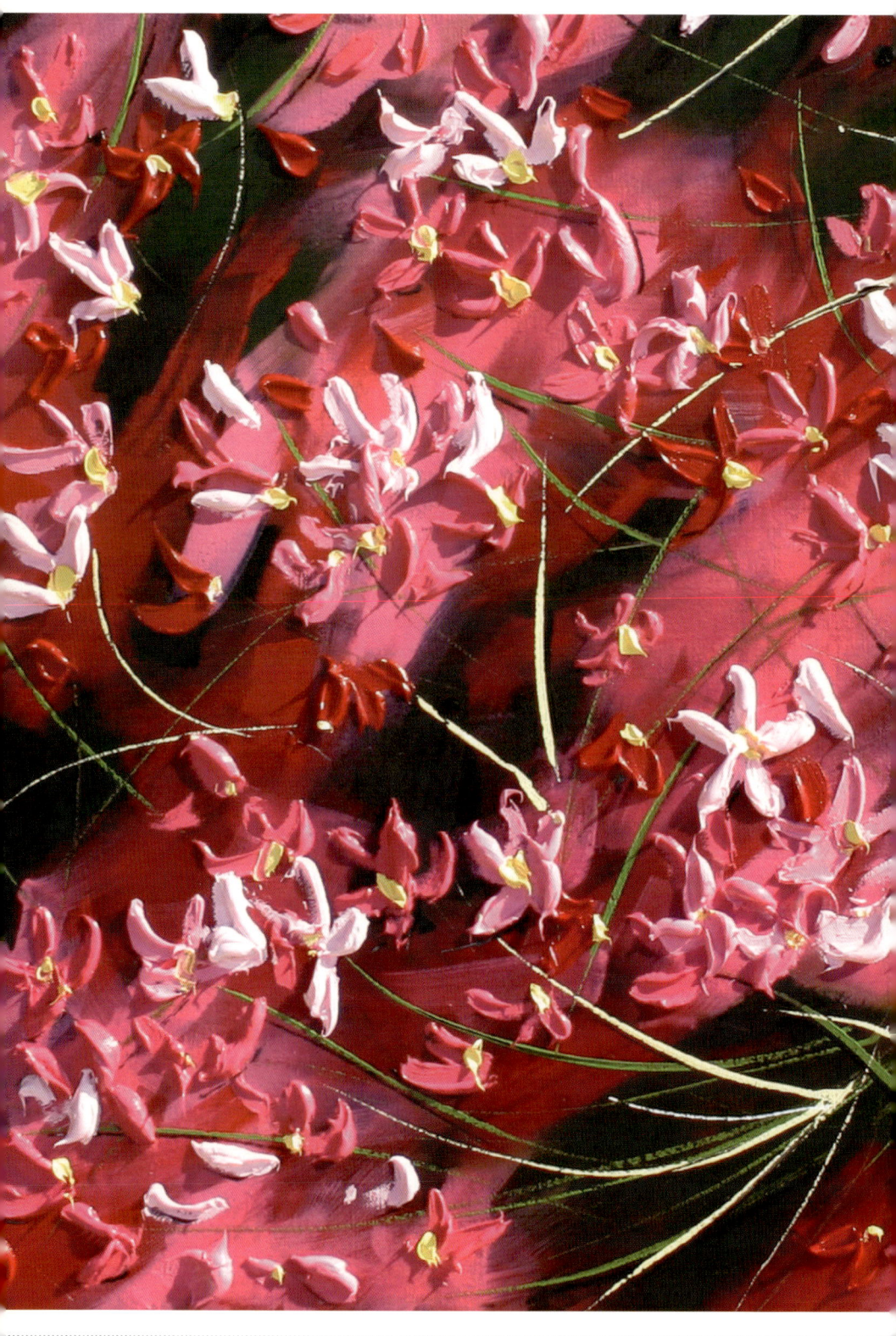

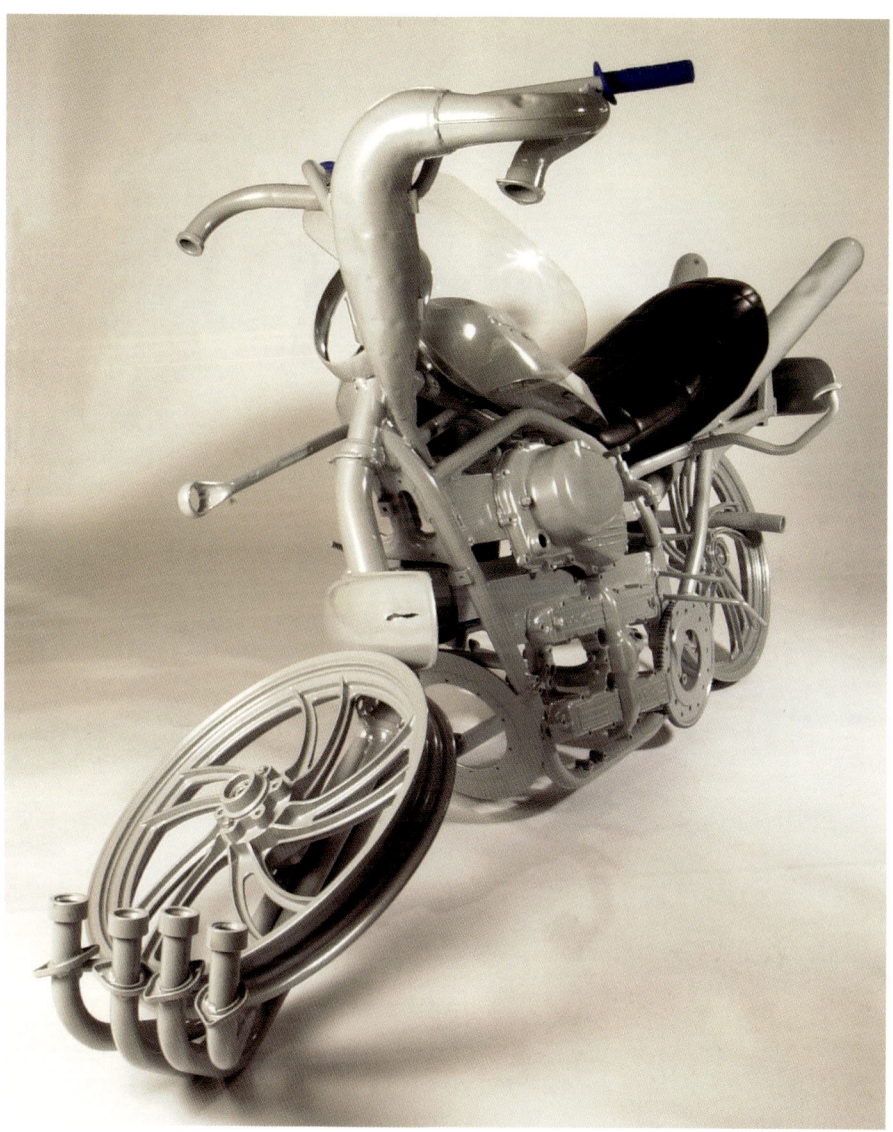

Left:
'The Cutting Storm'
Resin, stainless steel brass taps, saw blades 1480 X 1030 mm
Saw blades and sharp streaks of lightning in *The Cutting Storm* represent the pain suffered during his motorcycle accidents and the depression that came later. They also signify the terrible cuts Greg received as a result of the accidents – several major surgical procedures that left his neck, legs and arms badly scarred.

Above:
'Grey Days'
Clear coated, sealed and painted motorbike parts, seat and visor, tap 1130 x 2470 x 850 mm
'When you have depression you see life as greys, there's no colour, it's almost like the colour is taken out of life.'

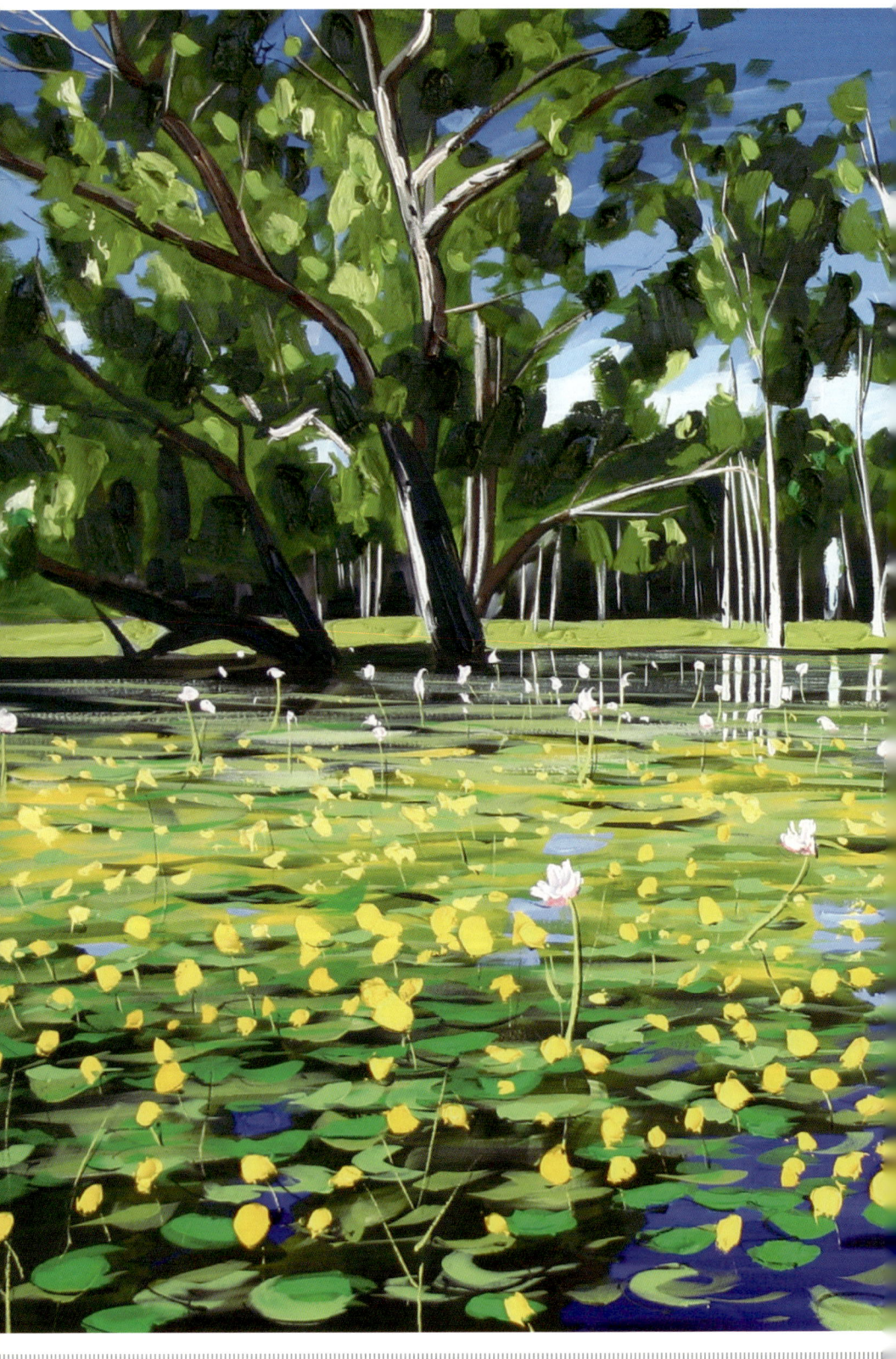

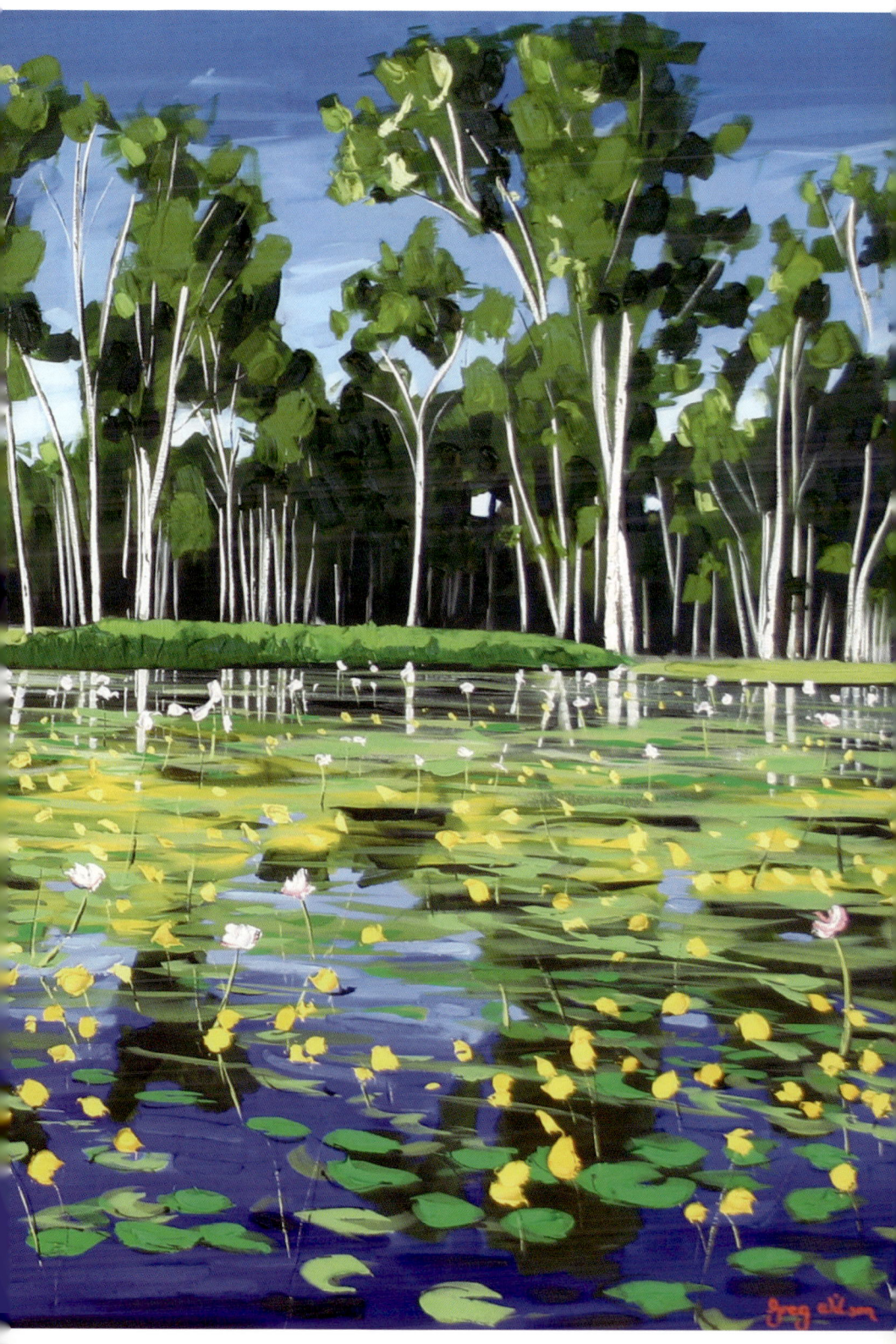

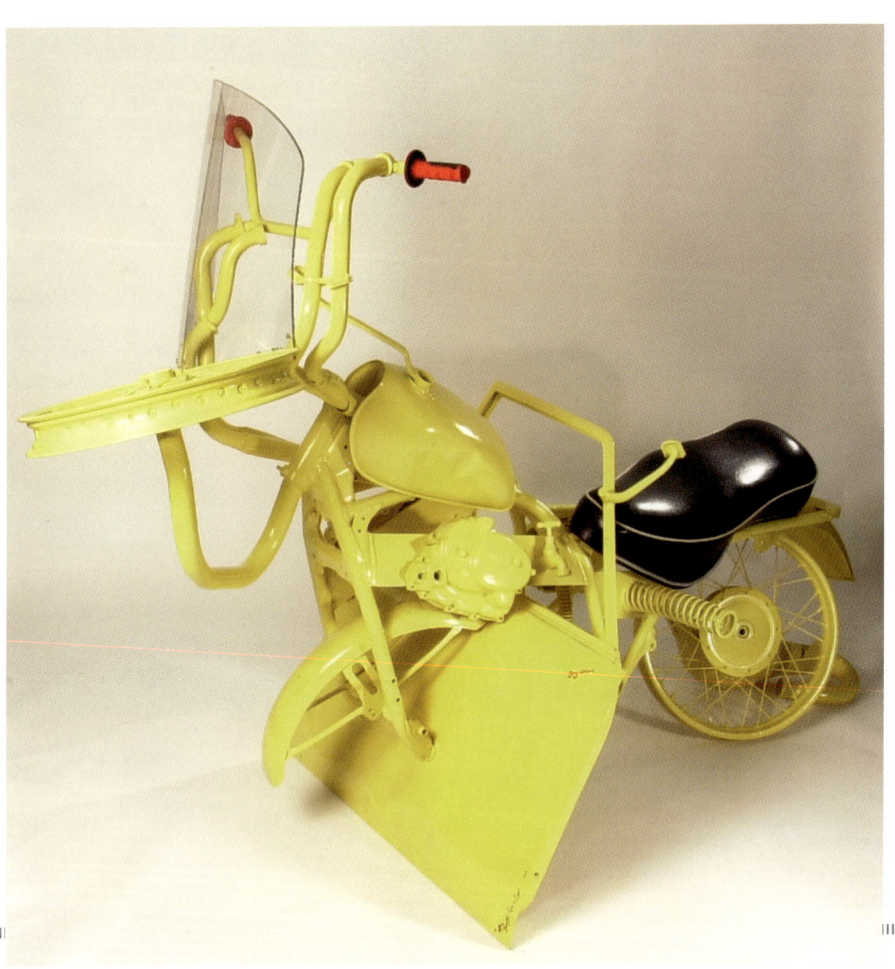

Above:
'Through the Taxi and into Another Life'
Clear coated, sealed and painted motorbike parts, seat and visor, tap, and car door.
1530 x 2220 x 910 mm

Previous page:
'Wetlands'
Oil on linen
1010 x 1520 mm

Opposite page
'Three Irises'
Oil on linen
1520 x 760 mm

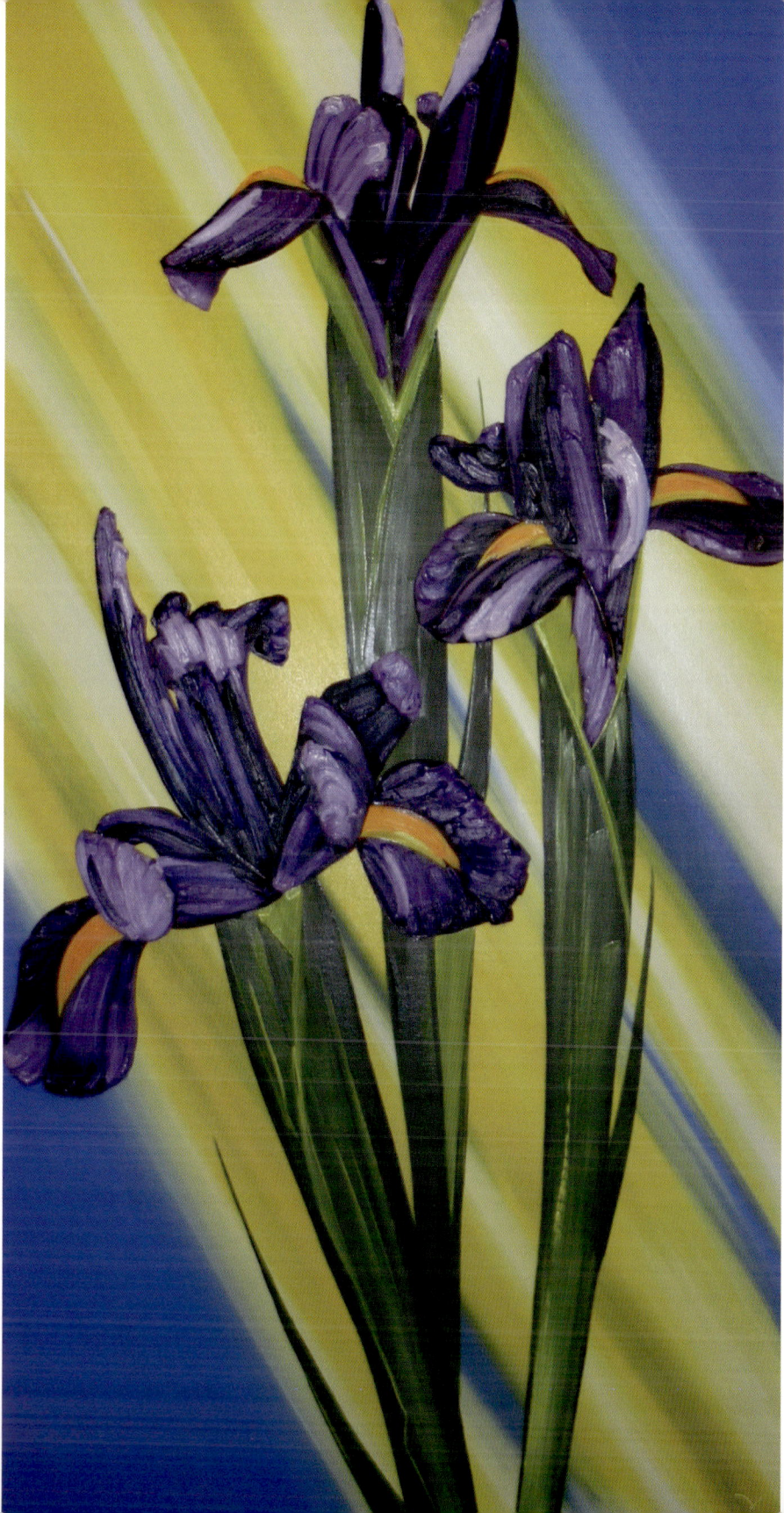

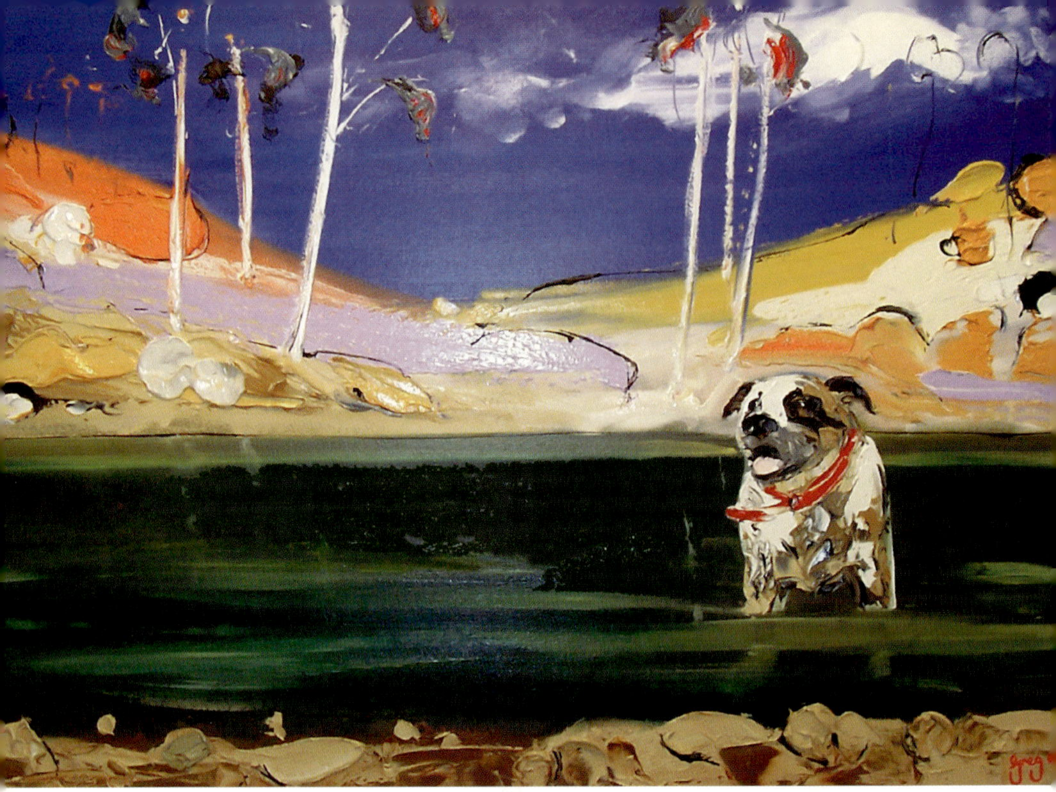

Above: **'Jackson'** – Oil on linen 510 x 760 mm
Greg's faithful and trusting companion: unwavering, unquestioning, unconditional loyalty. Truly, he is one of his best friends!

Below: **'Life Force'** – Oil on linen 1010 x 1520 mm

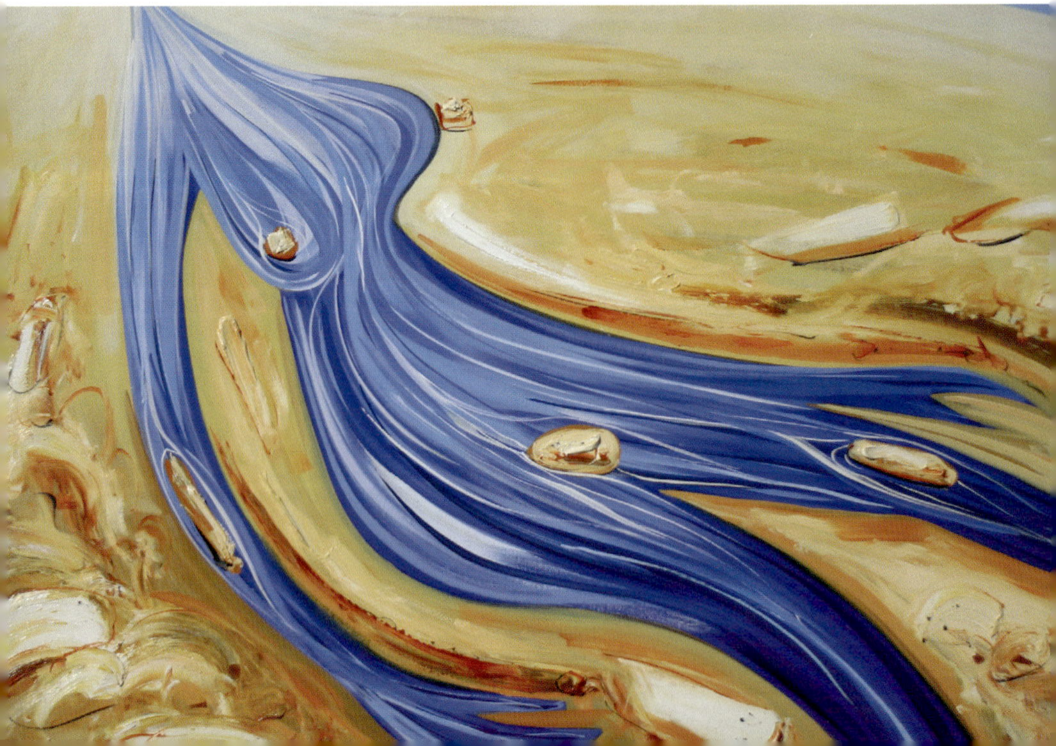

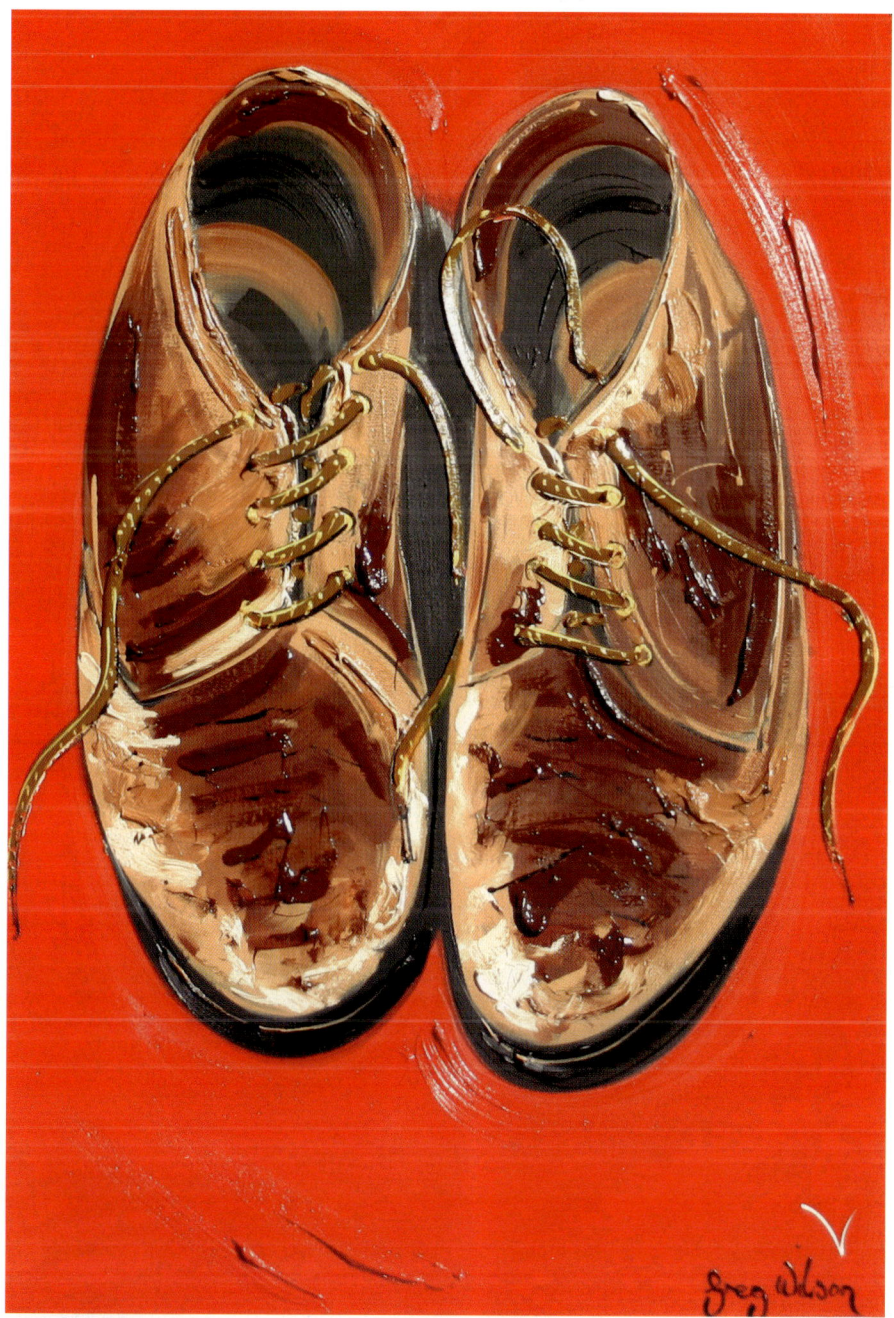

'**These Old Boots**'– Oil on linen 760 x 510 mm

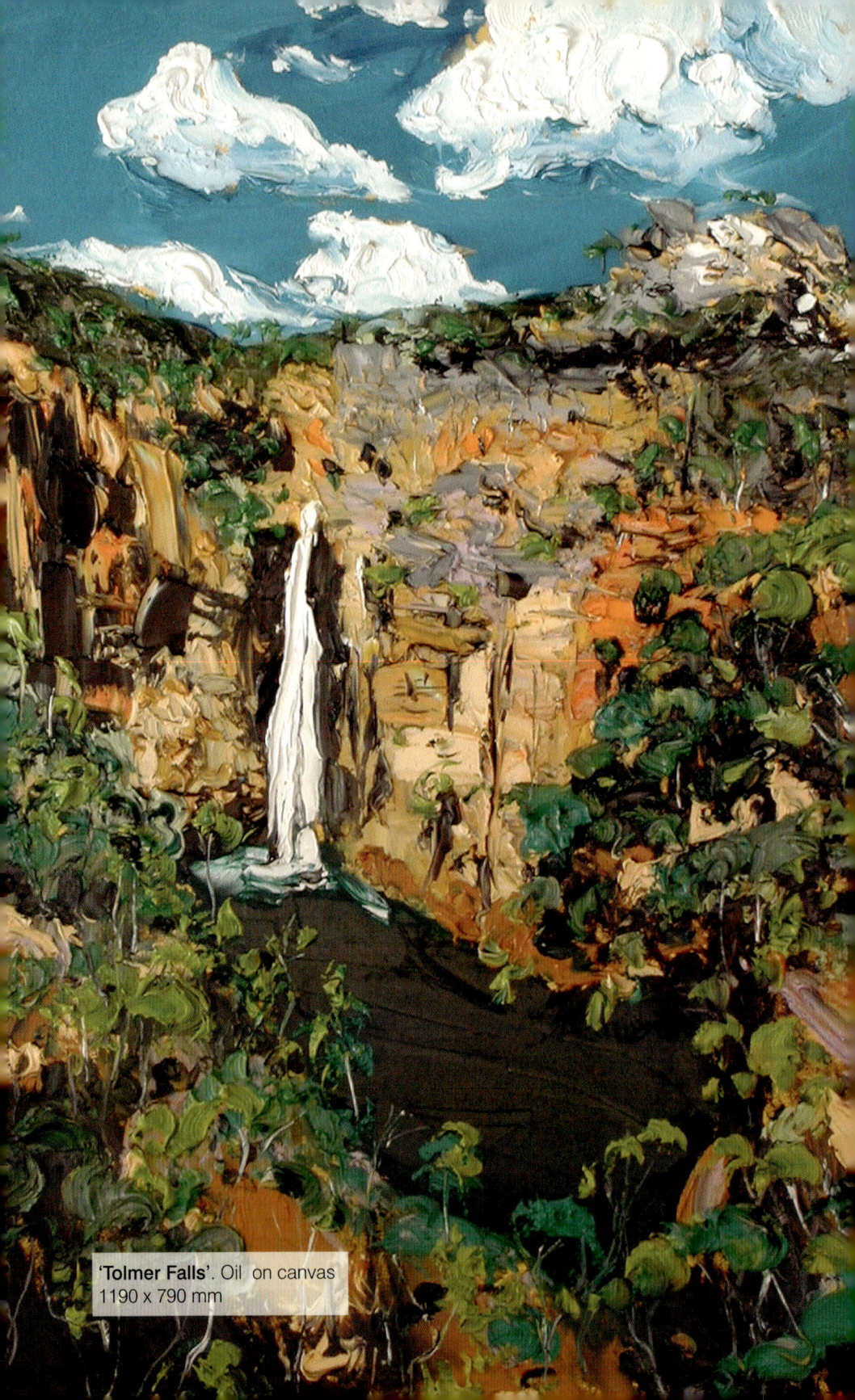

'Tolmer Falls'. Oil on canvas
1190 x 790 mm

contents

Foreword/18
A Few Words from the Authors/20
Chapter 1 The Edge of the Abyss/22
Chapter 2 Return to Eden/27
Chapter 3 The Early Years/38
Chapter 4 Adolescent Angst/42
Chapter 5 Sun, Snow and Speed/47
Chapter 6 The Parental Rift/51
Chapter 7 The Apocalypse/55
Chapter 8 The Depths of Despair/62
Chapter 9 The Hand of Loving-kindness/67
Chapter 10 Lightning Strikes Twice/75
Chapter 11 Hearts and Rainbows/81
Chapter 12 A Life-Changing Encounter/86
Chapter 13 The Understanding/92
Chapter 14 Art Mirrors Life/101
Chapter 15 A Tower of Strength/114
Chapter 16 Nailed/119
Chapter 17 Leaden Skies/124
Chapter 18 The Hard Yards/130
Chapter 19 Resurgence/139
Chapter 20 Early Exhibitions/154
Chapter 21 Trials and Tribulations/168
Chapter 22 Finding the Promised Land/173
Chapter 23 The Greg Wilson Gallery/197
Chapter 24 An Unforgettable Encounter/215
Chapter 25 Sharing His Inspirational Story/221
Chapter 26 Lights, Camera, Action/228
Chapter 27 International Recognition/234
Chapter 28 The Rainbow's End/244
Appendix One: Endorsements and Testimonials/256
Appendix Two: How Can You Help …?/264
Index/279

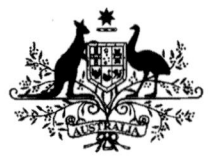

MINISTER FOR EDUCATION, SCIENCE AND TRAINING
THE HON DR BRENDAN NELSON MP

In Australia over 2000 Australians commit suicide each year and many more deliberately harm themselves. These acts, often triggered by depressive episodes, have a profound effect not only on the individuals themselves but also on their families, friends and community.

The Australian Government is committed to supporting efforts to improve mental health outcomes for all Australians. I am pleased to support *My Brush With Depression – The Greg Wilson Story* which explores Greg Wilson's brave journey through depression as described by his close friend, Aaron Cootes.

I was impressed by this book's sensitive portrayal of a young man fighting, and eventually overcoming, the debilitating effects of depression. In this story, the ordeals that Greg faces in trying to live his life, and the at times overwhelming responsibilities placed on his close friends as they supported him, were clearly articulated.

The experiences leading to Greg Wilson's recovery are also detailed here, along with his talents – particularly his great passion for painting and sculpting. I was impressed to learn that Greg now speaks at schools and to community groups in order to help others, particularly young people, to overcome this debilitating illness. He has recently become the Patron for Lifeline in Newcastle, New South Wales.

However, in addition to a courageous story, you will also find in this book an exploration of the practicalities of this disease. It identifies the triggers for self-harm during depressive episodes and, in particular, highlights the critical importance of an individual's support network for

foreword

his or her immediate and long-term wellbeing. This book also includes valuable information in the Appendices on how you can help if someone has depression.

I commend *My Brush With Depression – The Greg Wilson Story* to you, both as a doctor and a parent. I strongly believe that it is the power of individual stories such as these which can best assist the community to understand the complexities of depression and provide its sufferers with hope that, like Greg Wilson, they will eventually overcome it.

BRENDAN NELSON

Parliament House, Canberra ACT 2600, 10 February 2005

my brush with depression

greg wilson

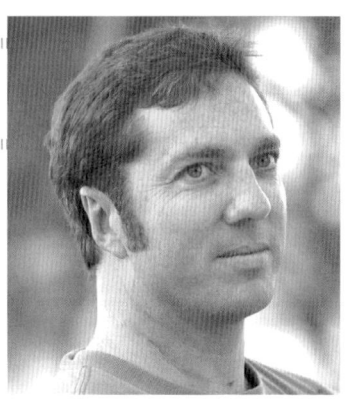

by Aaron Cootes

For as long as he can remember Greg Wilson felt as though he didn't belong in this world. Grappling with the feelings of depression, he wondered why he felt so abnormal, so alone, and so worthless. Sometimes he would experience temporary relief from these troubling emotions; however, his anxiety and despair would soon return for no apparent reason.

Desperate to find happiness, he tried to be part of life and was determined to fit in: he spent time with friends, was active at school, threw himself into his work, and had a keen interest in sport. Unfortunately, nothing seemed to alleviate his destructive feelings. No matter how hard he tried, he could not find meaning in his own life, and a feeling of doom followed him wherever he went. He couldn't picture a happy future for himself and it wasn't long before he was asking: Why bother? Why try and build a life when he really didn't want to be here?

Growing up, he didn't talk to his friends about his experiences because they didn't seem to have the same feelings as he did. Unable to speak to his mother and father about his emotions he was soon caught up in a downward spiral. He held everything in.

Greg remembers saying to himself that if he ever got over his depression he wouldn't talk about it, want to hear about it, or even think about it ever again. However, after having learnt to cope with the illness that almost killed him his feelings gradually began to change. He didn't want others to suffer the way he did and he decided he would like to help. He started by giving motivational talks, and when his best friend Aaron approached him with a proposal to write about his story, he was eager to do so. Maybe his learning would assist others who were currently in the midst of serious depression. His most fervent wish was that his story would deliver an important message to people – as long as there is life then there is hope.

about the authors

aaron cootes

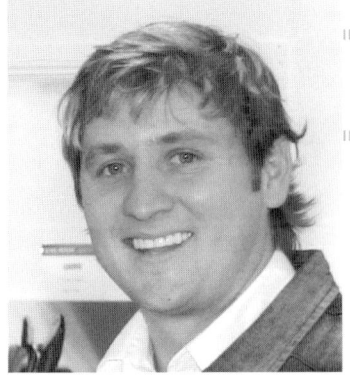

Born in Newcastle, Australia, on the 18.10.1974, he moved to Marsfield in Sydney several years later where he started primary school at Our Lady Help of Christians at Epping. He attended Marist Brothers Eastwood before transferring to boarding school at St. Josephs College at Hunters Hill for his final two senior years. After leaving secondary school he received a diploma in social science from the College of Applied Psychology in Surry Hills. He went on to study natural medicine and received a diploma in naturopathy from Nature Care College in Sydney. He currently has one subject remaining before he obtains a science degree from the University of New England in Armidale. Aaron has held a variety of jobs over the years from furniture removalist in Sydney to grape-picker in the Hunter Valley. He is a certified ski instructor and a self-confessed rugby league enthusiast. A keen fisherman and surfer when he gets the opportunity, he currently lives in the wine region in NSW where he divides his time between writing and working in the Greg Wilson Gallery.

Aaron hoped that, by sharing the story of his inspirational and courageous friend, it would demonstrate to others how to overcome depression or at least learn to manage the insidious disease.

chapter one
the edge of the abyss

'According to the World Health Organization, almost 1 million people take their lives each year, a figure which exceeds the annual death toll for war and murder combined. For every suicide, there are between ten to twenty failed attempts.'

Source: *ABC News*

It was six o'clock on a cool spring morning. I'd gone to bed late the night before after a serious study session for my forthcoming university exams and had been looking forward to a long and restful sleep.

Suddenly I was woken by a strange disturbance coming from the next room.

For a moment, as I struggled to identify the source of the commotion, I was tempted to roll back over and remain under my warm blankets. But as the nature of the sounds became a little clearer, I realised that something was seriously wrong. Greg was being violently ill.

In an instant I was fully alert as the sound of his vomiting intensified and became unusually loud, disturbingly loud. Now I was truly alarmed. Maybe something was critically wrong with Greg, and I had an overwhelming premonition that he may have tried to hurt himself yet again.

the edge of the abyss

That would be just too outlandish, especially for someone who now had so many reasons to live.

I found it inconceivable to think that someone with so many skills and talents to share with the world, someone whom I regarded as a talent bordering on genius with a huge future ahead of him, should have any reason to terminate his own life.

I jumped out of bed and headed towards my flatmate's room. Although my thoughts tried to convince me that he was going to be just fine, deep down I knew I wasn't quite persuaded. In fact, I became quite apprehensive.

My pulse rate had increased noticeably and I felt sweat on the palms of my hands and my forehead. All my senses were on full alert.

The sight before me confirmed my concerns. Greg was curled up in the foetal position and his bed was covered in thick and viscous vomit. But what added to my concern even more was that what he had thrown up appeared heavily tinged with blood. As I approached the bed, his body continued to be racked by harsh and convulsive dry retching.

His face was distorted and expressionless. He looked at me through eyes that were bloodshot and glazed, and although he appeared unable to talk properly he muttered something about tablets.

My thoughts raced back to the previous evening. I remembered Greg returning home with 100 prescription pills for some pain he had complained about. I warned him of the dangers of taking more than three pills at any time. I even told him these particular tablets caused liver failure and could cause death if taken in excess.

I ran to the kitchen to see if I could find the packet. On top of the rubbish was an empty box and container, but no white pills. I raced back to the bedroom and began waving the carton in front of his face.

'Where are the tablets?' I shouted. The trembling in my own voice startled me.

'I've taken them,' Greg slurred.

'How many have you had?' I yelled.

'All of them,' he replied.

I looked on the dressing table next to the bed and saw a note. I picked it up and hastily read its contents. It was addressed to his partner Josie who had gone away for a few days. It said:

'I am sorry, Josie, but I cannot go on living here any more. I am tired of this life. I am sorry to have caused you any problems. Please don't be upset for me, I just have to go. Take care of yourself and remember that I love you. I don't know how I would have lived this long without you. Look after the dog for me. Goodbye.'

I looked back at Greg. We were both crying. 'An ambulance, I must ring an ambulance,' a voice desperately bellowed in my head. I ran to the phone and dialled the emergency number, still not quite believing that this was really happening.

The operator said: 'Hello.'

I struggled to organise my thoughts before I eventually blurted out: 'Please send someone quickly, my mate is dying. He's taken an overdose.'

The woman on the other end of the phone tried to calm me down, but even her best efforts couldn't arrest my feelings of panic and despair. I gave the faceless woman our address and contact details and urged her to send an ambulance straight away.

As I waited for help to arrive I felt powerless. I couldn't do anything except cover Greg with some blankets and watch him slip into unconsciousness. The entire colour had now drained from his face, and I found the resultant deathly pallor particularly disturbing. His life force seemed to be slipping away right before my eyes.

It was by far the most tragic moment in my young life. My best friend, who had cheated death on more than one occasion, even staging a courageous recovery from a horrendous motorcycle accident, had now become another statistic in the staggering list of attempted suicides … and there was every indication that his attempt may well have been successful!

My brain struggled to accept the bleak circumstances in which I found myself. I could not believe that such a promising life could end so terribly.

the edge of the abyss

It was an atrocious and deeply saddening realisation that raced through my mind: Greg Wilson was probably going to die today.

Tears flowed down my cheeks once more as it dawned on me there was a distinct possibility that I was unlikely ever to talk with him, laugh with him, or even see him alive again.

Greg Wilson's life was going to end prematurely right before my eyes, and with it would go all that remarkable yet unfulfilled talent. All his admirable qualities, his goodness, would soon be extinguished because of this desperate act. It was an incredible contradiction. Someone with so much to live for wanted so desperately to die.

I attempted to recall and analyse my reactions over the previous five minutes because I still couldn't quite believe that my life had taken such a horrifying twist. Even though I knew that Greg was feeling a little bit low, I had hardly imagined that this would be the outcome of his depressed mood.

Suddenly I was overcome with an incredible sense of guilt as I waited for the paramedics. I should have seen the signs, should have known he was going to try something like this. How could I have been so stupid?

The siren of the approaching ambulance interrupted my thoughts. I ran to meet the vehicle as it pulled into the drive.

'Come quickly, my friend's this way,' I yelled.

The two ambulance officers seemed composed. As we made our way back into the house they asked me questions about Greg to find out what had taken place, and to get his medical history. I told them about the pills and his bouts of depression.

Soon we were back in the spare room of the house and they addressed their questions to Greg, but he was not really alert.

'Greg, can you hear me? What have you taken?' the ambulance driver yelled.

Greg mumbled a reply, but his words were unrecognisable. He didn't respond to any further questioning, so they gave him some type of injection to help counter the effects of the medicine he had taken.

'We need to get him to hospital quickly,' said one of the paramedics.

I helped the ambulance officers put Greg onto a bed they had just assembled and wheel him out of the house. Then we put him into the back of the ambulance.

'Will he be all right?' I asked the driver, as he shut the doors.

'We'll do what we can.'

The ambulance reversed down the driveway. It made an awkward U-turn in our narrow street and left hurriedly. I watched the white vehicle, sirens blaring, manoeuvre along the winding roads leading to the hospital. Soon it had disappeared from sight.

I fell to the ground and put my head in my hands, crying again now. I was overcome by uncertainty and fear. Would he live? Why would he do such a thing?'

Surely, a friendship as strong as ours, with so much promise, couldn't end like this! As I tried to come to terms with the dreadful turn that my life seemed to have taken, I couldn't quite believe that so much had taken place in just a few short years.

chapter two

return to eden

It was February 2004. I was in my office in the back room of the Greg Wilson Gallery. I removed my name badge from my white business shirt and placed it on the desktop.

'Who would have thought that Aaron Cootes would end up here as an art gallery director?' I asked myself. It all seemed a bit unlikely, given my background in science.

It was getting late and almost time to stop working for the day. As I sat at my desk, the screen of my computer cast a pale light across the room. I looked up from my keyboard and stared out the window in front of me.

I watched as dark clouds dropped a gentle rain over the vineyards that cover the hills in the distance. The trees to my right were leaning over, suggesting there was a strong breeze outside.

I still couldn't believe that I now lived and worked in the Hunter Valley, one of the great wine-making areas in Australia. It was harder to believe that Greg was my new business partner. For a time I hadn't been sure that he would have any future at all. My legs pushed the grey office chair away from my new L-shaped desk and I stood, turned and began walking across the carpeted floor to the entrance of the building.

I could smell the oil paint that had recently been thickly applied to his canvases. The walls of the gallery were covered with bright and colourful scenes: landscapes, picturesque floral and some abstract works. Several metal sculptures were displayed throughout the gallery.

I glanced at the clock on the far wall. It was now five o'clock on a drizzly Monday afternoon. As I placed the 'Closed' sign on the door of the gallery I couldn't help but think how different things could've been; how fortunate we were to have come this far. Even though the weather outside was a little miserable, I felt happy and content. My best friend was alive, living his dream.

For a moment my thoughts returned to Greg's attempted suicide and the ensuing heartache that it caused. I am always troubled and disturbed by these awful recollections. I tried to distract myself by picking up the red vacuum cleaner at my feet. I switched on the machine and began cleaning the floor. As the noise of the machine filled the studio, I hoped that my troubled thoughts would be sucked away along with the dirt.

My positive thinking technique soon worked, because after a short time my sad recollections were replaced by more pleasant imagery. I began looking forward to the delicious evening meal of tender chicken schnitzel and steamed vegetables that would soon await me. The thought of the succulent chicken breast and potatoes dripping with homemade gravy caused my stomach to rumble, and prompted me to finish some last minute jobs hurriedly: I emptied the vacuum, put on my coat, turned off the lights, locked up the gallery, and walked out to my silver four-wheel drive. I jumped into the car and began the five-minute drive home.

It was a new and exciting lifestyle that we were now enjoying. As I manoeuvred up our gravel driveway, Greg's loyal dog Jackson, part Red Cattle and part Labrador, with a distinctive black patch over his left eye, ran to greet me. He was barking frantically, the way he does whenever I return home. I undid my seatbelt and turned off the ignition before stepping from the vehicle onto our 40-acre property. 'This place is paradise,' I thought to myself as I looked around.

Both the house and Greg's nearby studio rest against the side of a large mountain. The tin structures are dwarfed by the towering mountain range behind them. I looked up and noticed a gentle mist had now come to rest on top of one of the distant peaks, hiding it from my view. The rain had eased and the air was fresh.

I bent down and scratched Jackson behind the ears. I noticed many of the eucalypts on the outskirts of the property were still black because of the bush fires that had ravaged the Pokolbin area months earlier. Even though large tracts of the surrounding bushland were burnt, it was still a majestic scene.

The wattles to my left grew profusely around our dam, and their stunning tiny yellow flowers coloured the landscape. Behind me, an acre and a half of Semillon grapes that we were growing were lush and hanging low from the vines, hinting they were nearly ready to be picked. The view at the front of the property was equally beautiful: rolling hills of vineyards, dams that mirrored the countryside, kangaroos grazing on the lush grass, and a small cottage set amongst rows of red grapes.

Greg's huge frame emerged from his studio. His short brown hair carried traces of yellow and blue paint. His normally pale complexion was looking more brown and red because his hands and face were also covered in paint. He was wearing his navy King Gee overalls, with bright splotches of paint freckled over them. I laughed uncontrollably when I noticed that even Jackson's tail had turned yellow!

'G'day mate,' he said, as he walked towards me.

'How are you?' I asked. 'How's the new painting coming along?'

'Just fine, Aaron,' he replied with an obvious air of satisfaction. 'And oh my, aren't you looking a picture of style in your new suit,' he jested.

Greg still found it unusual to see me in a suit, and welcomed any opportunity to joke about the seriousness with which I seemed to take my new role as his manager.

'I'm taking a leaf out of your fashion book,' I replied. (Greg dresses quite smartly when he isn't working.)

'Reluctantly, I've had to trade in my old pair of faded blue Botany Bay tracksuit pants for this attire, to project a professional image for you.

my brush with depression

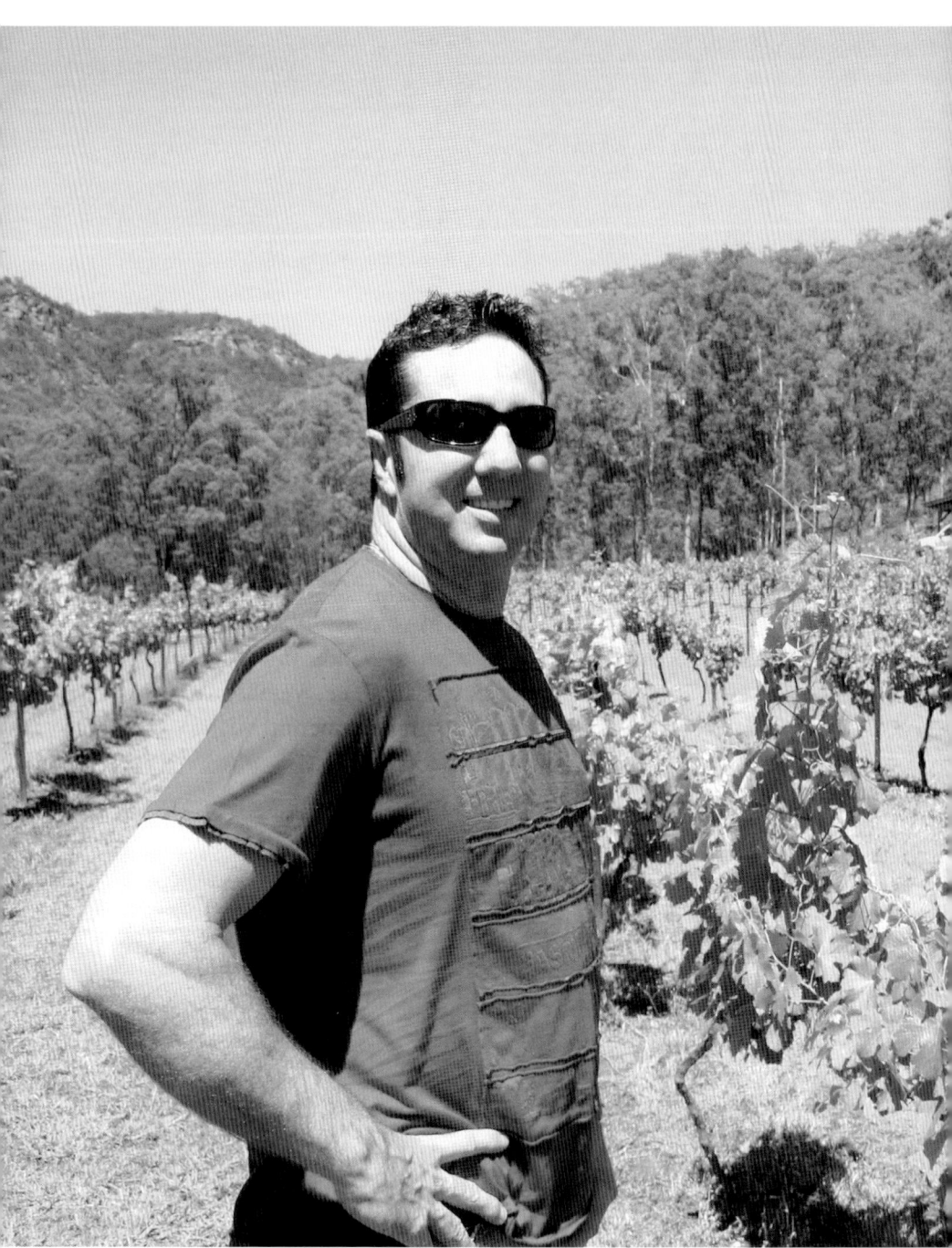

return to eden

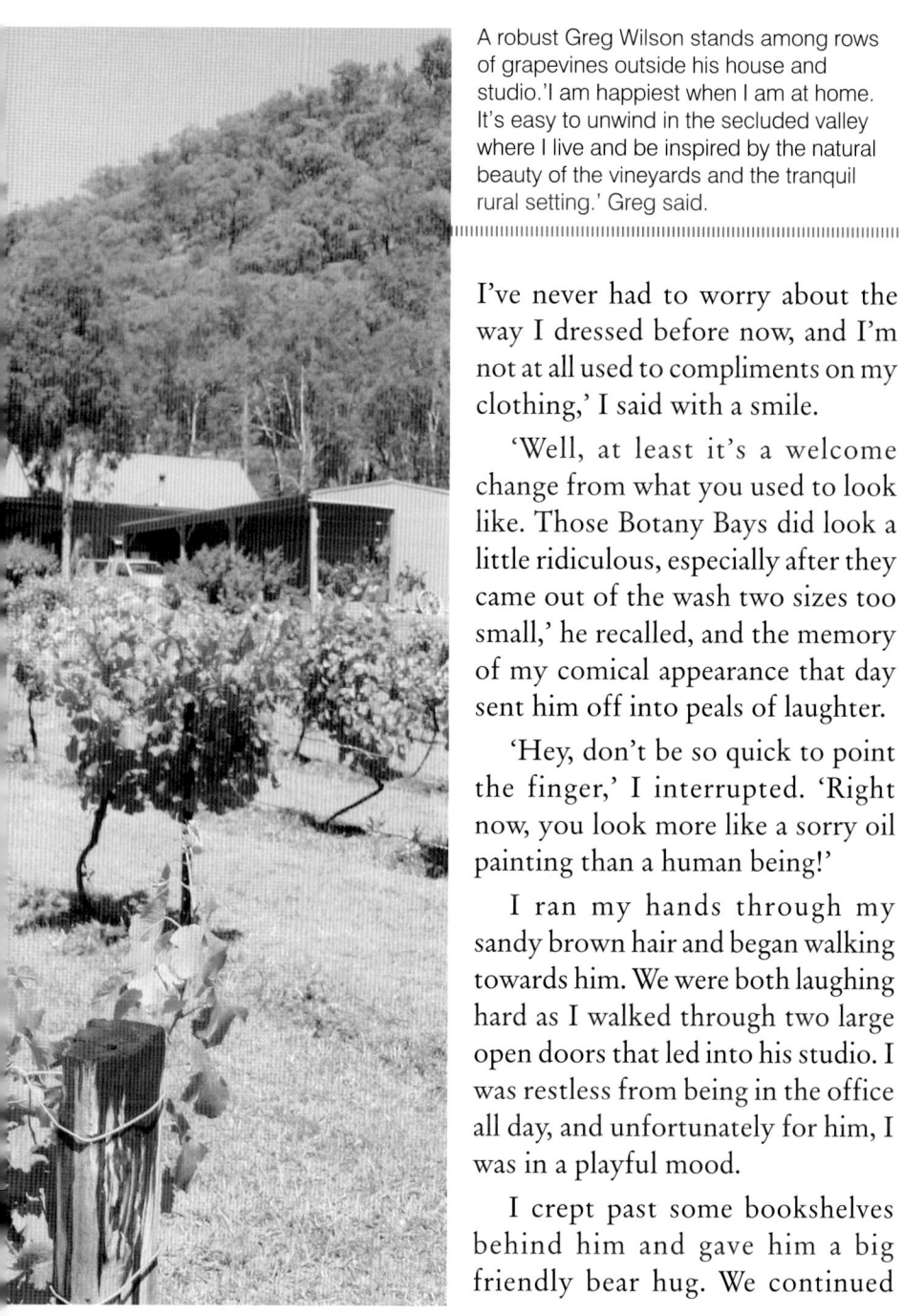

A robust Greg Wilson stands among rows of grapevines outside his house and studio. 'I am happiest when I am at home. It's easy to unwind in the secluded valley where I live and be inspired by the natural beauty of the vineyards and the tranquil rural setting.' Greg said.

I've never had to worry about the way I dressed before now, and I'm not at all used to compliments on my clothing,' I said with a smile.

'Well, at least it's a welcome change from what you used to look like. Those Botany Bays did look a little ridiculous, especially after they came out of the wash two sizes too small,' he recalled, and the memory of my comical appearance that day sent him off into peals of laughter.

'Hey, don't be so quick to point the finger,' I interrupted. 'Right now, you look more like a sorry oil painting than a human being!'

I ran my hands through my sandy brown hair and began walking towards him. We were both laughing hard as I walked through two large open doors that led into his studio. I was restless from being in the office all day, and unfortunately for him, I was in a playful mood.

I crept past some bookshelves behind him and gave him a big friendly bear hug. We continued laughing. Even though I was twenty-nine and he was thirty-three, we were both kids at heart. Greg was not too surprised by my action – he was, after all, more like my brother than a friend. We wrestled for a while before I released him and inspected some of the work he had finished during the day.

He had been making canvases during the past week and they were neatly positioned on timber shelves around his workroom. There were over fifty tins of paint positioned carefully on a bookshelf to my right, and a number of opened tins on his large glass palette. His palette was

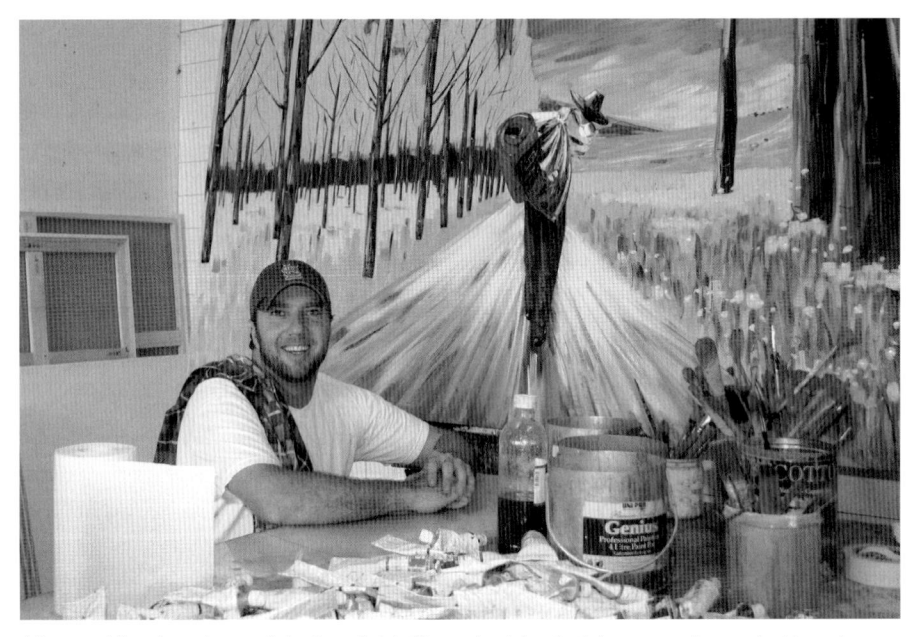

After working long hours into the night, Greg decides to take a much needed break from his latest creation.

much bigger than the hand-sized palette used by many artists. It was about the size of a large dining table. Blobs of paints were scattered all over the glass top, making them easy to access when he was painting. Brushes and tubes of paint were also spread across the tabletop. Near the far wall was an easel with a painting on it. It was a landscape of a swaggie walking along a beautiful sunlit walkway.

return to eden

'That looks brilliant!' I said, genuinely amazed once again by the magic in his hands and his ability to create such wonderful art.

'Talk me through it, talk me through it,' I said. That was my way of asking Greg to explain the painting to me. He chuckled at my expression before he described the scene and the colours that he was using.

When he had finished giving the details about the painting he picked up a paintbrush and returned to his unfinished artwork. He moved his brush effortlessly up and down the canvas, putting the final touches to the landscape.

He then put his paintbrush into a tin, half-filled with water, to clean his brush. 'I'm going to get Jess out of her cage,' he said.

He disappeared out the door and returned a short time later with our beloved pet cockatiel. The grey bird was sitting on his shoulder as he walked into the studio. I watched as the little animal, with brilliant yellow and orange feathers on its cheeks and on its head, nuzzled into his chin and lowered her head. This behaviour indicated one thing: Jess wanted her neck rubbed. Greg noticed the familiar posture and began scratching the bird.

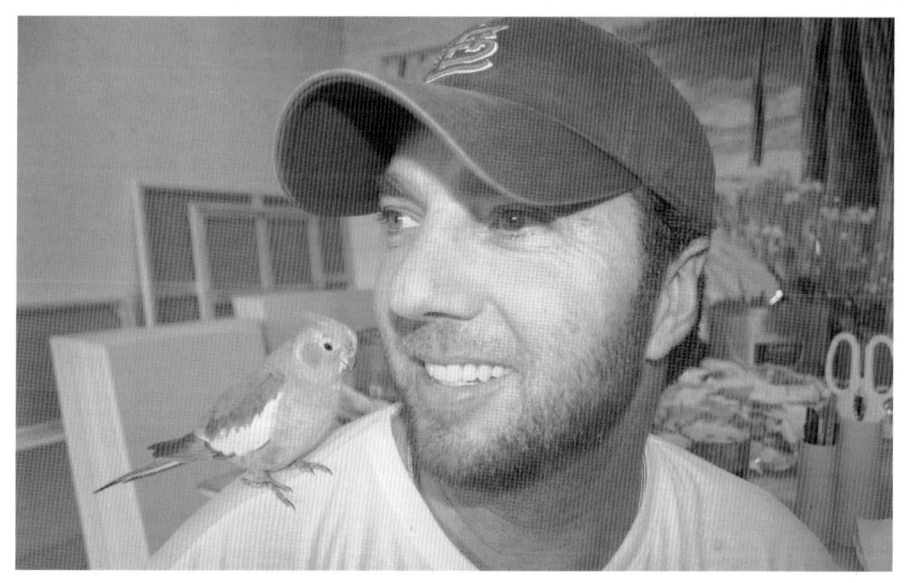

Greg and Jess consult over their next project.

greg wilson — 33

my brush with depression

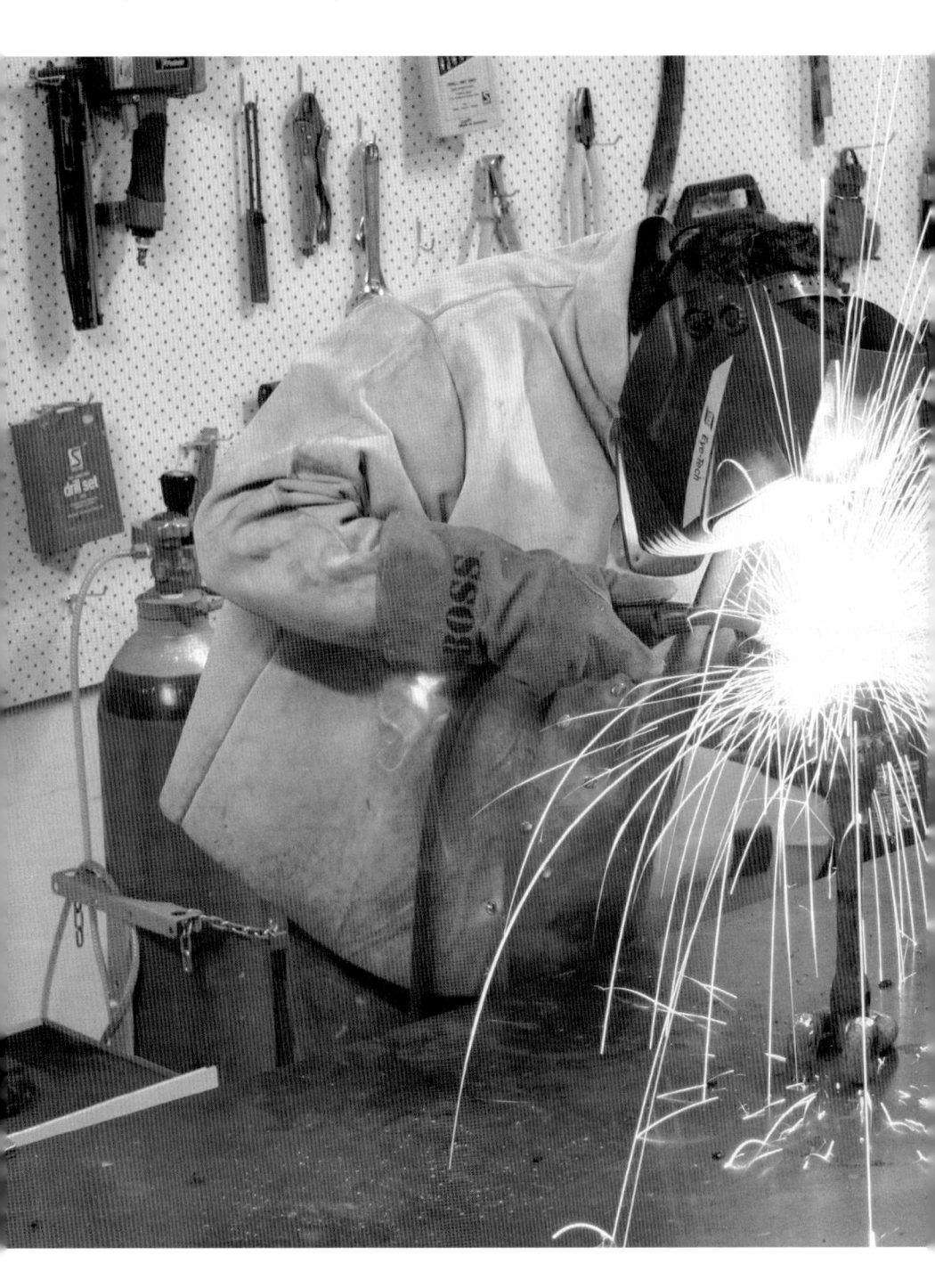

return to eden

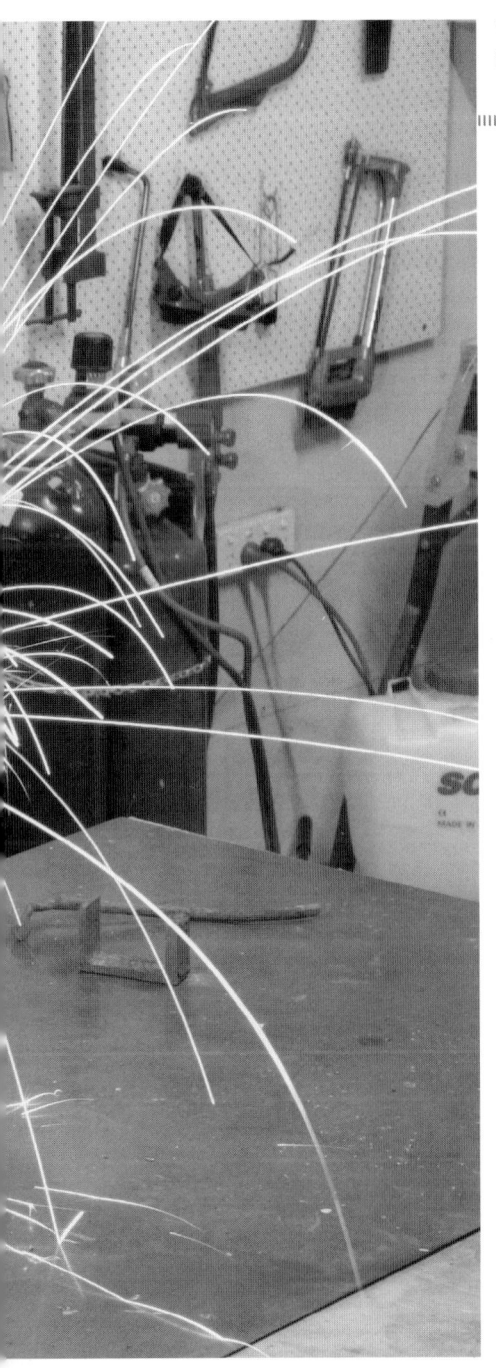

When inspiration dawns the sparks begin to fly, literally.

As soon as he stopped she flew from his arm and into the open air. She circled the house and vineyard a few times before she tired, then turned back towards Greg and landed on his outstretched arm. (Visitors to the studio were often treated to the delightful vision of the artist working on a new canvas, and Jess casting a critical eye over the unfolding masterpiece from her excellent vantage point on his shoulder.)

She launched herself once again off Greg's shoulder and landed on top of a bookshelf. She started pecking at one of his books on Pablo Picasso. She then fluttered out the door, made a left turn and came to rest in an adjoining room where he did all his sculptures. We followed Jess into the room.

Greg's sculpting room that he had set up on the property was certainly impressive. Over thirty tools were hanging strategically on the wall: saws, mallets, nail guns, hammers, pliers, and screwdrivers. Neatly aligned on the floor there was a welder, an air compressor and a torch that could heat and bend metal. In the middle of the room was a large worktable.

The left-hand side of the room had a bench that extended half a metre from the wall and ran the entire length of the fifteen-foot room. In the middle of the bench was a large drop saw that he used for cutting timber. Above the bench were four large metal brackets with pieces of timber and metal resting on top of them.

At the rear of the room there were a number of timber shelves that had paint and more tools stored on them.

I walked to the middle of the room and leaned on the worktable. I began to laugh again as Jess chewed playfully and rather awkwardly on some timber off-cuts lying on the floor. Then Greg picked up some metal cuttings from the surface of the bench. I watched as he rotated a few of the square shapes and tilted his head. It was almost as if he were trying to figure out how to incorporate these pieces in his next sculpture.

An urgent summons from Joyce, our housemate, interrupted our discussion: 'Dinner's ready, guys,' she called from the veranda of our house.

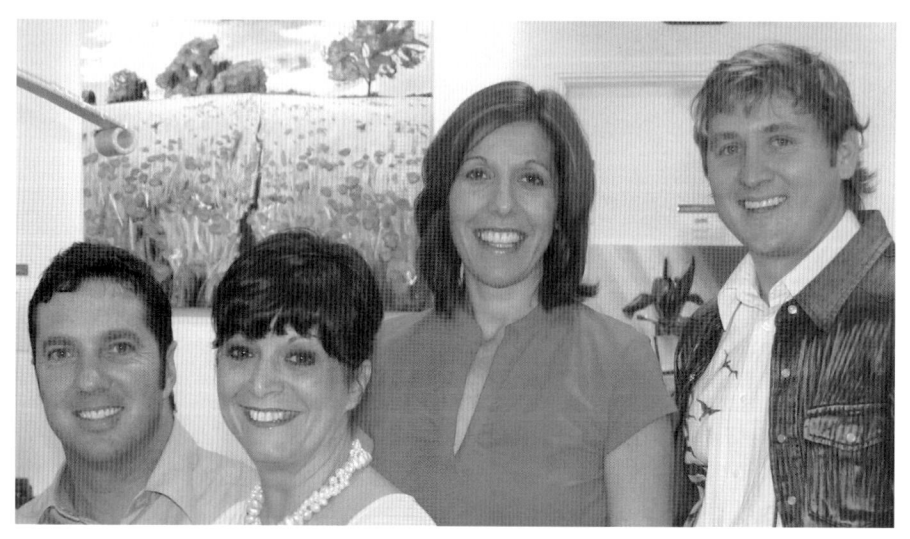

Inseparable friends: Greg Wilson (left), with Josie Alder, Joyce Biviano, and Aaron Cootes in the Greg Wilson Gallery.

return to eden

I popped my head out of the studio and looked at Joyce. Her brown shoulder-length hair neatly framed her face and she was wearing a big smile. There was flour, obviously used to make dinner, over her yellow shirt.

'Thanks, Joycie,' I replied. 'We'll be there in a minute.'

We called out to Jess, and soon she landed on my shoulder. I put her back in the cage.

I sat down at the timber dining table, with Greg, Josie, and Joyce – all members of my unstructured family. The smell of the chicken made my mouth start to water. Without further hesitation I piled the delicious selection of food high on my plate and prepared to enjoy the meal.

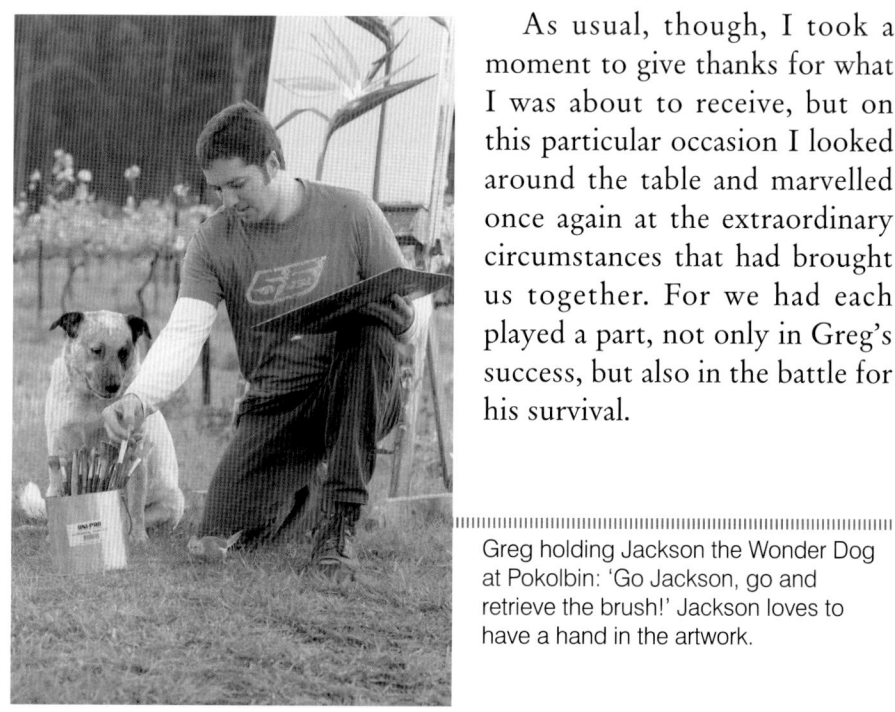

As usual, though, I took a moment to give thanks for what I was about to receive, but on this particular occasion I looked around the table and marvelled once again at the extraordinary circumstances that had brought us together. For we had each played a part, not only in Greg's success, but also in the battle for his survival.

Greg holding Jackson the Wonder Dog at Pokolbin: 'Go Jackson, go and retrieve the brush!' Jackson loves to have a hand in the artwork.

chapter three
the early years

Greg Wilson's life began on 15 June, 1970, at Mona Vale Hospital, when he was born to parents Marnie and Bob. He grew up in Davidson, an outer suburb on the Northern Beaches of Sydney, with his two sisters, Robyn and Lynda.

Their home was a marvellous house, an Australian colonial design with a long driveway in a delightful leafy suburb. Greg loved the pool in the backyard and he would spend countless hours swimming in it during the hot summer months.

The neighbourhood was filled with friendly people, so it was relatively easy for Greg to get to know and form strong bonds with his own contemporaries. His best friend was a popular youngster named Peter John-

Where the road began. 'Gee Grandad, do you think my hair will be like that one day?'

38 — aaron cootes

the early years

son. They would often play cricket together with other children in the street. Peter was far more solidly built than Greg, and he used this to great advantage whenever the pair met to decide the Ashes Series.

Peter had a really fast delivery, which meant that scoring runs against him was difficult. Whenever Greg did happen to make contact with his fast ball it normally went high into the air. For this reason, the pair always used a tennis ball. Although it didn't go as far as a cricket ball, it didn't break as many windows either!

When they weren't cricketing they would often turn their attention to the other love in their life at the time, BMX riding. They would pick up their bikes lying on the side of Twynam Road and head for the bush. Scamp, Greg's pet dog, whom he adored, always managed to follow them through the dense trees and along the worn dirt pathway.

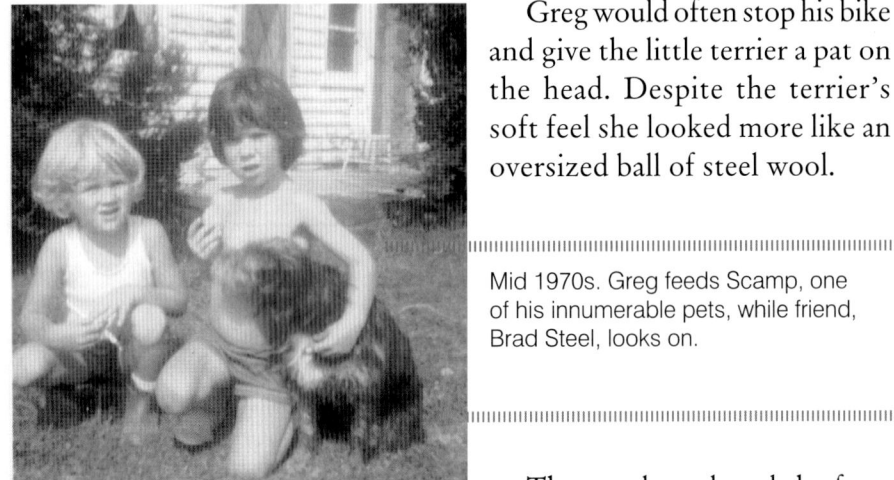

Greg would often stop his bike and give the little terrier a pat on the head. Despite the terrier's soft feel she looked more like an oversized ball of steel wool.

Mid 1970s. Greg feeds Scamp, one of his innumerable pets, while friend, Brad Steel, looks on.

The two boys loved the freedom of the bush where they felt independent of rules and adults. They would build jumps for their bikes and would spend hours launching from them into the air. Life for Greg, in the early eighties, was great: uncomplicated and full of new adventures.

Greg's parents liked Peter and would often invite him to share lunch at their place during the holidays. Marnie would prepare sandwiches for both the boys, who would invariably bolt them down as quickly as possible so they could resume their outdoor activities.

Whenever Greg had to return to Mimosa Public at Belrose after the holidays it was always with mixed feelings. While he regarded it as a great school and looked forward to being with his other classmates, it also meant he would be unable to spend the daylight hours playing with Peter, building skateboards, or constructing animal houses for his birds and guinea pigs. Like most kids, too, he didn't exactly relish the thought of being burdened with the daily ration of homework!

After Year Three at Mimosa, Greg's parents approached him with an unexpected proposition. A new primary school called Kambora Public was opening much closer to home. They wanted to know if he would like to transfer to the school the following year. When he learned that Peter and several other friends would be changing over as well, he agreed. Greg enjoyed the next three years at his new school and remembers this phase of his life as a period of strengthening bonds with his peers.

Many new friendships were also formed through his involvement with sport. He was really active at this time. On weekends he played soccer and rugby league and also began surfing.

Rugby league and surfing had come naturally enough. However, soccer and distance running were sports at which he excelled. He played right wing for his soccer team, the Wakehurst Tigers, who went undefeated in many of their competitions, winning an impressive six titles from the time Greg joined the under-sevens until he reached the under-thirteens. For four seasons they went undefeated and during the seven years he was associated with the club, they never lost a grand-final. Greg believes the secret to their success was the fact that every member of the team got on extremely well with each other and they simply loved playing together.

Distance running wasn't as much fun as soccer for Greg, although his tall frame and long legs proved a distinct advantage and he nearly broke the school record for the 800 metres event. Despite this success, Greg missed the team spirit and involvement that he'd enjoyed while playing soccer, and 'retired' from distance running at the tender age of fourteen! Greg's final year in primary school, which began with Peter being named School Captain, was a happy and carefree time for him and went all too quickly.

the early years

Greg was a little apprehensive about starting high school the following year. He loved the time he had spent at Kambora and was nervous about going from the top of one school to the bottom of another. His only comfort was that Jacob and Peter, two of his closest friends, would also be going to Davidson High with him, and this would make the transition a lot easier.

It came as quite a shock when his mother informed him that he was to be enrolled at Frenchs Forest High. Greg was devastated. He didn't want to go to 'Forest' as it was known: Peter and Jacob and all his other good friends were going to Davidson, and he wanted to be with them.

His persistent requests to attend Davidson, however, fell on deaf ears. His parents believed there would be better opportunities available to him at Forest. He would start at the school the following year.

It would prove to be one of the real hardships of his life.

chapter four

adolescent angst

Greg's first day in his new school environment was daunting. The small and friendly environment at Kambora had been replaced by a huge, imposing building that towered overhead and hundreds of kids – total strangers – playing in the school grounds and on the adjoining football fields. This unfamiliar and overwhelming environment made Greg feel uneasy. He became increasingly anxious and had butterflies in his stomach as he walked into his first class.

Greg was acutely aware that he had been separated from all his good friends when he went into secondary school, but unlike his primary years, he found it difficult to make new friends. The other kids at Forest had all grown up together in the local area, and Greg felt that he was the outsider.

Although he made a few acquaintances at Forest, it wasn't the same as the friendships he had with Peter and his other companions from primary school. They had enjoyed a long and happy history together, they had shared so many experiences, and it was easy to talk with them. He had always felt so comfortable with his former friends, whereas now he always felt awkward around others.

He felt isolated and alone during much of his first two senior years. For the first time in his life he felt as though he didn't belong; he felt

adolescent angst

like a misfit. It was the most disturbing and distressing emotion he had ever experienced.

As a result Greg became a bundle of nervous energy. He began talking excessively, trying to win others' approval. He tried so hard, in fact, that in the end he would often say something stupid or act stupidly and his actions would only serve to distance him from the other children.

There were times when he would try to assume different personalities, to become different people, just to make a more favourable impression.

In time, not only did others not know who he truly was, but Greg himself became confused about his own identity He felt that he had no sense of purpose and no real self-confidence at all.

Not even sport could break down the barriers. The friendly atmosphere that had characterised his team involvement during his primary years had been replaced with a fierce competitiveness that felt foreign to him. Winning at all costs became more important than fair play. When abuse began to be hurled at him if he ever made a mistake, Greg gradually withdrew from the sporting teams for which he was selected.

Greg threw himself into his classes to try and shift his focus. Art and Woodwork were his favourite subjects in his junior years. It was during these classes that his creative flare really began to blossom. In many ways, his creative side helped him to escape from many of the unpleasant times that were never too far away: the critical comments, his awkwardness, his inability to form any meaningful relationships. Instead of thinking about such things, he would be distracted and he would no longer feel alone and so self-conscious.

Fortunately, his ability in these areas did not go unnoticed by his teachers, especially in Art and Woodwork. He was able to announce quite proudly to his parents that Mrs Brusalo had awarded him a perfect mark for one of his major art works, and that Mr Clarke had described him as one of the most talented students he had ever taught in Woodwork.

Despite these achievements, Greg was still deeply troubled.

Try as he might, he was never able to shake his troubled emotions. He knew that there was something that he wasn't happy about. Something just wasn't right. He had persistent feelings of sadness and anxiety. He felt hopeless and worthless much of the time. He used to think: 'Next year I will feel better, or the year after.' But next year would arrive and he would discover that the feelings remained unchanged.

He was extremely sensitive at this time and would over-react to things that made him unhappy. Any encounters with dishonesty, bullying or cruel people were exceptionally hard to bear. It was this sensitive side in particular that made his time at school so difficult.

He felt that he couldn't be himself around his classmates. He feared that if he told people how he was feeling that he'd be ridiculed. When he did say a few things, people told him not to worry and just to get on with life. He would squash the feelings, almost trying to ignore them altogether so that he would fit in. People didn't seem to have the same feelings as he did, and they didn't seem to care about how he felt.

It was no surprise then that Greg would crave the school holidays. It gave his mind a break from study and the other students. During the wintertime he would go skiing with his parents. They would set off for either Perisher or Thredbo, and he even went to Colorado in America and spent some time at Aspen when he was sixteen.

There was one holiday that he took when he was an adolescent, however, where even staying at school would have been better alternative. The tropical Fijian paradise, stunningly beautiful with its palm trees, white sandy beaches and coconuts, revealed a darker side of its character that left Greg with a terrible and painful memory. During the school break, Greg stood on a deadly stonefish and was severely poisoned. Highly venomous, stonefish poison attacks the nervous system and has been known to kill people within three hours.

Remarkably, not only did Greg step on the fish but he also had a premonition about one of those poisonous creatures before he even got to the island. He told his family, who were his travelling companions, about his fear. They thought his concerns were ridiculous.

'Don't be silly. You won't step on one. We haven't even heard of stonefish,' they said.

adolescent angst

The entire time he was swimming in Fiji he wouldn't put his feet on the bottom of the ocean, as he was terrified he would stand on one. But even his best efforts to try and avoid the fish didn't work. He trod on one near the shoreline just four days into his holiday, while walking out of the ocean. It caused his leg to swell to three times its normal size.

Greg remembers a group of Fijian men laughing uncontrollably when he began jumping about and yelling on the beach. Never before had Greg experienced such excruciating pain.

Fortunately there was a medical convention on a neighbouring island, and one of the subjects for study was stonefish poisonings. As Greg continued to scream, the Fijian men who were laughing soon realised the seriousness of the injury and helped him to the doctor. Specialists then spent three days managing his condition before the swelling subsided. He counts himself lucky to have survived.

After he recovered, the doctors told Greg that stonefish were the most poisonous of all fish. They also told him that he was lucky to have recovered because one sting could be life threatening. It certainly wasn't the holiday Greg had imagined it would be!

When he returned to Forest after his disastrous vacation, it took Greg years to rid himself of the feeling that he was a stranger. Eventually, however, he started to make some new friends. Years nine, ten, and eleven were a lot easier.

Paul Williamson was one of the few good friends that Greg made in the later years of high school. Their friendship grew steadily, and it was their mutual love of skiing and surfing that saw them spend more time together. Greg really liked Paul, and the pair would often spend their lunchtimes discussing sport and their other common interests. The laughter that was such a familiar element of his primary school years gradually returned as Paul and Greg exchanged funny stories and comical incidents from their own lives.

Even though school got easier as Greg formed new friendships, it also became more difficult in other areas. He began to neglect his studies, and over time there was a steady decline in his performance at school. Regrettably, he paid less and less attention to his teachers, and soon his grades plummeted. In a short period of time he moved from near the top of his class to the bottom. Scholastically, Greg struggled in his final senior years.

The consequence of this behaviour meant that he grew increasingly restless and agitated. Eventually, he began to rebel.

Even though he had an extremely sensitive nature, quite often he projected an entirely different image. He started to pretend that he was tough and mean and hard. He tried to put on a thick skin to protect himself.

But even though he acted this way on the outside, underneath it was an entirely different picture. He was actually fragile, and there were many times when he would go to his bedroom, close the door and cry for hours after difficult days at school.

Although he still had two years to complete for his Higher School Certificate, when Greg returned to school in Year Eleven, he grew increasingly disinterested in studying. His lack of effort meant that he was getting poor results. With his failing grades, he came to the conclusion that continuing with his schooling was pointless.

When this realisation hit home, Greg started having serious problems with some of his teachers and his disillusionment resulted in an abrupt and premature termination of his High School education.

Ironically, the final moments of his schooling came during an art class, undoubtedly his favourite and most successful subject. He wasn't following his teacher's instructions and was reprimanded. There followed a heated exchange after which he simply stood up and walked out of the classroom – out of the school, and into the next phase of his eventful life.

chapter five

sun, snow and speed

Not long after Greg walked out of school he began looking around at work opportunities and decided that carpentry would be the most suitable profession for him. It would allow him to pursue his real love in life, which was creating things with his hands.

At age seventeen Greg began his apprenticeship with Colin Haste Services as a trainee carpenter and enjoyed one of the better periods of his life. His memories of those years are still quite vivid.

'I remember my first day at work, turning up on a building site ready to start making a house. It gave me a real buzz to watch the concrete slab being poured and helping to put up the timber beams. It was so exciting, but best of all, there was no more homework!

'Even though we worked in quite a disciplined environment – no radio was allowed on the site, for example; we had to be responsible for all our tools; we had to be punctual; we had to make sure we put in a determined effort; and at the end of each day we had to make sure we cleaned up any mess – it was still easier for me. I really enjoyed it and I got tremendous satisfaction from seeing a house go up. It was a great feeling to stand back and admire the work you had done and see the end product.'

For Greg, who had built things for most of his young life, carpentry was a natural progression. He used to spend time as a youngster in the garage making things with his dad's tools: cupboards, small sculptures, billycarts, and tables. His familiarity with tools and woodwork made it easier when he started his apprenticeship. Many of his fellow employees were impressed with the easy transition he made into carpentry.

At his TAFE course, he usually topped the class in anything that was practical. His boss was a perfectionist and his thoroughness made a big impression on his young apprentice. Greg began to approach his work with the same meticulous attention to detail, and this was a trait that was to continue to develop for the rest of his life. It was not long before Greg had developed an enthusiasm for hard work. He learned a great deal during those times as he built houses and did many renovations. It was a new and exciting environment, and he found it far easier than being at school.

But there was one obvious advantage to being employed that Greg really enjoyed – he was being paid, and this opened up new and exciting opportunities and benefits.

It was during his apprenticeship that he bought his favourite car, a faded yellow Kombi van. It was older than he was, but he got great enjoyment from it, even though it kept breaking down regularly and occasionally running out of fuel. Fortunately, its battered looks belied its power, as many other motorists were to observe as it sped away from them, and there was plenty of room for luggage and sporting gear.

When he wasn't working as a carpenter, he would throw all his skiing equipment into the car, pick up his mate, Paul Williamson, and together they'd set out on in search of adventure. Nearly every weekend during the winter months, they would head to the NSW snowfields. In the summer months, they would throw their surfboards into the car and head for their favourite surfing beach Dee Why. They really enjoyed their time skylarking together.

On the surface it appeared that all was well with Greg's world: he was gainfully employed with a job that he enjoyed; he was mobile and active with his newly acquired motor vehicle; he had time to indulge in his love of sports; and he spent quality time in the company of his friends.

His reflections on this period of his life, however, reveal an underlying conflict that had been foreshadowed by the unrest and uncertainty that plagued him in his final years at school.

During his adolescence he felt as if he were riding a merry-go-round. He was on a quest, looking for a lifestyle that would make him happy, but his emotions were constantly going up and down and he felt he was just going round in circles. He threw himself into sport and became an accomplished surfer and skier. But although he would meet and exceed the goals he set for himself he would still feel unfulfilled, and a sense of emptiness would soon return.

When he almost despaired that he would ever really be happy the way he was going he began looking for alternative solutions. Towards the end of the first year of his apprenticeship he started going to parties even though he still felt rather awkward around people. He had noticed that some of his contemporaries thought that drugs or alcohol would solve their problems, and he became desperate enough to pursue that line of enquiry himself.

Initially, taking the drugs seemed fun, but it was not long before the cocktail of drugs and alcohol was making his life far worse. There was a significant risk associated with these substances, as Greg was about to discover.

When he was seventeen he attended a party that was a little light on solid foods when Andrew, one of his friends, suggested they go and get something to eat. They were both pretty much under the weather, and Greg remembers they even had difficulty deciding which car to take. His had a really good stereo system and Andrew's was really fast, so they had to choose between power and sound. Sadly, as it turned out, they chose power and jumped into his mate's Ford Cortina.

Despite the fact it was raining quite heavily, his friend took off at a brisk rate and continued to accelerate – faster and faster. Greg remembers asking himself what on earth his mate was doing, driving so fast. He started to panic as he watched the Speedo reach one hundred and forty kilometres an hour. Andrew had the accelerator to the floor as they approached a difficult corner. The car began to slip in the wet conditions, and when Greg looked at him to see how he was going to react, he could hardly believe his eyes – he had passed out behind the wheel!

When Greg looked back to the road he saw that they were headed straight for a parked car. There was nothing he could do to avoid the inevitable collision and he was convinced that they were both going to die. He braced himself for the impact as the car slammed into the stationary vehicle.

He still remembers the sound of the collision – an ear-shattering blast that haunts him to this day. The car that they hit flipped several times and landed upside down in a driveway ten metres away. Their car was a write-off. Amazingly, neither of them suffered any serious or long-lasting injuries. They were all right, with the exception of a few cuts and bruises. People who lived nearby heard the accident and ran outside to see what had happened. It was obvious that the two lads were under the influence of alcohol, so the police were called – and his mate was arrested.

Firefighters who later turned up to the scene couldn't believe that they had survived the crash. They talked to Greg for a while, warning him of the dangers of drink-driving before he was allowed to go home. He was terribly shaken up by the whole experience and ready to acknowledge that drugs and alcohol were certainly not the answer to his predicament.

His search for happiness took another turn as he began to focus on what he regarded as the 'trappings' of life. He reasoned that maybe looks and image were the key to success, so he began to spend most of his hard-earned wages on clothing and accessories. Designer labels and jewellery became the order of the day, and he devoured the fashion magazines to keep informed of all the latest trends.

They did little to prepare him for the further trials that lay ahead.

chapter six
the parental rift

Greg had just turned twenty-one and had nearly completed the final year of his apprenticeship when he got some extremely sad news: his parents had decided to get divorced.

He still remembers with perfect clarity the day he found out. He walked into the house just as his mother finished packing.

'Greg, please sit down, I have some sad news to tell you,' she said. 'Your father and I are separating.'

Although previous outbursts and a number of minor altercations in the home had given Greg an inkling that there may have been problems with the marriage, he was nevertheless devastated by the news and just sat there, stunned. He had no idea how to reply to his mother's announcement.

He had been aware for some time that there was a growing tension between his parents, but it was a subject that was never openly discussed. The sudden termination of the relationship after twenty-five years was a distinct shock, and prompted Greg to seek additional ways to cope with the disturbing news.

After he had helped his mother settle into accommodation in Manly, his anguish and confusion resulting from the separation boiled over and he decided he needed to escape for a while, to seek further distractions that would take his mind off his sadness and confusion.

As soon as he had completed his carpentry apprenticeship he decided he would travel overseas, and chose the ski fields of Chamonix Valley, France, as his destination. He was astounded at the sheer size and beauty of the French slopes, which were many times higher and longer than anything he had known in Australia. He hoped the thrill of skiing would compensate for the sense of loss he was feeling, and spent every day on the slopes for the following two weeks. But try as he would, even in such a winter wonderland, he was unable to shake his despondency.

From France he headed to Austria, and worked as a ski instructor at Otto's Ski School in Saint Michel. For a few months, he devoted himself to the task of teaching children how to become better skiers. He discovered that a kind and caring approach to teaching seemed to produce the best results, and the kids really enjoyed his classes.

Unfortunately, however, when the ski season was over and he had exhausted his savings and reached the limit on his credit card he felt he had to return home. It was time to go back to work.

For the next two years he made kitchens in his father's business, where he spent most of his days in the factory while his dad was on the road organising quotes and taking measurements for the various jobs.

When they did spend time together, the subject of the separation was rarely discussed.

Before his artistic career took off, Greg ran a successful carpentry services business at Manly Vale.

the parental rift

Because Greg was living with his mum in West Manly, he was anxious to preserve the bonds between himself and both parents, and handled the situation as delicately as he could.

Most of his spare time was spent with Paul, surfing and enjoying the beach hotel scene. He had a number of attractive girlfriends, but felt some reluctance to develop these relations further. His parents' separation still had a profound effect on his thinking, and there was always the nagging doubt that any strong relationship he might form could end in a similar fashion.

Working in his dad's business helped Greg to become exceptionally efficient and skilful in his trade, and he was soon acknowledged as a respected craftsman and kitchen maker. He built and installed hundreds of kitchens, most of which were in the Northern Beaches district.

After he had gained further experience he left to establish his own business. He started working as a registered carpenter a short time later, and for the next year he repaired decking, built kitchens, and renovated bathrooms. When the fledgling business had grown sufficiently he rented a workshop in Manly Vale. He was now working sixty hours a week, and at busy times it was often more.

Greg's life finally seemed to be on track. To all intents and purposes, he had established a successful business; he was doing something he enjoyed; and he had time to spend with his friends. What he found difficult to come to terms with, therefore, was a sense of foreboding that he experienced when he attempted to look towards the future and determine his own place in the world around him.

As his workload gradually increased, Greg saw himself becoming a slave to the demands of his business. The pressures of meeting his customers' demands, the humdrum nature of his daily work routine, the longer hours that he had to spend at his workbench, the relative 'sameness' of the products he was now making and the minimal demands that these products made on his creativity, all convinced Greg that he needed another outlet to relieve the stress and break the monotony of his now rigorous schedule. His choice proved to be one of the most disastrous of his life.

my brush with depression

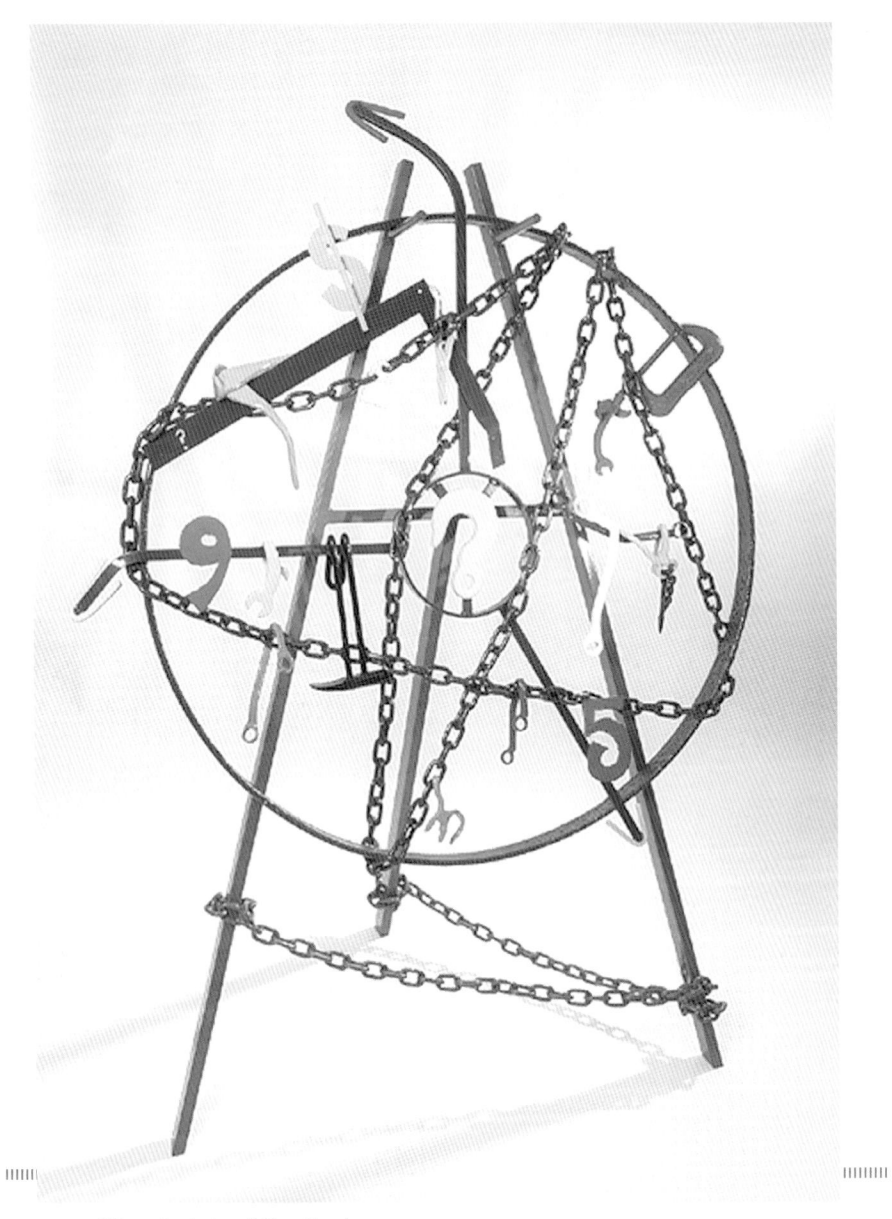

'Constraints of Routine'
Metal, carpentry tools, gemstones
1970 x 1420 x 590 mm
'The demands of the daily grind, the struggle for survival in an increasingly material world threaten to enslave us unless we break free of their shackles.' – Greg

chapter seven
the apocalypse

During his apprenticeship Greg had saved enough money to buy his first motorcycle. He developed quite a passion for bikes and loved the exhilaration and the sense of freedom they gave him. His first bike was a Honda 250cc. As his riding skills improved and he grew more confident he gradually moved to faster and more powerful machines.

His favourite bike was a black Ducati 900SS, which he would often ride to Eastern Creek Raceway and watch the stars of motorcycle racing in action. His hero at the time was Mick Doohan, Australia's five-time world champion. He seriously considered taking up competitive racing and would sit in the stands dreaming about getting out on the track and emulating the performances of his idol.

Greg admits that he first developed an interest in motorcycles because they were regarded in some circles as a sign of rebellion. He was a self-confessed 'adrenaline junky' after he left school and openly acknowledges that he would only ever feel good about himself if he were chasing thrills in one form or another.

He found that the resultant exhilaration was able to distract him temporarily from the feelings of pessimism and despondency that would often plague him. He was prepared to do whatever was required to take his mind from the turmoil that was going on inside his head: running faster, skiing faster, choosing dangerous roads, or riding his motorbike were all his ways of trying to escape.

When quizzed later about some of these dangerous pursuits, Greg admits that during this 'rebellious' period of his life his recklessness bordered on an almost fatalistic attitude towards danger. 'If I die, I die,' he was once heard to remark. 'So what?'

He almost answered that question for himself when he was just twenty years old. He had been shopping at Warringah Mall on Sydney's northern beaches and jumped onto his motorbike to ride home. Just minutes into the trip, after throwing his bike into a tight corner, he suddenly realised that, not only was he going too fast, but a motorist in front of him was on the wrong side of the road!

Instinctively he thrust the bike towards the gutter, pushing himself clear and skidding along the ground in the middle of his lane. He had closed his eyes and braced himself for what he thought was an unavoidable collision with the car. When he finally skidded to a stop and opened his eyes, he was staring up at the car radiator, his head just centimetres from the front wheel.

As the horrified elderly gentleman helped pull Greg out from under the vehicle and muttered his profound apology, he marvelled that the young rider had escaped with little more than a few cuts and bruises.

Strangely enough, this close call didn't deter Greg from continuing to ride his bikes.

He remembered being told that the best thing to do if one ever fell from a horse was to remount immediately, and he applied the same advice to his motorcycle accident. In no time at all, he was back in the saddle.

A second accident, with far more drastic consequences, occurred a year later and resulted in far more serious injuries. What was intended as a leisurely ride suddenly took a turn for the worse on the way to a friend's house for dinner.

It was dusk and Greg was making his way down a fairly steep hill

the apocalypse

heading towards Manly when he noticed a car coming in the opposite direction. As it started to slow down and pull over to the side of the road, he assumed it was going to stop. However, as he continued down the hill he couldn't believe his eyes when the car did a complete U-turn directly in front of him!

Greg thought it was 'game over'. He was travelling at around eighty kilometres an hour when he smashed into the side of the car. After the impact he went spinning through the air, conscious the whole time until his back slammed into the gutter. An elderly gentleman, who was an eyewitness to the accident, said that Greg did five cartwheels before his momentum was stopped.

Greg's first concern was that he had broken his back. He couldn't feel anything in his legs. He was convinced that he was going to be a paraplegic and that he would never walk again.

Fortunately, this was not the case, although he certainly did not escape lightly. Injuries from the accident included: a broken wrist, two broken thumbs, several gashes in his legs, severe bruising of the groin, which had ripped the petrol tank from the bike, and back and neck problems. The car was extensively damaged and the bike was a complete write-off.

The police were called to the scene and discovered that the driver of the vehicle that caused the accident was an unlicensed 15-year-old, taking his mates for a joyride in his father's car. As the teenager was taken to the police station for questioning, an ambulance took Greg to hospital where he had to undergo several surgical procedures to fix his broken bones. He had to have a bone graft, where a portion of his hip was removed and transferred to his wrist. Surgeons then had to insert metal pins into his shattered wrist and enclose it in plaster.

Despite these severe setbacks, Greg could not be persuaded to stop riding. In mid-1994 he had just turned twenty-four and was on his way to a friend's house in the city on his Ducati 900SS motorcycle. It had been raining in the streets of Paddington, an inner city suburb of Sydney, and the road on which he was travelling was wet and slippery. He felt cold, and the black and red leathers that he was wearing were becoming soaked. The driving rain was seriously hampering his vision.

As he made his way down Oxford Street he noticed the eclectic mix of people huddling under shop awnings and umbrellas to escape the rain. Others warmed themselves by sipping coffee at the trendy cafes and restaurants that lined both sides of the roadway.

A short time later, as the road climbed higher, he approached the crest of a hill and suddenly found himself yet again in a life-threatening situation. There had been a minor accident, and the traffic had all stopped, slewed across the street, with a taxicab blocking the road just metres in front of him. It was glaringly obvious that Greg was in serious trouble, and he panicked. There was no time to brake, nowhere to turn, and a violent collision with the cab was inevitable.

The Ducati slammed into the taxi's bumper bar, and Greg was sent flying through the air into the cab's rear window. His head and neck shattered the glass and, as the rest of his body rebounded from the boot of the cab, remaining shards of glass tore deeply into his neck, severing the main artery. His unconscious body fell backwards and dropped awkwardly to the ground, bleeding profusely. It all seemed to

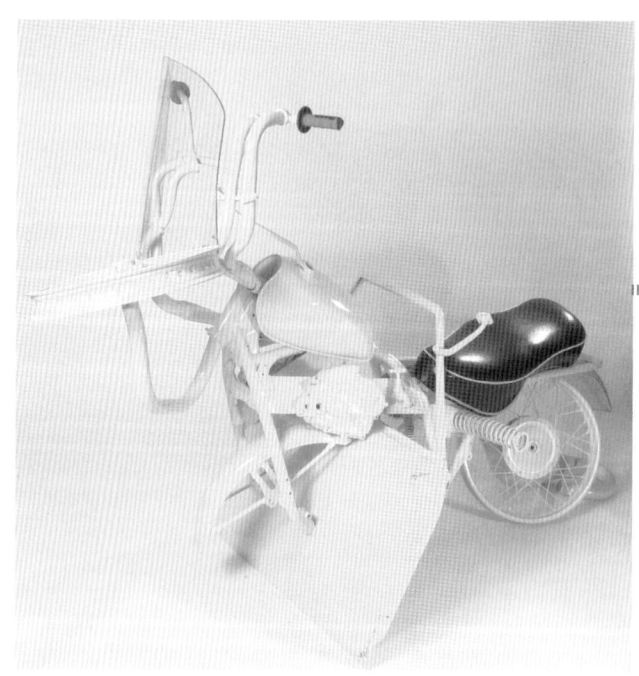

'Through the Taxi and into Another Life'
Clear coated, sealed and painted motorbike parts, seat and visor, tap, and car door.
1530 x 2220 x 910 mm

the apocalypse

happen in a split second, according to observers, who rushed off to call an ambulance.

It was not long before the police had arrived at the scene, and they were quick to seal off the area with a security barrier. They did not want bystanders to witness the horrendous sight of Greg's body bathed in blood by the roadside.

Next to arrive at the scene of the carnage were the paramedics, who rushed to his side. Given that Greg had just cut a major artery, it's not surprising that they feared for his life. They could tell by the amount of blood he had already lost that the situation was critical. By the time they began their examinations his blood pressure had fallen alarmingly, and his pulse was barely discernible. They later confided, in fact, that at one stage Greg's heart had actually stopped beating and that for a short time he was clinically dead.

Their first concern was the excessive bleeding, which they managed to stem. Then they began CPR to try and start his heart once more. As a result of their efforts, Greg began to breathe again and a weak pulse returned. Before they could move Greg, however, his rescuers had to apply a splint to a badly broken left leg.

Despite their best efforts, his life was still hanging in the balance, and his brain was being starved of both nutrients and oxygen due to the lack of blood flow caused by the damaged artery. If he were going to survive the crash, he needed medical attention at a hospital, and he needed it urgently.

Doctors were not sure if he would live when he arrived at St Vincent's hospital. They rushed him into the Emergency Department and began operating immediately. They had to seal the artery and stitch the large gash in his neck to prevent any more bleeding, and several litres of blood were needed to replace what he had lost. Finally, they repaired his leg by inserting a surgical rod to hold together his broken femur. It took several hours of intensive medical care before his condition finally stabilised.

However, some disturbing questions still needed to be answered. Would his leg fully recover? More distressingly, would there be any long-term brain damage? Doctors were seriously concerned that the cut artery had stopped vital oxygen from reaching his brain during the accident, possibly injuring brain tissue. They would have to wait until Greg regained consciousness to know just how bad these injuries were.

Greg opened his eyes a few hours later. He had no idea what had happened to him or where he was. When he tried to move his arm, it was restricted by a drip and there was a large bandage on his elbow. The bed he was lying in was much firmer than the one he was used to. A large curtain enclosed the bed, and there was a strange woman standing before him in a white uniform.

'Where am I?' he asked groggily.

'You're in St Vincent's Hospital and you've been in a serious motorcycle accident,' replied the nurse who was caring for him.

Greg had no recollection whatsoever of the events leading up to his admission.

When Greg's distraught mum came to visit, she told him what the hospital had learned from the attending police officer.

'You crashed your motorbike into the back of taxi and were pronounced dead at the scene of the accident,' she informed him. 'The paramedic team had to do heart massage, and you needed a full blood transfusion at the hospital. The doctors told me it had been a life or death situation, and the policeman said he couldn't believe that you had survived. It took two fire engines to hose away the blood you lost. You're lucky to be alive.'

'I don't remember a thing,' Greg said. 'I woke up with forty stitches in my neck and drips in my body; it was frightening.'

Even though he was unclear about what had happened, one thing had already become evident – the life he once knew was now gone forever. He was in extreme pain; his neck throbbed; his leg was swollen and aching badly; and his body was riddled with cuts and bruises. The doctors who examined him told him his injuries were quite serious and that it would be some time before he would be well enough to leave the hospital.

The next two weeks were pure agony. Despite regular administrations

the apocalypse

of morphine, Greg found the pain unbearable, and each day seemed to drag on interminably.

Finally, one month after his admission to St Vincent's, he was allowed to return home.

As he left the foyer on his newly acquired crutches, he thanked the nurses sincerely for their wonderful care, and boasted jokingly that, because of his accidents, he probably knew more nurses and paramedics in Sydney than any other patient.

His jovial demeanour was to be short-lived, however, as Greg's battle with the demons of depression posed the most serious threat yet to his survival.

chapter eight
the depths of despair

From St Vincent's Hospital, Greg was taken by maxi-cab to his mother's house in Marsfield, a pleasant, leafy suburb in Sydney's inner west. Both his mum and her new husband, Rob, had agreed to accommodate Greg for the term of his convalescence, knowing full well that it could extend over a long period.

It turned out to be well over twelve months, and was one of the worst phases of Greg's entire life.

The metal rod caused his leg to ache excruciatingly, and the great gash in his neck hurt every time he moved his head. For a time the pain killers prescribed by his doctor brought temporary relief, but the dosage was restricted and there were long stretches where the pain was almost unbearable.

The stillness of the house and the absence of other persons was such a contrast to the hospital environment that he had so recently left. There had been doctors, nurses, other patients and visitors to occupy him and engage him in conversation during the day; now there was no-one.

Despite the best efforts of his mother and Rob, Greg felt as if he had been sentenced to solitary confinement in a suburban prison. There was

the depths of despair

no escape, not only from his physical boundaries, but even worse, no escape from the mental anguish that was to plague him.

Each day he would hear the sounds of the boys making their way to the nearby high school at Epping, the sound of busy commuters on Vimiera Road, and on weekends he could detect the sense of anticipation as supporters of the local rugby team, the Woodies, made their way to the nearby oval at T.G. Milner Field. All of this activity and bustle only served to make him feel more isolated and frustrated.

There were none of the distractions that had been so available in his life before the accident, and he began to wonder if he would ever be able to pursue them again: would he ever catch another wave on his board at Manly; would he ever run the slalom gates again at Mount Perisher; would he ever know the sense of freedom that riding his motorcycles always seemed to produce; would he ever again play skins with his mates down at the local golf course; dear God, would he ever be able to walk without a limp? Would he ever be able to look in a mirror again without feeling a sense of revulsion at the great scar that he feared would disfigure him for life?

His surroundings did little to relieve the sense of apprehension that he had about his future. For hours at a time, day in and day out, he would stare at the gyprock ceiling of his bedroom, seeing it as a giant screen on which he began to replay the tragic circumstances that had led to his present situation. They were all classified M for misery.

Whenever friends would visit, their talk of all the good times they had enjoyed together depressed him even further. Here they were, getting on with their lives and making the most of their opportunities; his life was static, if not actually going backwards!

He found himself being so negative and so pessimistic that their visits would become less and less frequent, until eventually they gave up altogether. He began to prefer the relative quiet and isolation of the night time to the daylight hours, and withdrew even more markedly from human contact. All the outside daytime activity was too painful a reminder of what 'normal' life used to be like, and all the things of which he was now being deprived and which he missed so sorely.

There were other times when his thoughts became so destructive that he felt he was going insane. He would eventually come to terms with the physical scars that would forever disfigure his body, but there was no cosmetic surgery to remove the mental scars that remained.

At times he tried to replace these negative premonitions with much more optimistic affirmations, trying to convince himself that yes, he would overcome, he would get over it, and that he would make a determined effort to shake off his depression. Problem was, he didn't know where to start the journey to recovery, and had no idea how to achieve his goals.

One evening, just on dusk, as a southerly buster brought its welcome relief from the summer heat, Marsfield was visited by a sudden downpour. Greg hobbled across to the window of his bedroom and gazed out at the sullen, grey landscape. He slowly became aware of his own reflection, pale and drawn, staring back at him in the fading evening light.

He remembers remarking to himself how closely the weather resembled his own feelings and condition. All the light seemed to have been drained from his world; grey was now the predominant hue. He was unable to contain the tears that slowly ran down his cheeks as he closed his eyes and mourned the loss of all the vibrant colours from his life.

He recalls that in that one, desperate moment he actually railed at God in an uncharacteristic burst of irreverence. Why had he been targeted and chosen as the victim for all this adversity? Why did he seem to have all the bad luck? Why did the future suddenly seem so abysmal? What was the purpose in trying to resurrect a life that now had so little promise? Why didn't God just take him without delay and put an end to all this misery!

When Greg found himself seriously considering death as an 'easy' solution to his problems, he instinctively knew that he was in need of professional psychological help. Up to this point all of his treatments had consisted of visits to a physiotherapist, where any references to depression had been put aside while attention was given to his physical rehabilitation.

the depths of despair

Because of the long period of inactivity that his broken femur had required while it began to heal and mend itself, a certain amount of muscular atrophy had occurred. As soon as he was able, Greg attended a clinic at Chatswood, where he was painfully acquainted with the agony of coaxing his battered body back into working order. He almost screamed when his wasted leg muscles were massaged for the first time, and bending his knee produced a searing spasm that shocked him with its intensity.

The recovery periods after his physiotherapy sessions proved an extremely difficult time for Greg, and as he laid his aching body to rest after each session, he found it impossible to dispel the despair he felt at the slowness of his progress and the price he was being asked to pay. When doctors later confirmed that he would have to undergo a total knee reconstruction, his flagging spirits reached rock bottom.

So now, more than ever, he felt an urgent need to seek professional assistance for his mental well-being. He was being visited by nightmares that brought back some of the remembered details of his accidents, but above all he was assailed by a sense of being abandoned, of being alone, of being misunderstood, of being … worthless.

His tiredness and disgust, his depression and trepidation, his own hopelessness and mental weariness, had all stripped his spirit of its defences. When he shut his eyes, there was nothing but darkness. His thoughts were in disarray and he had no idea which way to turn. He was numb. He remembers thinking that maybe there was no solution to his problem.

Even his attempts to seek assistance and guidance from a number of local psychiatrists proved fruitless. He describes the visits as clinical and impersonal. The doctor would hit a clock to start timing the sessions, Greg would give a brief account of his life, and no one really offered any explanation as to why he felt the way that he did. On none of these occasions did he feel that there was any real empathy or understanding of his problems. These conclusions, naturally, did nothing to alleviate the anxiety and desperation that he was feeling.

In a last frantic attempt to find out what was wrong with him, Greg sought to gain admission to a psychiatric hospital at Manly. His first impression of the clinic was not favourable: it felt like being in a place that time had forgotten! It felt like a holding pen where he was going to remain until someone deemed him fit to be returned to civilisation. Seemingly normal people wandered around aimlessly without appearing to have any real purpose; taking their medication; attending the odd counselling session; but, most surprisingly, hardly ever discussing their feelings or their own particular problems. Greg felt desperate, abysmally low, and his life seemed hopeless as he endured the agony of true depression in that place.

When Greg described these concerns to his sister Robyn, she listened carefully to what he had to say and then quietly told him: 'I know somebody whom I think you should meet!'

chapter nine
the hand of loving kindness

Josie Alder was born in the south of Italy, the second of seven children in the family, and came to Australia with her parents when she was two years old. Her mother had been well regarded in Bella, their Calabrian village, and had been a highly respected natural therapist and midwife. Much of her wisdom had been faithfully handed down from generation to generation and her knowledge of herbal remedies and medications was extraordinary.

When the family settled in Melbourne, Josie grew up as a typical Australian youngster, attending school at Moreland and eventually deciding on a career as a beautician. No doubt influenced by her mother's interest in natural medicines, she also decided to further her own knowledge in that field and eventually went to Canada, where she attended the Old Montreal Health and Healing Centre.

Returning to Australia, Josie began sharing her newly acquired knowledge and skills with friends and acquaintances, eventually building up an extensive range of clients on Sydney's North Shore. It was in this capacity that Robyn, Greg's sister, had come to know Josie and benefit from her professional advice.

When Robyn dropped him off at Josie's place in Fairlight, neither of them had any idea of the remarkable impact that this meeting was to have on Greg's life. Greg limped up the narrow staircase leading to the front of the house, steadied himself on the railing, and knocked on the door.

He remembers being pleasantly impressed by the attractive, olive-skinned woman who greeted him. Her warm, brown eyes and her welcoming smile put him immediately at ease. He noticed that her bright blue and yellow outfit provided a stark contrast to his own. He was dressed in sombre black – shirt, jeans and boots.

'Come in,' she said. 'Welcome to my humble abode!'

Josie's impressions of their first meeting are still quite graphic. She recalls being scrutinised by a pale and hesitant looking individual with a haggard face, who had dark shadows under his eyes. There was a troubled look about him, almost as if he were afraid. His whole carriage and bearing seemed to represent a silent plea for help.

She ushered him quietly inside to a neat and tidy lounge room. He noticed a glass coffee table with a number of books on natural therapies resting on its surface. A large bookshelf overflowed with natural medicines, pills and tinctures. A framed wall chart showing the anatomy of the human body was prominently displayed near one of the windows, and two chairs had been positioned in the middle of the room.

Something about the décor and Josie's demeanour gave Greg an almost immediate sense of relief. Josie's diminutive figure was anything but intimidating, and the genuine warmth with which he had been welcomed told him that he was in the company of someone who genuinely cared. His first impressions were so positive that he knew he would have no trouble discussing his feelings and problems with this woman.

He began by apologising for his dark and sombre outfit, but explained to her that it really reflected how he was feeling inside. He told her that he felt simply terrible, confused and lost. He had no energy, and because of his injuries would be unable to return to his carpentry work for some time. He was desperately seeking answers to the meaning of his life, the reasons for his battered existence, and a way to overcome or manage his depression.

the hand of loving kindness

He told her how he felt that no-one really appreciated what was happening inside his head, not even the doctors who professed to understand his symptoms and their causes. How could anyone who hadn't experienced depression themselves hope to understand what he was going through, let alone treat his problem or cure it?

He said he felt like a punch-drunk fighter, who had been put into the ring blindfolded. He kept throwing punches but could never land a blow or even make contact with his opponent. He just felt so powerless and so inept. As he related his innermost feelings he was so stirred up by the desperation of his plight that he stopped for a moment and confided to Josie that he felt that he would be better off dead; that it seemed so unfair to his family and friends that he should inflict his suffering and pain upon them as well; that he should be such a burden to those that he loved.

Greg was stunned when Josie quietly assured him that she understood perfectly what he was going through. She informed him she had been visited by the demons, had suffered from depression and had managed to overcome the threat that it posed to her life. She told him that she believed she had emerged from her ordeal a much stronger and more confident person. For that reason, she said, she felt she could help him and would be happy to continue to assist him.

At that instant, Greg experienced the birth of a glimmer of hope. Here was someone who had been through the torment that he had experienced. Here was someone who really cared, who did understand what empathy was. Here was someone who wasn't going to pass judgement on him. Here was someone, at last, whom he felt he could trust. Here, please God, was the answer to his desperate prayers.

During the following month, Greg continued to visit Josie each week. She continued to reassure him and repeat her positive affirmations about the future. She was able to advise him about his dietary needs, and supplemented his daily intake with a number of herbal preparations that she felt would assist him. Above all, she was there to listen to him when he needed to express his thoughts and describe his emotions and fears.

After each visit he felt a little clearer in his own mind, taking great comfort from the fact that there was one person in the world who seemed to understand him. Josie was a person whom Greg felt was totally credible and she helped him understand that his life was important. Greg believed he could trust her, a feeling that had eluded him in many of his relationships up until now.

Slowly he perceived a rekindling of his own sense of worth … slowly, slowly he began to appreciate that progress was being made, although he still felt himself periodically dropping back into the depths of his own despair.

He was delighted when he felt a resurgence of interest in his old pastimes and hobbies. When he opened his mail at Marsfield one morning and found a cheque from the insurance company which had provided coverage on his motorcycle, he was even confident enough to go back to his favourite cycle shop and pay for another Ducati.

His growing optimism was shattered, however, when he woke one morning and, for no apparent reason, felt once again the overbearing oppressiveness of depression crushing his spirit. The most pessimistic of thoughts suddenly began to assail him, and again he despaired of ever finding the cure for his problem.

He returned to his room, sat himself in front of his television and tried to lose himself in the Oprah Winfrey show, where he sometimes found a small measure of encouragement from the success stories that were usually featured there. But his dreadful premonitions continued to plague him, and he found himself sinking irretrievably back into the pit.

He began to panic as he also realised that his support network was starting to disintegrate. His mum had made plans to move to Queensland, his sister Lynda was now living in Jindabyne, and Robyn was travelling overseas. Even his friends seemed to be deserting him: many of them had expressed their scepticism about the real nature of his illness. They failed to understand that Greg could not simply 'pull himself out of it' as they so glibly suggested. Greg decided that he had to see Josie and hear her reassuring voice. When he dialled her number, however, all he heard was the answering machine asking him to leave a message. He slammed the phone down in exasperation.

the hand of loving kindness

His thoughts then followed an all-too-familiar pattern. Why should he continue to be a burden to his friends and family? What had he to look forward to when it was apparent there was no cure for his problem? What was the point of continuing a life that was becoming devoid of all meaning?

Donning his leather riding gear, Greg decided on a course of action that would solve all of his problems. He wheeled the Ducati out of his mother's garage, started the engine and headed across town for the pharmacy on Manly's Corso, as a desperate plan started to crystallise in his mind. He would end this wretched existence once and for all!

Fortunately, because he had no prescription for the medication he would have preferred, Greg was only able to purchase a much weaker sleeping tablet than the ones he wanted. However, he felt those that he obtained would be adequate for the plan he had in mind. There were twenty-five tablets in the packet that the pharmacist handed to him across the counter.

From the Corso it was only a short ride to his destination: the cliff-tops above Shelley Beach. As he brought his motorcycle to a halt in the nearby car park, he stopped himself from following his usual procedure of padlocking his bike. He told himself that he would never need the machine again, so what was the point of taking precautions?

After making sure there was no-one else around, Greg climbed over the wire safety fence that surrounded the car park and he found himself a vantage point out of sight from above. Satisfied that no-one would be able to witness his last despairing act, Greg perched himself precariously on a large rock that was hanging out over the steep drop. He could hear the waves crashing onto the rugged shoreline far below. He opened his box of tablets and swallowed all of the contents, one by one. He calculated that it should only take about twenty minutes or so for drowsiness to overtake him, he would then gradually fall asleep, tumble forward off the rock … and gravity would bring down the final curtain on his miserable life!

He felt the weariness begin to seep into his body. It wouldn't be long now – just a few minutes more. Then, in what he thought were to be his last moments, Greg became aware of an inner voice that had been silent up until now. It was a jarring, contradictory message that it was attempting to deliver. He tried to silence it, but it was insistent. Gradually he was able to discern its message: 'Don't do it, Greg. Don't do it!' That was all he heard, just that simple, monotonous mantra: 'Don't do it, Greg. Don't do it!'

He barely remembers what happened next, but somehow he managed to scramble back from the edge of the cliff, clamber over the safety fence and find his motorcycle in the car park. He didn't know how much longer he could stave off the tiredness, but Josie's place was only ten minutes away if he could stay awake that long. When she greeted him at the door, he pushed roughly past her and barely made it to the bathroom before the contents of his stomach disgorged into the toilet bowl.

'Josie, I'm so sorry, but I'm in desperate need of help,' he pleaded when he returned to the lounge room. Josie was only able to hear sketchy details of the suicide attempt before Greg finally succumbed to his weariness and collapsed, exhausted, on the couch. Josie put a pillow under his head, wrapped him in a blanket, and kept a watchful eye from the kitchen as he fell into a deep, troubled sleep.

During the vigil, Josie took her mobile phone outside so she would not wake him and called Greg's mother in Marsfield. She explained that she was deeply worried about Greg's welfare, and that she feared he might make another attempt to take his own life if he were not supervised. Marnie was deeply upset and not sure what to do. She could ill afford to take time off work, and her busy schedule prevented her from spending extended periods of time supervising Greg. Josie offered to let Greg stay with her and promised she would keep a watchful eye on him until he got back on his feet. Marnie expressed her grateful thanks and asked Josie to keep her informed of Greg's progress.

By the time Greg awoke the following morning, Josie had already made some enquiries and found that a psychiatrist in the Manly area would be available to see Greg despite the short notice, and she went with him a few days later. It was to be an unfortunate experience for both of them.

the hand of loving kindness

They later described the atmosphere in the consultancy as cold and intense. The psychiatrist who greeted them reclined in his chair and stared intently at Greg as he entered the room, carrying a number of forms and questionnaires that he had been asked to complete in the waiting room.

Greg seated himself nervously in a chair, and when he was asked by the doctor to outline his problem, he thought long and hard about how best to describe all the anguish that he had suffered, all the heartache and pain he had endured ... and with some hesitation finally volunteered: 'I feel as though my heart has broken!'

The reply from the doctor stung both of them: 'I am also a surgeon,' he said, 'and to suggest such nonsense is ridiculous. During all my years in the operating theatre I have never once come across a broken heart!' This outburst was delivered with such unexpected vehemence that both Greg and Josie flinched noticeably.

Greg got the distinct impression, as the consultation continued, that the doctor had formed the unshakeable conclusion that Greg had somehow fabricated his symptoms, and that there was no real case of depression to consider. He began making comments like: 'Come on, now. You're a fit young bloke, capable of getting on with your life. There's really no reason for anyone to have depression! Look outside, it's such a beautiful day. It's time to grow up, son, and start living!' Greg felt completely dejected!

A lengthy and almost self-congratulatory list of the doctor's own credentials and qualifications did little to impress Greg. The doctor may have understood the physiological reasons for depression, but it seemed blatantly obvious to Greg that he had no idea what it was like to suffer from it. Greg could detect no empathy whatsoever, and interrupted the doctor's comments by asking him: 'Have you ever had depression?'

The doctor replied: 'That has nothing to do with my job or my diagnosis!'

Greg could not tolerate the man's rudeness any longer. He leapt up, shaking his head in disbelief and scattering the papers that had been resting in his lap.

'It has everything to do with your job and your diagnosis!' he snapped at the surprised medico.

Unable to stand another moment of such treatment, he brushed Josie aside and fled from the room.

Josie was deeply upset by what had transpired, and she said sadly to the doctor: 'I don't think you realise what you've just done!' She left to find Greg, and then drove with him back to Fairlight.

She let Greg out at the front door and went to park the car. When she entered the house she froze as she came through the hallway and saw him in the kitchen. He had picked up a large carving knife that she'd been using to fillet some fish earlier, and he was slowly brushing his finger across the sharp edge. He raised the knife and gently began stroking the scar on his neck with the blade. She called out to Greg, softly so that he wouldn't be startled by the sound of her voice.

'Don't do it, Greg. Don't do it!'

He turned slowly with such an incredulous look on his face that Josie was completely taken aback. The tears started to course down his face as he replaced the knife on the kitchen bench and went as if in a trance to the spare room at the back of Josie's house. He stayed there for four days.

chapter ten
lightning strikes twice

It appeared to Josie that Greg's situation couldn't get any worse. It was just too bizarre, too inconceivable, to entertain such a thought. However, this is precisely what happened when another cruel twist of fate impacted on his life a few weeks later.

Josie had eventually been able to coax Greg from his self-imposed isolation. She told Greg that he was welcome to use the spare room of the house until he improved and that she had okayed this arrangement with his mother.

Greg divided his time between moping around the house and lying in bed. With his recent disastrous visit to the psychiatrist still fresh in his mind, Greg believed the only thing he could do was to find the most comfortable room in the house, the most comfortable bed, prop up the pillows and resign himself to the fact that depression was going to be an inevitable part of his life. He really believed that this was his lot and was firmly convinced that no outside help could ever alter his predicament.

One fateful afternoon, out of sheer desperation, he decided he had to get out of the house and take his mind off the gloomy introspection that constantly plagued him during this period.

Josie had a number of appointments that day, and was treating a patient for some digestive disturbances when she noticed Greg leave the spare room and head out the door. Her heart skipped a beat when she heard the unmistakeable sound of the Ducati being kicked over in the garage. Before she could do anything, the engine roared into life and the bike took off at a great rate down the driveway with Greg hunched over the petrol tank.

Greg sped from the Fairlight house and zigzagged from side to side down the street. He began shaking his head as if the wind whistling past his helmet could sweep away the troubled thoughts that haunted him.

Gradually, he steadied the bike and began making his way into Manly. Reaching the conclusion that perhaps an afternoon in the sun, strolling along the walkway in front of the ocean, would ease his beleaguered mind, he headed towards the beach.

He was cruising through a familiar traffic island in Balgowlah, looking forward to the respite that he hoped his beach walk would provide, when the rear of the bike was suddenly jerked to one side. Some part of the bike had clipped the raised edge of the concrete. It threw the Ducati into a death wobble that rendered the bike completely uncontrollable. He wrestled with the handlebars, desperately trying to regain control. His efforts were in vain. The front tyre clipped the pavement on the side of the traffic island and, with a horrible sense of déjà vu, he was catapulted violently into the air.

Everything became a blur as he tried desperately to push himself away from the bike, which had now become a lethal projectile. His body spun over the handlebars and went flying out into space. He came back to earth head first, and as he crashed back onto the road everything went black.

An off-duty police officer who had been driving a short distance behind Greg was the first to arrive at the scene. He later informed us that the stand which Greg used to prop up the bike had dropped down as the bike turned into the roundabout. It hit the road and caused the rear wheel to shoot up into the air.

The policeman called an ambulance, and Greg was again rushed to hospital.

lightning strikes twice

Josie had been worried since Greg had left and when the phone finally rang, she raced to see if it was him. Instead it was the Manly hospital. A staff member had contacted her to let her know that Greg had been admitted after a serious motorcycle accident.

She reached the hospital shortly after Greg had regained consciousness. When he came to, he could not believe he'd been involved in another accident. This time he had broken a shoulder, and the pain was severe. His body was lacerated with cuts, and his head ached excruciatingly from his collision with the road surface. The tremendous emotional pain that he was suffering proved far worse than his physical injuries. He was convinced that life was some sort of cruel joke, and that he was the victim of a quirk of fate yet again.

As depression descended on him once more, he began to feel sorry that the accident had not claimed his life. He was angry that he had survived and disappointed that the accident hadn't killed him. Josie listened patiently as he poured out his frustration and despair.

When the hospital staff overheard some of his outbursts and realised that he was bewailing the fact that he had survived, they approached Josie and asked her how he had developed such a morbid state of mind.

When she informed them of Greg's previous accidents and his attempted suicide, they recommended further treatment, and made arrangements for him to be admitted to the Psychiatric Unit at the Manly Hospital. She also informed doctors that she thought the herbal remedies she had introduced into his diet weren't strong enough to produce the desired results, and that maybe they should enquire about the availability of stronger medication to assist in his recovery.

When the doctors approached Greg in the clinic and asked why he had decided to take his own life, he welcomed the opportunity to vent his frustration. He told them that he believed suicide was the only way he could stop his pain and his feelings of despair. There didn't seem to be any way that he could deal with his life any more. There was so much uncertainty that surrounded him at the time that he didn't believe he could get over the episodes of depression that he was feeling.

He felt that life was too disturbing, too hard to take. He had nightmares when he slept, and absolutely no peace of mind. During the day it was as if he was living the same nightmares. He thought that if he killed himself he could escape them. The depression was relentless. Night and day were as bad as each other. He would try and distract himself by watching TV, but in the back of his mind he knew his depression was still there and that he would fall straight back into its clutches when the programme he was watching had finished.

When Josie suggested that Greg inform his parents of his admission to the clinic, he was not in favour of the idea. He told her that he did not want to cause them any undue concern and did not want to interrupt their busy lives. Besides, he felt that no one could understand his situation as well as Josie, and she was the only one in whom he wished to confide.

One week after he had been admitted Greg was feeling a lot calmer, and the doctors were sufficiently satisfied with his state of mind to allow him to leave the clinic. Greg was now faced with a practical dilemma: he had nowhere to stay, no money to afford accommodation, and no job prospects. Once again, it was Josie who came to the rescue, offering to let Greg use the spare room at her house in Fairlight until other arrangements could be made.

Josie was well aware of the enormous task that was ahead of her. She knew that her decision to care for Greg would bring with it some serious disruptions to her life, but she accepted the responsibility none the less. She was still shaken by the attempts that Greg had made on his life and was aware that there was no guarantee it would be the last. She just wanted him to live, and her inner voice told her that if she failed to look after him there was nobody else who would.

And so she took him from the hospital to her Fairlight home where she fed him and helped him recover from the trauma that his attempt to end his life had produced. Greg is convinced that had Josie not become his Good Samaritan he could never have survived.

There were a few other bright lights on the horizon, and they helped correct a rather jaundiced opinion that Greg had formed of the medical profession. Greg reluctantly agreed to Josie's request for him to see doctors to help with his depression. What other course of action was there for him to take? They were Dr Bruce Westmore from Sydney, and Dr Greg 'Becker' Norris from Mona Vale. Dr Norris earned his nickname because of his dry mannerisms that reminded people of Ted Danson of the TV sitcom Becker fame. (Dr Norris had a great sense of humour and light-heartedly told Josie that he loved seeing Greg, as he was the only bloke he knew who was almost as crazy as he was!)

When Greg was later asked why he liked these two specialists, he replied simply: 'Because they cared, and because I had confidence in them.'

Greg was able to explain to them how he was feeling, how life lacked any real purpose for him, and that he was in extreme emotional pain. He told how he was not able to sleep; how he would lie awake constantly at night; how he would cry without any provocation; how he would become irritable; and how the thoughts of suicide never seemed to completely vanish from his mind.

The doctors outlined some of the reasons these things were happening to him. They told him that his depression was caused by a combination of many circumstances, genetic factors and possibly inadequate supply of chemicals to the brain. When they learned the details of the motorcycle accident, they explained that the stress caused by the accident could also have aggravated his depression.

Dr Westmore helped him to understand that depression was an illness, no different from any other. With medication, it could be controlled. He never blamed Greg for having the depression and actually gave him a lot of hope during his consultations. The visits progressed favourably, and eventually the doctors suggested a course of different medications to help Greg during this critical period. These would be replaced by preventative medicines further down the track. Greg confided that he would take anything that would help ease his pain.

It was during this time, also, that Greg really began to understand how important was the production of adequate chemicals in the brain. Lack of these chemicals in his brain actually caused him to have emotional swings. This new medication was going to help stabilise his moods so that he didn't experience the extreme highs and lows over which he seemed to have no control.

Initially, the side effects were too strong, and he suffered bouts of nausea and stomach upsets. Eventually, through a process of trial and error, a satisfactory balance was achieved and Greg began to notice not only a marked improvement in his physical condition, but a most welcome change for the better in his mental outlook.

Another important element in his gradual recovery was the re-awakening of his interest in sport. His knee had now healed completely from the reconstruction that he'd had to have as part of his recovery from the accident, and the continued physiotherapy had improved his flexibility to such an extent that he was ready to make his way back onto the golf course. After several visits to the driving range at Narrabeen, he eventually felt confident to take his clubs out onto the course. He fondly remembers the great sense of relief and of wellbeing he experienced as he stood on the first tee at the Mona Vale Golf Club and quietly complimented himself: 'You have come a long way, baby!'

chapter eleven

hearts and rainbows

After the lease on their Fairlight house ran out, Josie and Greg moved to Bayview, where the local coffee shop soon became one of Josie's favourite haunts. Set in a tranquil sunlit courtyard, it was a great place to escape the bustle of Mona Vale Road and the busy shopping centre.

Not only did patrons enjoy the mouth-watering pasta dishes that were on offer each day, but they delighted in the company of the young woman who managed the business and who always greeted her customers with a beaming smile. Her name was Joyce Biviano, and she was an outstanding chef. Joyce's mother, Maria, had also earned a reputation as a great cook, and brought with her from Italy a host of wonderful recipes and culinary 'secrets'.

Josie would sometimes sit at the table closest to the kitchen, sipping her cappuccino and talking with Joyce while she cooked, prepared sandwiches and made a variety of salads for her customers. Their conversation was often interrupted as Joyce would race hurriedly from one pot to another, carefully stirring the contents, or taking money from her departing patrons.

It wasn't long before a feeling of trust had developed between the two women, and Josie gave Joyce some of the more personal details of her own life. She explained how she was using her training as a natural therapist to help care for Greg in his battle with depression.

For some time Joyce had been troubled by a nagging sprain to her left ankle that seemed to be taking forever to heal. The sensation of pins and needles in the joint did not stop her from working, but it was an unpleasant restriction to her movement, and she was worried that it did not seem to be improving. When she learned of Josie's background in therapy, she asked if she could make an appointment and have Josie examine the injured joint. Josie readily agreed and invited Joyce to visit her at the Bayview residence. During this time Joyce met Greg, and soon they too became friends.

Treatment for the injured ankle involved massage and liniments, and after some time there was a noticeable improvement and the pain began to recede.

In 1996, the owner of the coffee shop indicated that she wanted to move away from the district, and she offered Joyce the option to purchase the business. Joyce was eager to make the most of this opportunity, and after being given the promise of some financial assistance from her parents, she went ahead with the contract.

Joyce threw herself into her work with renewed vigour after she became the proprietor of the shop and when she recalled that Greg had a background in carpentry, she approached him with the idea of giving the premises a facelift.

They reached an agreement that was to be mutually beneficial: Joyce would provide the materials and Greg would take over the renovations, in return for which he was promised free breakfasts 'for the rest of his natural life!'

For Greg, the freedom to redesign the shop and replace the fittings was an opportunity to give expression to his artistic flair, and he threw himself into the work with great enthusiasm. It also provided relief from his bouts of introspection.

Soon he was engrossed in the work, remodelling the bench tops and the cupboards in the kitchen, building new tables and seats, and

hearts and rainbows

upholstering the cushions with bright colours and sturdy materials. He made two new large chalkboards so that Joyce could highlight the daily specials, and built three large mirrors that gave the main room a new sense of space and light.

The finishing touches involved a fresh coat of paint for the whole shop, and when Greg had selected the colour scheme that he thought would work, Joyce was overjoyed. They were bright blues, oranges and yellows.

Three weeks of solid labour came to a happy conclusion when the new sign welcoming customers to the Café Bella Cino was emblazoned across the front windows.

Greg, however, still felt there was one final detail that needed to be addressed. There was one large blank wall inside and it was just a little too bare and unadorned for his liking. He decided that it needed a painting to break up the space, and began visiting the local art galleries to find something suitable.

When he began searching for the paintings he soon realised that the cost of the work was beyond Joyce's limited means. Not prepared to abandon his ideas, however, he decided to revive the skills that had helped him achieve such distinction during his school days. A quick visit to the local art supply shop and he was ready to get to work.

It was only as he stood before the blank canvas stretched across his easel, that Greg began to have second thoughts. Maybe he'd bitten off a little more than he could chew! As soon as the first few strokes of the brush began laying down the colours, however, Greg was engrossed in his project. He felt a surge of adrenaline course through his body, his spirits soared and he realised that he was doing something that gave him an enormous amount of joy and satisfaction. He was painting again! He was creating something worthwhile, something of beauty! He almost laughed in sheer delight as he squeezed the brilliant colours from the small tubes of paint. He really felt alive again!

The following week is one that Greg will always remember. As he immersed himself in producing what he wanted to be a work of art, he began to realise that during all that time he found a sense of peace and

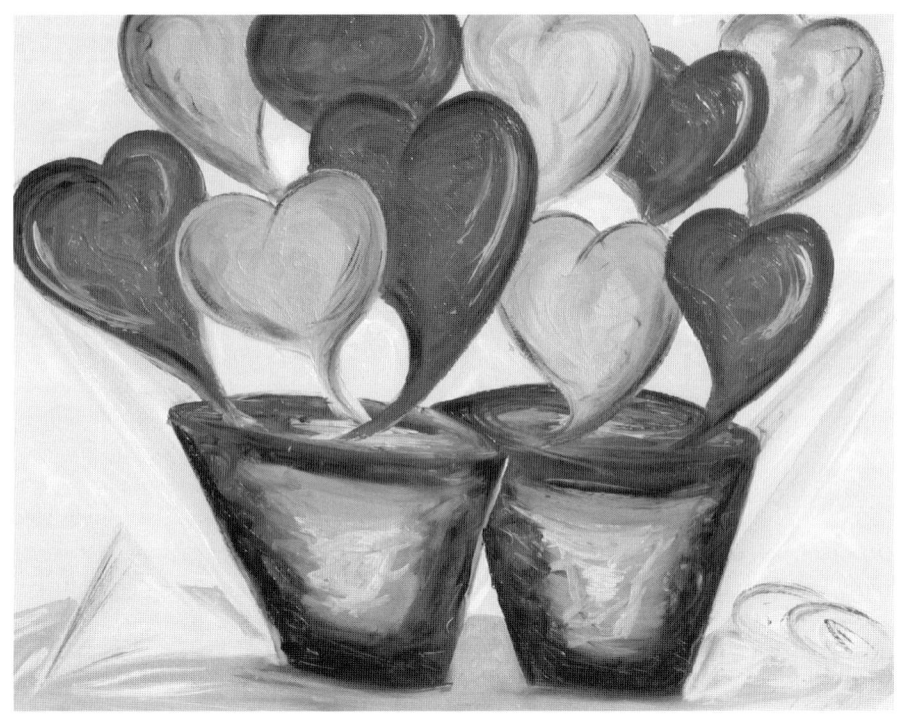

'My First Work' – 910 x 1210 mm
'When a friend asked me to design a motif for her coffee shop it started a few of my own creative ideas percolating as well!'

fulfilment that temporarily replaced his concerns about his depression. It was a glorious respite from the constant stress of wondering just how he would survive each day. It was a release from so much worry and anxiety, and he wished the feeling could last forever.

The subject of the painting was two dark blue coffee cups, set against a lighter blue background on a bright yellow base. Wafting from the cups, the steam and aromas had formed a series of hearts which Greg had rendered in reds and creams. The design filled the space quite attractively, and he had encased his work in a yellow frame to match the cups.

When the time came to unveil his work and hang it in the café, however, he had a few momentary misgivings – was it good enough for public display; would Joyce like it; was it too amateurish?

hearts and rainbows

He was relieved when Joyce squealed with delight when she first saw it and said she couldn't wait to display it in the shop. They hung the work with great aplomb, and both politely and formally applauded when it was fixed in place on the wall, pretending they had just witnessed the unveiling of the latest masterpiece to grace the halls of the Louvre in Paris!

He was pleasantly surprised when Joyce regularly informed him in the following weeks of the number of compliments she had received for the new décor of the shop, and how often she was asked if the painting of the coffee cups was for sale.

At last Greg felt that he had earned his free breakfasts!

But above all, he was overjoyed that for the time he was involved in painting the coffee cups he had found a way of holding his demons at bay. He had enjoyed a period of relative peace and tranquillity that was precious to him. He had rediscovered the colours that had been absent from his life for so long.

He wondered how long his euphoria would last. To help prolong it as much as he could, Greg responded to the requests of a number of Joyce's customers and began to paint other pictures that he made available for sale. He was pleased that few of his works stayed on display for more than a week before eager patrons snapped them up.

During all this time, Greg could feel emotions beginning to stir that had been absent for a long time. He was doing something that he genuinely enjoyed, and his work was appreciated. Was it possible that he could actually make a living from his talent for painting? There were so many ideas that he suddenly wanted to share, so many subjects that he wanted to portray, so many beautiful landscapes that he had witnessed that he now wanted to commit to canvas. The colours that had come back into his life were turning into a rainbow!

chapter twelve
a life-changing encounter

I met Greg Wilson at a surprise birthday party that my parents had arranged for Josie. She had helped them with the catering for a number of family functions, and when they learned that she was going through a difficult phase of her life, they decided to try and give her a lift.

A young man a few years older than me, whose large frame, athletic build and bearing were in strange contrast to his pale and haggard complexion, accompanied Josie. He appeared reserved and quiet, more of a bystander and observer than an active member of our group. When I mentioned to Josie that he seemed somewhat ill at ease, almost sad, Josie told me a little about his background. She also informed me that she had decided to take care of him while he struggled to overcome his depression.

I felt sorry for Greg, suddenly finding himself amidst a group of strangers and probably not feeling at all like joining in the group singing and general happy banter that our family so enjoyed. When I singled him out I told him that I used to feel that way, whenever I would find myself in a similar situation.

As we continued to converse, however, I found it difficult to under-

a life-changing encounter

stand how someone like Greg could suffer from depression. He was athletic, personable, and an engaging conversationalist especially when we discussed our shared enthusiasm for sport. I had never before come into contact with depression, having grown up in a relatively secure and stable environment with loving parents. My father John worked extremely hard in his furniture business so that he could give us a good education. He was a priest before he met my mum, but they were able to marry after he received a papal dispensation from his vow of celibacy. I often joked with Dad telling him that he'd done the right thing by choosing to get married. His decision was critical for my birth!

My dad had also been an Australian representative rugby league player, and often regaled us with stories of his experiences in New Zealand, France and England. It's not surprising, therefore, that rugby league was one of my favourite sports. We would often go to games, and Friday Night Football was almost compulsory weekly viewing. It made me feel good sharing those moments with him.

As a boy I would sit listening to funny stories he would share about his playing days. He told me that on his first trip away with the Australian side, he was so proud of his Australian blazer that he wore it on every possible occasion. On the flight to New Zealand, therefore, he left his black suit and Roman collar in the hanging space at the rear of the plane. The Australian fullback Graeme Langlands, never one to let an opportunity go by, suddenly appeared walking up the central aisle, blessing all and sundry as he made his way towards the front of the aircraft.

When he approached one of the stewardesses and asked if he could meet the Captain, she nodded in agreement and took him through to the cockpit. A short time later, when 'Changa' was making his way back to his seat, he created quite a scene when he gave the most attractive stewardess a much too familiar embrace and a cheeky kiss on the cheek! She was immensely relieved when the other players informed her of Graeme's reputation as the team's jester!

My mother Gina is a real sweetie. She has a wonderful smile and the greatest sense of humour that any mum could have. She finds amusement in the simplest of situations, and has a chuckle that is so infectious it is irresistible. Something about her encourages even perfect strangers to engage her in conversation.

Our parents imbued all my sisters and me with a sense of worth, and we knew that they would be there to support us come what may. Depression was something to which I'd never been exposed and something that I simply did not understand.

However, the more I learned from Josie, the more interested I became, and I began to see Greg in a new and compassionate light. I was interested to learn more about his depression and why Josie had decided to help him.

When I later asked her why she had taken on such a major responsibility in helping Greg, she told me that I, of all people, should know the answer to my own question. Hadn't my family taught me that helping another human being in trouble was one of the most worthwhile things we could do?

I was fascinated when she told me that if she hadn't offered to care for Greg then his life would have been in serious danger. She didn't want anything to happen to him – she wanted him to live.

My mother informed me the day after the party that Josie had taken Greg in because he had depression and nowhere else to go. It was then that she encouraged me to spend some time with Greg, to try and help this young man out. Soon afterwards, I arranged to play golf with him at Mona Vale. Not only did we have a great time that day, we began a friendship that has stood the test of time and has endured to this day.

I had an immediate liking for Greg. I found him sensitive, kind-hearted and funny. Conversation flowed easily between us, and we both shared a lot of common interests. Even though Greg and I aren't exactly the most talkative or garrulous individuals, we never experienced any of those awkward silences that I'd endured with some people. After that first round of golf, it was as if I had known him my whole life. I felt really at ease in his company.

It wasn't long before I was visiting Greg and Josie regularly at the new house they were renting at Church Point. I still remember the first time

a life-changing encounter

I entered their place. As I walked through the front door and into the lounge room, I thought I'd wandered into an art gallery. His paintings were striking. The colours, the range of subjects, and the depth of his work were quite remarkable.

Art was my favourite subject at school, and I received a great mark in my final year. While I have shown no real ability in painting, I will always be grateful for the development of my art appreciation, and I believe it was my study of art that at least gave me an ability to evaluate Greg's amazing talent.

Sometimes I would sit quietly in the background and marvel at the concentration and focus which Greg applied when he was at work. There were times when his creative juices were in full flow, and on those occasions I was afraid to break the spell.

Not only did we both like art but we also shared a similar sense of humour. We would break into fits of spontaneous laughter at the same things. Whenever we'd watch a movie together, we'd both respond in perfect unison to all the funny lines. Because we loved golf so much, Happy Gilmore with Adam Sandler was one of our favourite videos.

Greg was a great help to me in preparing for some of my exams. I was studying Science and Natural Medicine at the time, and had to spend an inordinate amount of time trying to memorise some of the more difficult botanical names of herbs. Greg would quiz me, reprimanding me roundly if he felt I wasn't performing.

He would love to ask me his favourite question: to give the name of the herb that people take to boost energy levels and help them deal with stress. It has a scientific name that even some of the second year students had trouble enunciating. Because of the frequency with which he asked me the question, in no time at all I was able to spit out the answer quite confidently: Siberian Ginseng is the herb, and its botanical name is *Eleutherococcus senticosus*!

Imagine how impressed I was when, one afternoon as we were driving back from the supermarket, we noticed a tired and frazzled looking driver who had pulled up next to us at a traffic light. Greg took one look and remarked, quite fluently, that he felt that particular individual could certainly use some *Eleutherococcus senticosus* to feel better! His comment reduced us both to hysterics of laughter, and the poor individual who was the subject of Greg's diagnosis must have thought we were a couple of simpletons!

I tried to match his talent for remembering exotic names by learning some of the quite complex descriptions of his paints. It gave me some satisfaction to wander through his home studio and casually observe that the 'transparent gold oxide' or the 'magnesium blue hue' might be more effective on some part of his painting! It was always good to hear him laugh, and we both made the most of any opportunity to add a little humour to our lives.

I learned a lot from Greg, just by listening to some of the things he had experienced and how he had handled some tough situations. He had some simple principles to which he always intended to be faithful: be honest with people, don't put on any masks; and stand by your friends through thick and thin. His friendship was something I came to treasure more and more each day.

I found him to be a thoughtful person, possessing a great deal of sensitivity. He also had a soft spot for animals, and was never able to ignore any creature that was suffering. In the short time that I had known him he had provided temporary shelter and/or an urgent trip to the veterinary hospital for two cockatoos, three injured dogs, four birds, a duck, a lizard that had been pecked and a baby possum.

This concern for animals led to a lighter moment shortly after I met him. He was walking around the block one morning, and was horrified when he noticed a gentleman in a battered old white Volkswagen open its door, let a dog out and then drive off. The brown spaniel, looking worn and dirty, ran up to Greg as the man in the VW continued to drive away. Greg was really upset that the dog had been abandoned like that. He decided to adopt the dog and began walking it back to his house.

When he arrived home he spent hours caring for the dog. He washed the pooch with shampoo, dried its coat with a hairdryer, trimmed its hair and removed burrs from its coat. Then he went and bought some dog food for the scrawny and apparently undernourished animal and gave

a life-changing encounter

it a large bowl of water. After completing all these tasks he decided he would take the dog for a walk.

He wasn't long into the walk when the same Volkswagen that had dropped the dog off hours earlier appeared. It stopped, and its door opened. As the dog ran back to the car, the relieved driver half-heartedly threatened the poor unfortunate creature with all sorts of reprisals for 'getting itself lost'!

Greg was left wondering what the owner would make of the newly washed and trimmed canine, smelling sweetly of apricot shampoo, and sporting a coat that had never looked so good. As he waved a wistful goodbye, he remarked that at least the dog would be happy!

Dogs enjoy a special place in Greg's affections, and his own constant companion, Jackson, is one of his 'best mates'. Not surprisingly, Greg rescued Jackson from the Animal Welfare League. He was to become a regular subject for Greg's paintings, and gives his owner an enormous amount of pleasure.

I would often turn up to the house to notice Jackson running down the driveway to retrieve a ball that Greg had thrown. Then we'd follow a regular routine: I'd make Greg a cup of chamomile tea with honey and I'd have a coffee. We'd then play with Jackson until he tired. He'd jump high in the air, catch a ball or a frisbee, and come to a skidding halt. He'd turn and run towards the concrete veranda where Greg and I would be waiting to compliment him on his great skills as a retriever.

Jackson is a dog with a remarkable personality and has developed his manners to an exceptional degree. He can be the most placid of pets as he shakes your hand or the fiercest of sentries as he growls and barks when strangers approach his territory.

chapter thirteen
the understanding

Although I spent time playing golf with Greg and visiting his Church Point home, it wasn't until two years later that I really began to understand his depression. I was in a transition period in my own life. My relationship of two years had just come to an end and I was looking for somewhere to live and make a fresh start. Josie suggested that I take the spare room in their house at Church Point. It was an invitation I couldn't turn down. For a modest rental each week I would be living in a house overlooking a part of the Pittwater coastal inlet, surrounded by lush bush land and only five minutes away from Mona Vale beach.

Nevertheless, as I made plans to rent a room with Josie, there was no way I could anticipate the dramatic turn that my life was about to take through this living arrangement. At that point I really didn't understand what I was getting myself into by choosing to live under that roof. I was poorly prepared for the emotional highs and lows that accompany serious depression. Even though I had seen some of Greg's insecurities I had no idea how bad his depression was until I moved in.

Not long after I arrived, Greg arranged his first exhibition. It wasn't until then that it became obvious to me how serious his condition was.

the understanding

The Pasadena Hotel at Church Point was where Greg had his first exhibition on 8 November 2001. Josie knew the owner of the hotel, and asked if she would mind if we put some paintings on display on the premises for one evening. Mary was happy to accommodate her request and we began eagerly preparing to make arrangements for the exhibition.

I was the self-appointed Public Relations Officer, and I contacted the *Manly Daily*, the local newspaper, asking if they would run a story on Greg. I was hopeful that this story would generate some interest in the exhibit and convince the local residents that it would be well worth a visit. A journalist rang Greg shortly after and ran the story the day of the exhibition.

We hired a truck to transfer the artworks to the hotel and carefully wrapped each painting to protect it during the journey. We completed the display the afternoon prior to the opening.

About seventy people attended the one-day exhibition, and at the end of the show we were ecstatic with the result. Seven paintings had been sold, and receipts for the sales made the bank balance a little healthier.

The following afternoon Greg and I went to collect the works that remained, carefully wrapped them in blankets, and made the short journey down the road back home. I could tell instinctively that something was bothering him. He was morose and gloomy and barely spoke on the way back to the house. I asked him if everything was fine, if he was okay, as we pulled into the steep driveway.

'Not really,' he answered. 'I feel as though I've let everybody down.'

I wasn't about to contradict him, even though I could hardly believe that he would rate the evening as anything but a wonderful success.

We opened up the metal roll-a-door and I jumped up into the back of the truck and started passing some of the paintings to Greg. The transfer was continuing reasonably smoothly: I would pass the works to Greg or Josie, and they would carry them up into the studio.

I handed a red landscape to Greg, and his mood suddenly worsened.

As he took the painting from me, he raised it high above his head and threw it onto the ground at his feet. Josie and I were dumbfounded as he picked up the damaged art work and hurled it like a giant frisbee down the drive-way.

'Greg, what are you doing?' Josie cried out in bewilderment.

Despite our best efforts we could not stop Greg from destroying more of his work.

He strolled inside the house and returned with one of his golf clubs in hand. We dared not interfere as he took two short swings and another two paintings lay in tatters on the ground. His eyes welled with emotion as he continued to break the frames, leaving gaping tears in the canvas.

'I knew I couldn't do it. I am a hopeless artist. I haven't got what it takes. What was I thinking? It takes years of study to become a talented painter and I haven't been anywhere near a classroom. My father was right about me.'

I wanted desperately to help ease my friend's heartache, yet I was unsure what to say. Josie was close to tears and did her best to try and calm him down. 'Greg, for your first exhibition you have done an outstanding job.'

'If I was so successful why do I still have all these paintings left?' he cried out.

Josie continued to talk with him calmly. 'A lot of Australia's most successful artists sold nothing at their opening shows. You sold seven works,' she said.

Greg remained silent for a moment. Eventually, he began to speak: 'Nobody liked my work,' he told us. He strained to contain his feelings; however, there was a lump in his throat, and a look of pain swept over his face as I watched on.

A short time later, he apologised for demolishing the pieces. When he had retrieved the broken art works and put them in an outside rubbish bin, he turned around remorsefully, staggered past Josie and me and went straight to bed.

My stomach had knots in it. I had been deeply upset when he started

the understanding

to swing the golf club and I had grown increasingly worried for Greg as his melancholy continued. I had never seen him get so upset for so little reason. Greg was normally such a gentle soul, and his behaviour of the past few minutes was completely out of character. The exhibition had been truly outstanding, and I failed to see how Greg could reason otherwise.

All our efforts to coax Greg from his room were to no avail. He refused to come out.

I had no idea how long it would take for Greg to recover from this setback. For the entire next day he was depressed. He stayed bed-ridden, although he at least allowed me in his room. I gave him as much encouragement as I could. He wasn't too interested in what I had to say but I continued telling him that I had never come across an artist with so much talent. I told him that I knew that he was disappointed, but that this exhibition was only the first faltering step in his career. I told him that we had handed out lots of cards in response to genuine enquiries, and it was quite possible that further sales could be generated from the showing.

Eventually, I sat down on the edge of the bed. 'Why are you so upset Greg?' I asked. When he didn't reply, I continued, 'Greg, I care about you. Please tell me the reason why you're so disappointed, tell me what you're feeling, so that I can help.'

'I'm useless', he answered. 'I feel as though I can't do it.'

'Of course you can.' I said. 'Your ability is obvious.'

'No, my father was right. I'm not good enough; I keep hearing my dad's comments in my head. He used to tell me repeatedly that I could've done better. It's like a record that is being replayed over and over in my mind. I should've done better.'

We sat together in silence, and for a moment I reflected on Greg's words. Ever since I had known Greg he had been so critical of himself. Either his work was not good enough, or there was some flaw in his character. This comment about his father offered the clearest insight yet to me as to where he had learned this self-condemnation. When

greg wilson — 95

Greg turned away from me I became sad. I had been encouraged by my own dad.

I desperately wanted Greg to get better. I hoped that by passing on some of the words of encouragement that my father had given to me it might help him.

I took a moment to collect my thoughts before speaking with my friend. 'Greg, I was taught that we must believe in ourselves.'

'Aaron, I told you I'm useless, I can't do it,' Greg interrupted.

'Greg, those harmful ideas, those words aren't helpful any more,' I replied.

'My artwork is no good,' he continued.

'Greg, you know that you can rely on Josie, Joyce and me to tell you the truth.' I told him. 'We believe in your talent, and we believe that you have a unique gift as an artist.'

Greg pulled the sheet over his head and said nothing more. It was then that I came to understand how fragile his mind could be, and what a fine line it was between his happiness and his depression. I also realised what a destructive impact words could have on someone's life.

Josie was waiting for me as I left the room. She explained that Greg's self-talk was quite debilitating and self-defeating, a pattern that had developed as he grew up. The consequence of this meant that Greg felt as though he was worthless much of the time.

I asked Josie what we should do to try and break these thought patterns. She suggested that encouragement was the best way to help. She assured me that if we fed Greg positivity, gave him hope, and lent him our support, then he could achieve his goal and become a successful artist. By following these steps she was confident that we could reverse his thinking.

Josie was right. However, her solution to Greg's problems would take time. I had an idea that might elevate Greg's deteriorating spirits and approached her with a proposition, hoping that my new plan might give Greg a little more confidence in himself.

I had fallen in love with one of Greg's paintings from the first moment

the understanding

he had applied the final brushstroke. I had secretly been wishing that his art work titled 'Bush Nativity' would not sell at his recent exhibition. In fact, I had always intended purchasing one of Greg's works so that I could put it on display in my own home one day, and decided now was an appropriate time to buy one of his pieces.

'Josie, I have a little bit of money saved. I am going to go to the bank and make a withdrawal so that I can buy a painting,' I said.

'You can't do that,' she protested.

'Yes I can, and you're not to tell Greg that I am the new owner of one of his paintings. Just say that a man bought it for a friend who attended the exhibition last night. Josie, the reason for Greg's reaction is that he feels as though he's not good enough, and this might just help convince him otherwise.'

I intended taking the painting to Joyce's house and hiding it so that Greg wouldn't know that I had made the purchase. Hopefully, that would give him enough encouragement to get out of bed and start painting some more.

'Aaron, I don't think you should do that,' she continued, as I put the canvas in my car, careful that Greg didn't see.

I told her that the situation we were in reminded me of the story of Vincent Van Gogh. Theo, who was Vincent's brother, cared for him so much that he went to extraordinary lengths to give him support and confidence. Greg had been like a brother to me. I just wanted to be there for him – after all, he would have done the same for me.

'Go and watch Greg, and remember, don't tell him that it was me who bought the painting.'

When I returned from the bank I gave the money to Josie and told her to pass it on to Greg. She rested it beside his bed soon after.

'Look, somebody bought a painting today,' she told him.

'Who was it?' he enquired.

'Oh, some man bought it for his friend. He came to pick it up while you were sleeping earlier.'

'Which painting was it?' he asked.

'The Bush Nativity,' she replied. 'It was the painting of the farmer and his family.'

'That's good,' Greg said.

His mood did improve, but he remained in bed. At least he began to talk after his latest sale.

When he did finally get up, he told us that he wasn't painting any more. For several weeks he didn't even go near his easel. Despite our encouragement his sombre mood remained.

Greg was still upset with the exhibition. 'When I put my work on display it's not easy. My soul is exposed for everyone to see. It was a big risk for me to show my work to others and I was hoping for a better response so that I could give something back to you guys.'

'I know you find it hard to believe, Greg, but for your first show it was a huge success,' I said.

Josie and I were upset by what had happened but deep down we hoped that Greg's love for his art would be strong enough to encourage him to start painting again.

Underlying his behaviour there was obviously a nagging doubt about his own ability. It was Josie who would calm him down, sitting with him for weeks, encouraging him, reinforcing his wonderful talent as a painter and sculptor. If it weren't for her support, there's no way that Greg would have even thought about continuing to follow his calling.

Josie kept on believing in him and giving the support he needed the most. Self-belief was something that Greg didn't know at that point in his life.

I remember one day he came into the kitchen while Josie and I were having our morning coffee. 'What am I doing here?' he said.

Josie replied, 'Greg, each of us has a gift. For some, that gift is to be a great friend, for others, a talented accountant, for some a good mother.'

'What am I supposed to do?'

the understanding

'Greg, you have an amazing talent for painting and sculpture,' she told him.

'I'm not going to be an artist any more,' he vowed, 'I need a new direction in life.'

He went back to his room more despondent than ever.

Sometimes Greg would consider the prospect of returning to work as a carpenter, but the thought of subjecting himself again to the rigorous schedule did not appeal to him at all. The injuries he suffered during the motorcycle accidents were mending slowly, but he was still getting pain in his neck, legs and back. Weakness also plagued him and prevented him from returning to any workplace that was physically demanding. Besides, he had serious doubts that he could adapt to such a restrictive and confining schedule ever again, now that he had experienced the relative freedom that painting had brought.

Still, he would taunt himself and pose the questions: 'Why can't I make my life work? Why can't I exist within a nine-to-five routine? Why is my leg still aching? Why am I constantly fatigued? And why am I so useless; why am I such a failure?' Then he would say, 'I am never going to be able to get over this depression.'

During the period of troubled introspection that would inevitably follow, Josie would then sit with Greg, sometimes until three or four in the morning, and tell him that the role he was being asked to play in the overall scheme of things was an important one. She kept highlighting the progress that Greg had already made and reassuring him that this improvement boded extremely well for his future.

'Greg, you're not useless!' she would assert. 'Look at your wonderful talent for painting. Just because you have depression doesn't mean you are a failure. We know that it's a chemical imbalance in the brain that's responsible for some of the reactions, but we can try to rectify that and get you some help.'

She did everything she could to exorcise the feelings of inadequacy and inferiority that possessed him in the throes of his depression. It was an ongoing battle.

'I don't want to go on living any more, Josie. I have had enough of this place,' he would moan.

'Greg, you must have faith. God has a plan for all of us, and we might not know the reason now but we have to have patience. You are gifted at what you do. It would be a terrible waste if you were to end your life. Let's put your gift to use. You're talented, creative, let's use those skills!'

Josie's optimism would slowly permeate his thoughts, and he would eventually pick himself up. She would continue to encourage him until he was ready to start painting again.

Then, thankfully, the joy of doing something he really loved would surface once again. I came home from university one afternoon a few weeks after the exhibition to find Greg sitting on his chair preparing a new canvas.

I was overcome with a flood of relief when I saw what he was doing. His attitude had obviously started to improve after our constant reinforcement.

'I'm really proud of you, Greg,' I said, as I walked through the door and put my bag on the ground.

'Thanks,' he replied, almost in a matter-of-fact way, 'I had a little setback, but I am under way again now!'

chapter fourteen
art mirrors life

While Greg returned to his painting, the depression that I had witnessed at our home recurred with predictable consistency. I began to notice a pattern emerging over the following months that gave me a fair indication of Greg's mental state. There were times when his demeanour was calm and controlled, and this was reflected in the work he would pursue. When he stood at the easel and stroked his bright colours on the canvas, I knew that he was in a buoyant mood and that the likelihood of an outburst was extremely remote.

At other times, he would leave his painting and concentrate on his sculptures. Often these works would incorporate motorcycle parts, and there was a sombreness to the compositions that made me just a little apprehensive. The early sculptures seemed to convey the mental anguish that would plague him. Saw blades, sharp streaks of lightning and taps were materials that he used. They hauntingly conveyed to me all the anguish of the mental illness that had resulted in his attempted suicide, and the horror of his motorcycle accidents. They provoked cold, sad and despondent feelings whenever I examined them. It was as if he were reverting for inspiration to those dark recesses of his mind that harboured all the fears and terror that the accidents had involved.

'Resurrection of the spirit', a freestanding motorcycle sculpture, was a grief-stricken piece. A muffler that resembled a giant outstretched hand protruded from the bike as if it were ready to grasp the onlooker in its clutches. A metal bar, the surgical rod that had been inserted into Greg's leg and later removed, jutted out from the front of the bike, acting as a chilling reminder of the pain to which he had been subjected during the time of his recovery.

It was such a relief when we observed him at work on a painting when the palette was filled with daubs of bright yellows and blues and greens. Such times were almost a signal for us to relax and enjoy a respite from the usual doubts and troubles.

'Resurrection of the Spirit'
Clear coated and sealed motorbike parts, seat and visor, stainless steel surgical rod (removed from the artist's femur after he had recovered from the accident), saw blade 1280 x 1400 x 950 mm

'Like the phoenix arising from the ashes, my spirit was resurrected from the debris of a near-fatal motorcycle accident.'

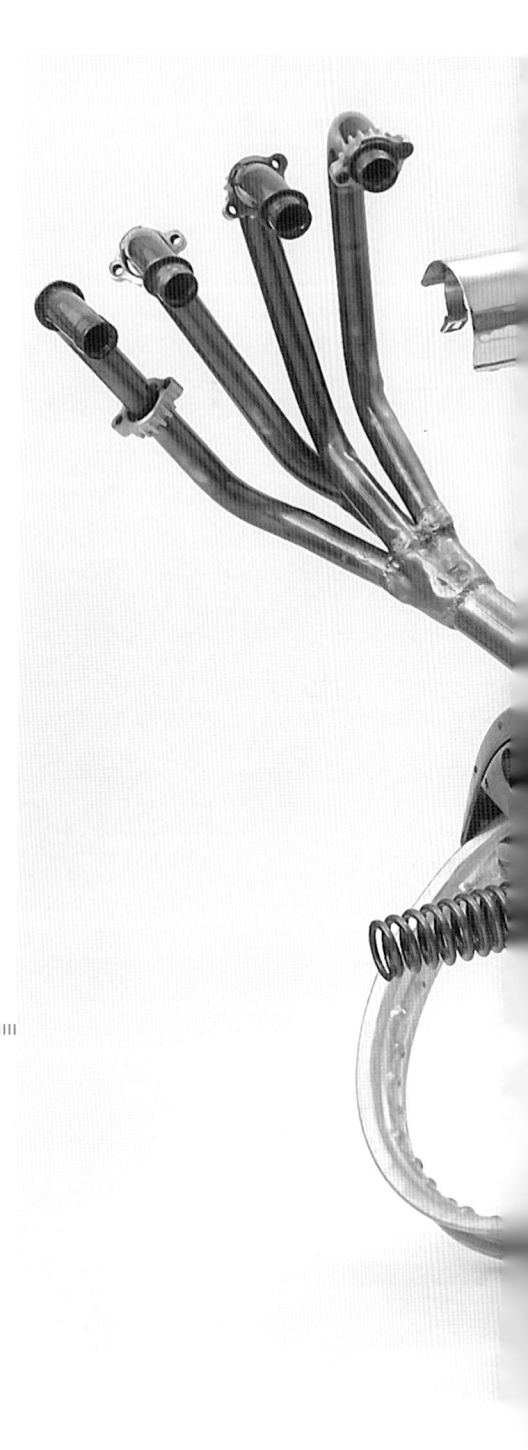

art mirrors life

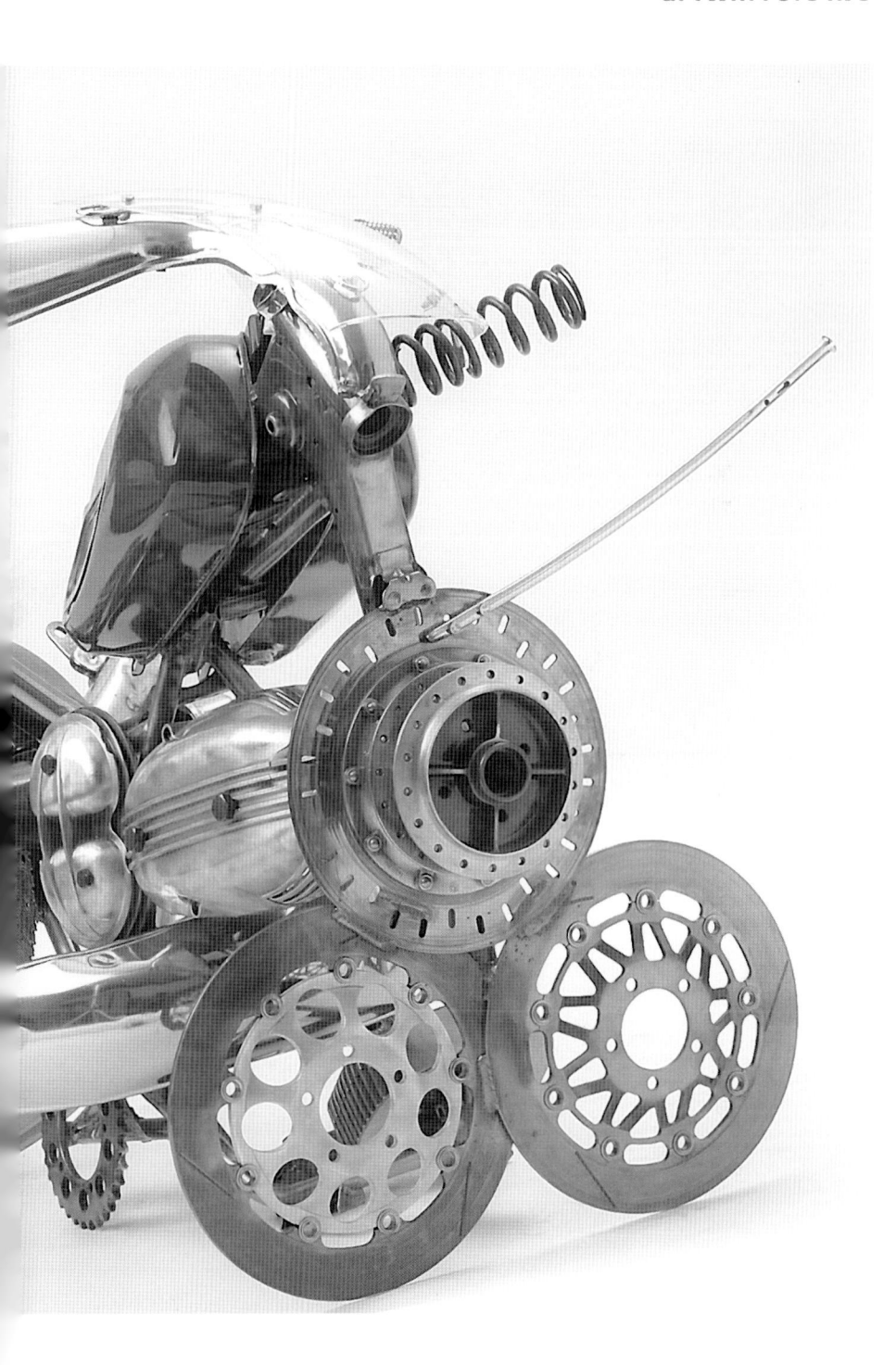

greg wilson — 103

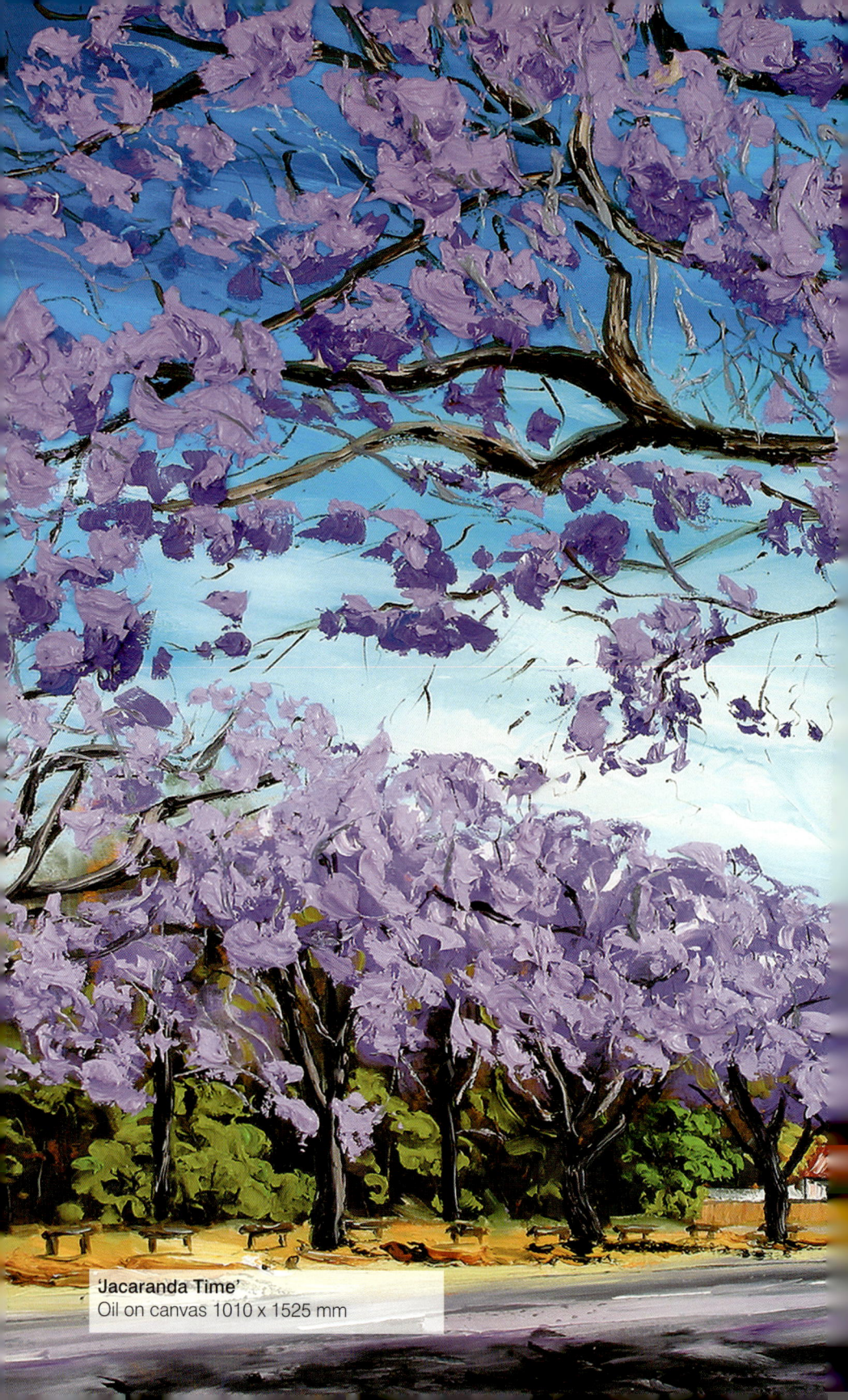

'Jacaranda Time'
Oil on canvas 1010 x 1525 mm

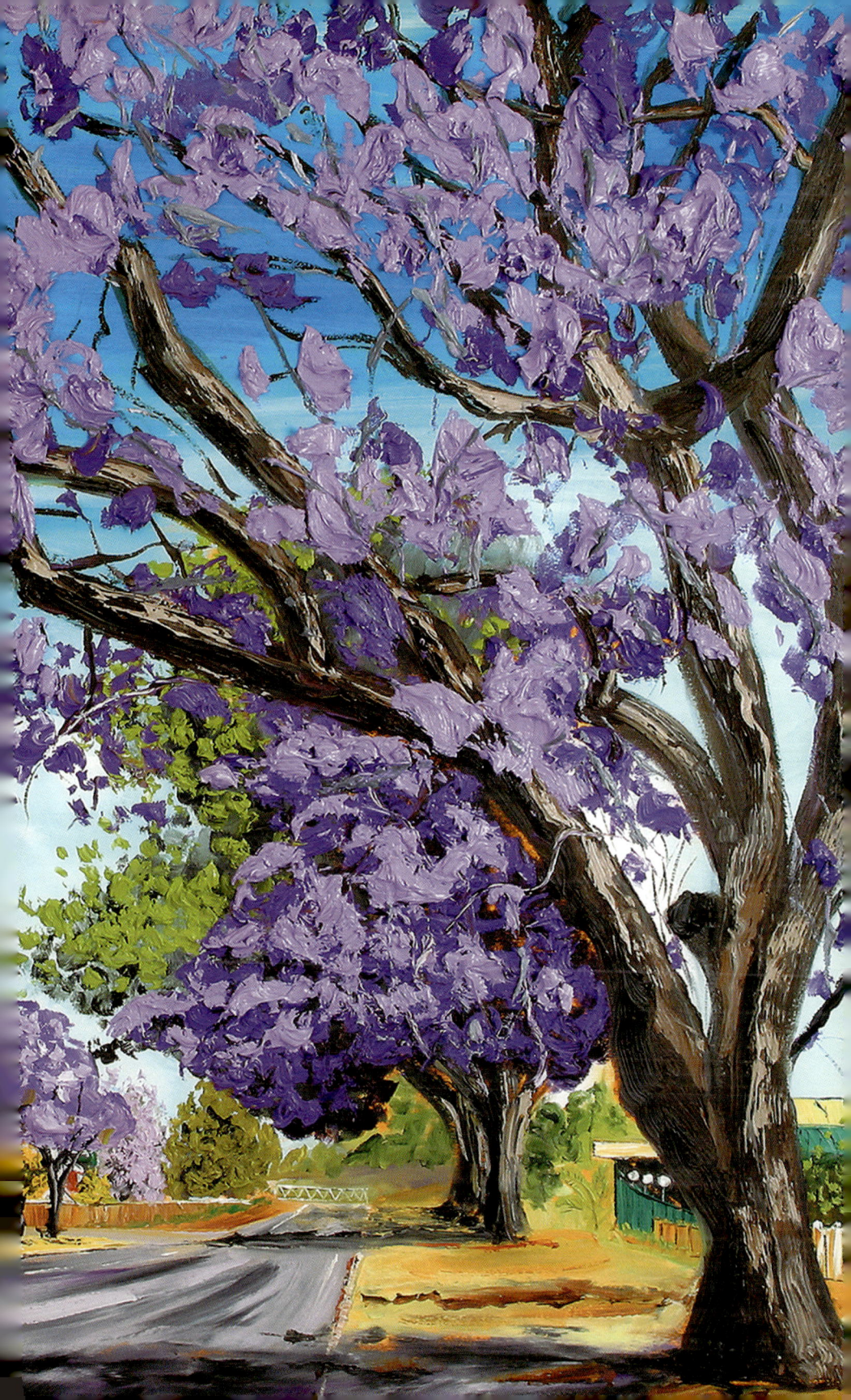

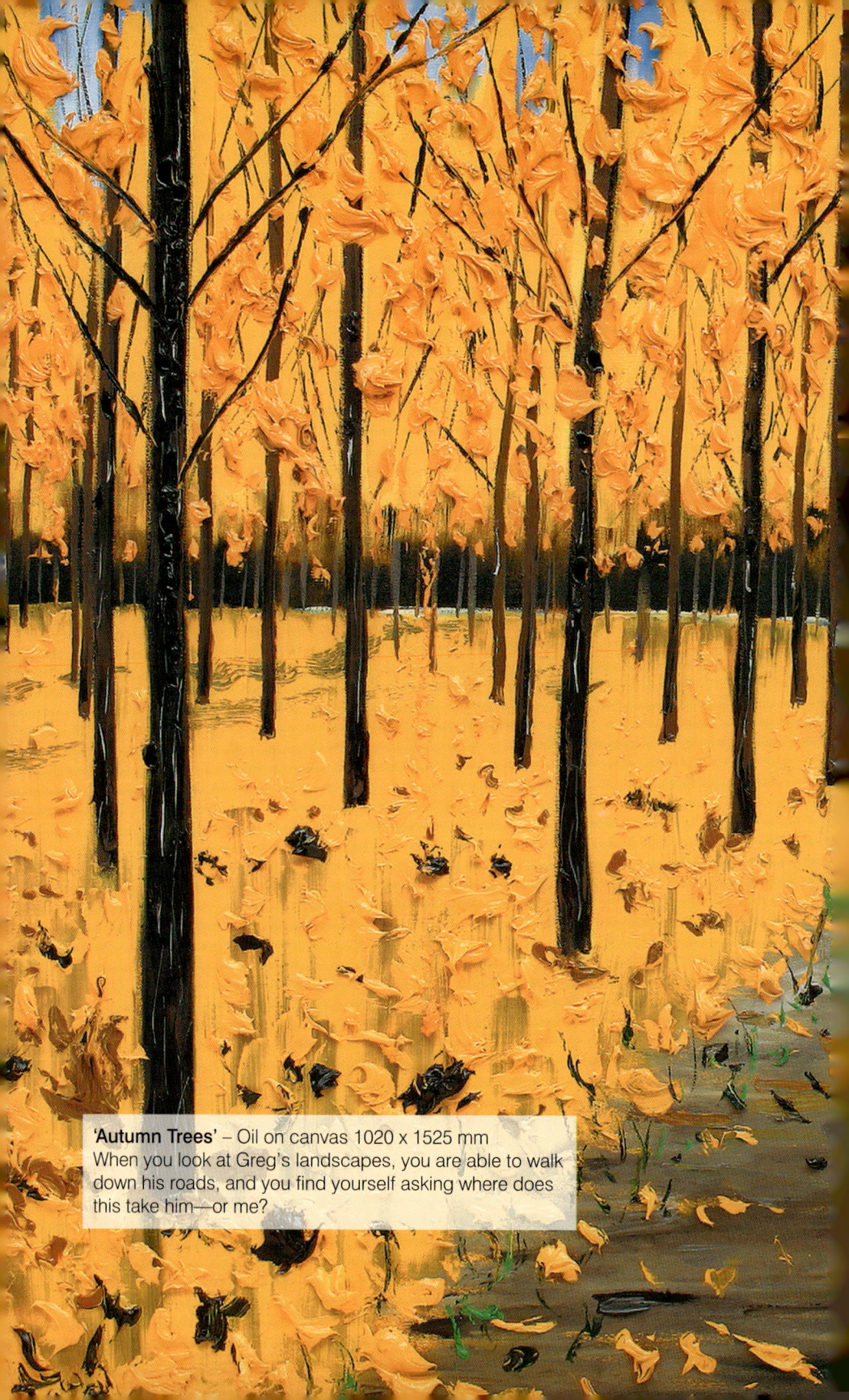

'Autumn Trees' – Oil on canvas 1020 x 1525 mm
When you look at Greg's landscapes, you are able to walk down his roads, and you find yourself asking where does this take him—or me?

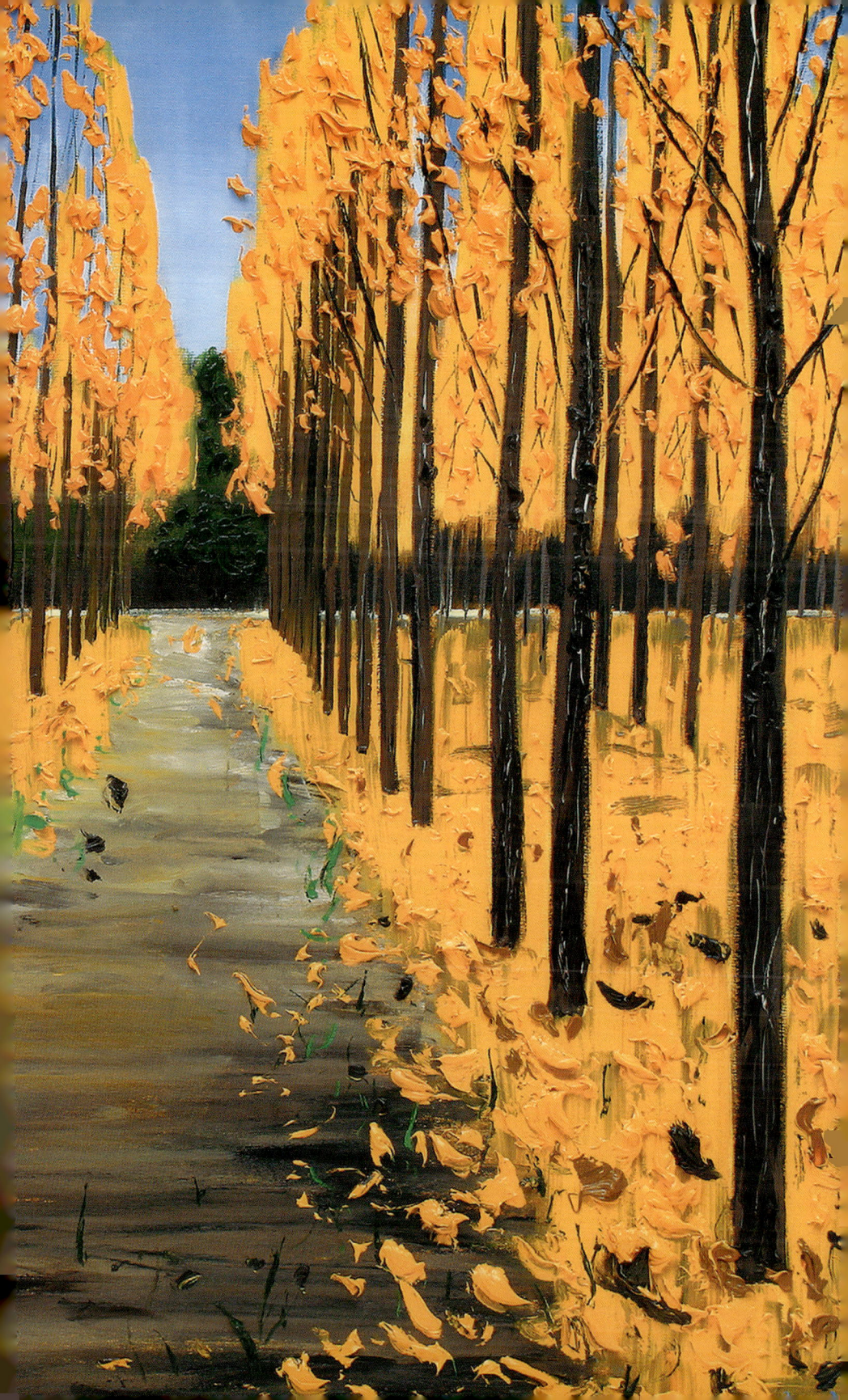

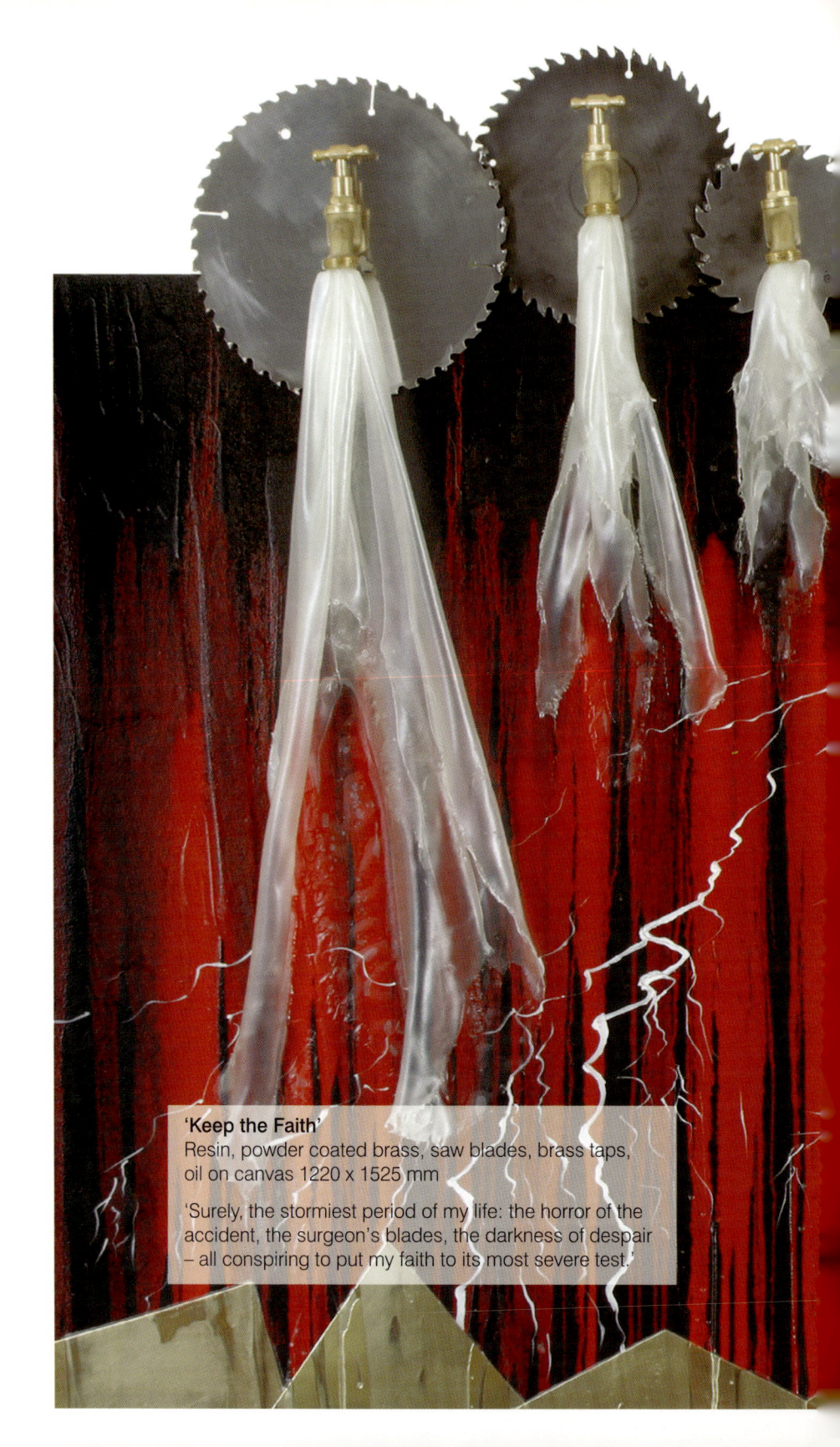

'Keep the Faith'
Resin, powder coated brass, saw blades, brass taps, oil on canvas 1220 x 1525 mm

'Surely, the stormiest period of my life: the horror of the accident, the surgeon's blades, the darkness of despair – all conspiring to put my faith to its most severe test.'

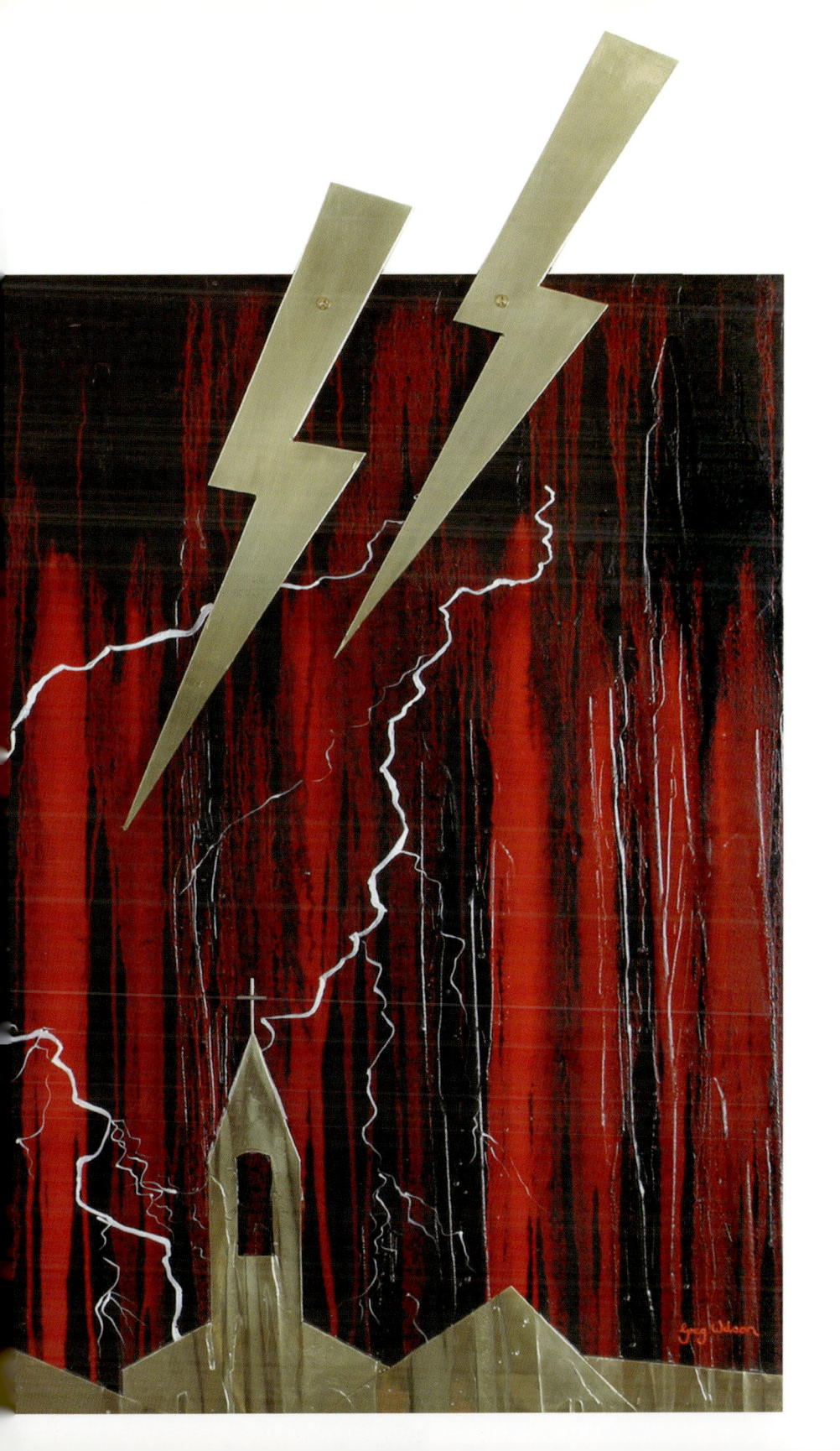

my brush with depression

'Drive … Spin Out'
Board, steel, clothes, resin, collage, chrome taps 920 x 920 mm

'Drive … Spin-Out' is an everyday reminder of the cycle of life and our constant struggle for renewal. Our vital forces are represented by the tap and the drive to succeed in our endeavours.

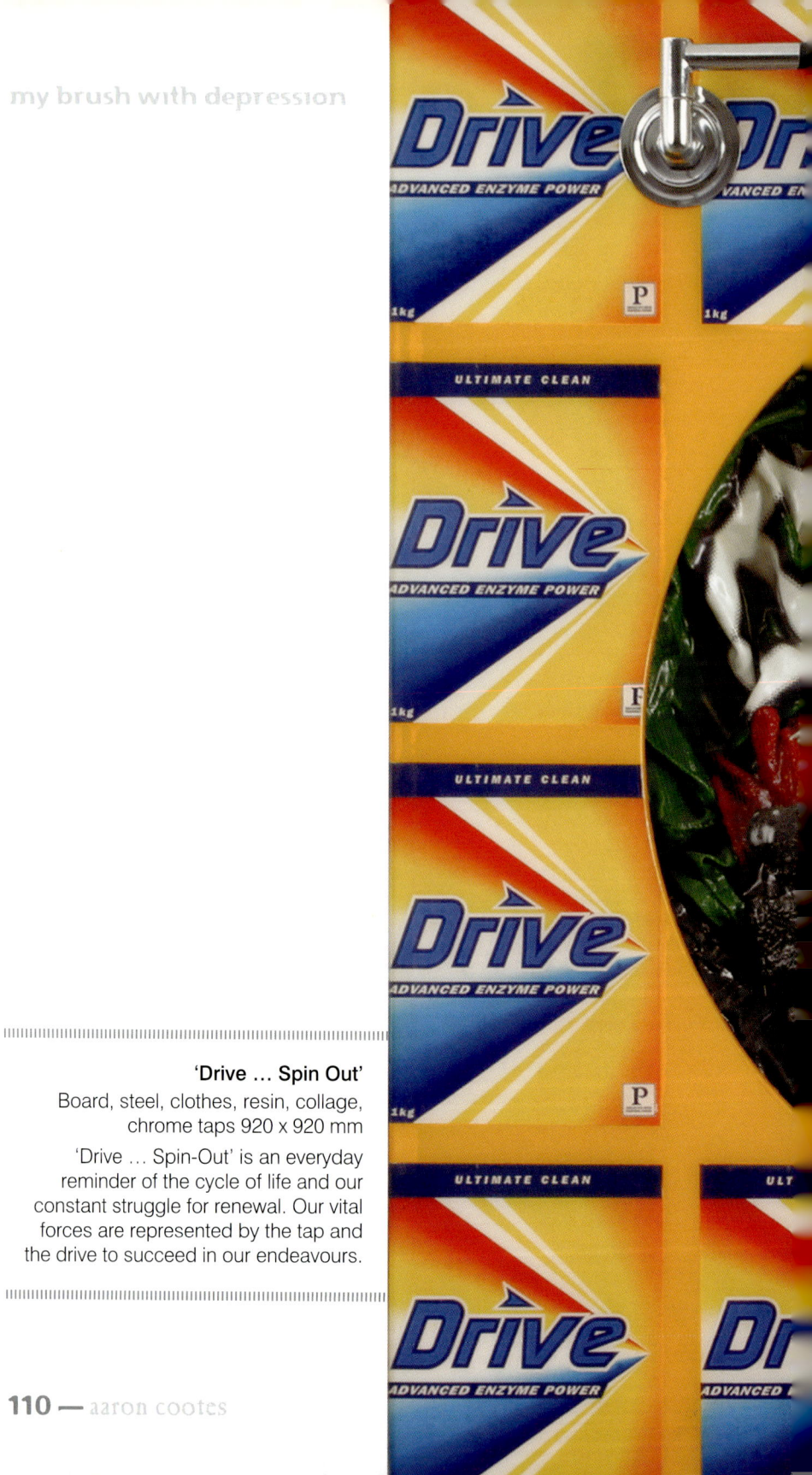

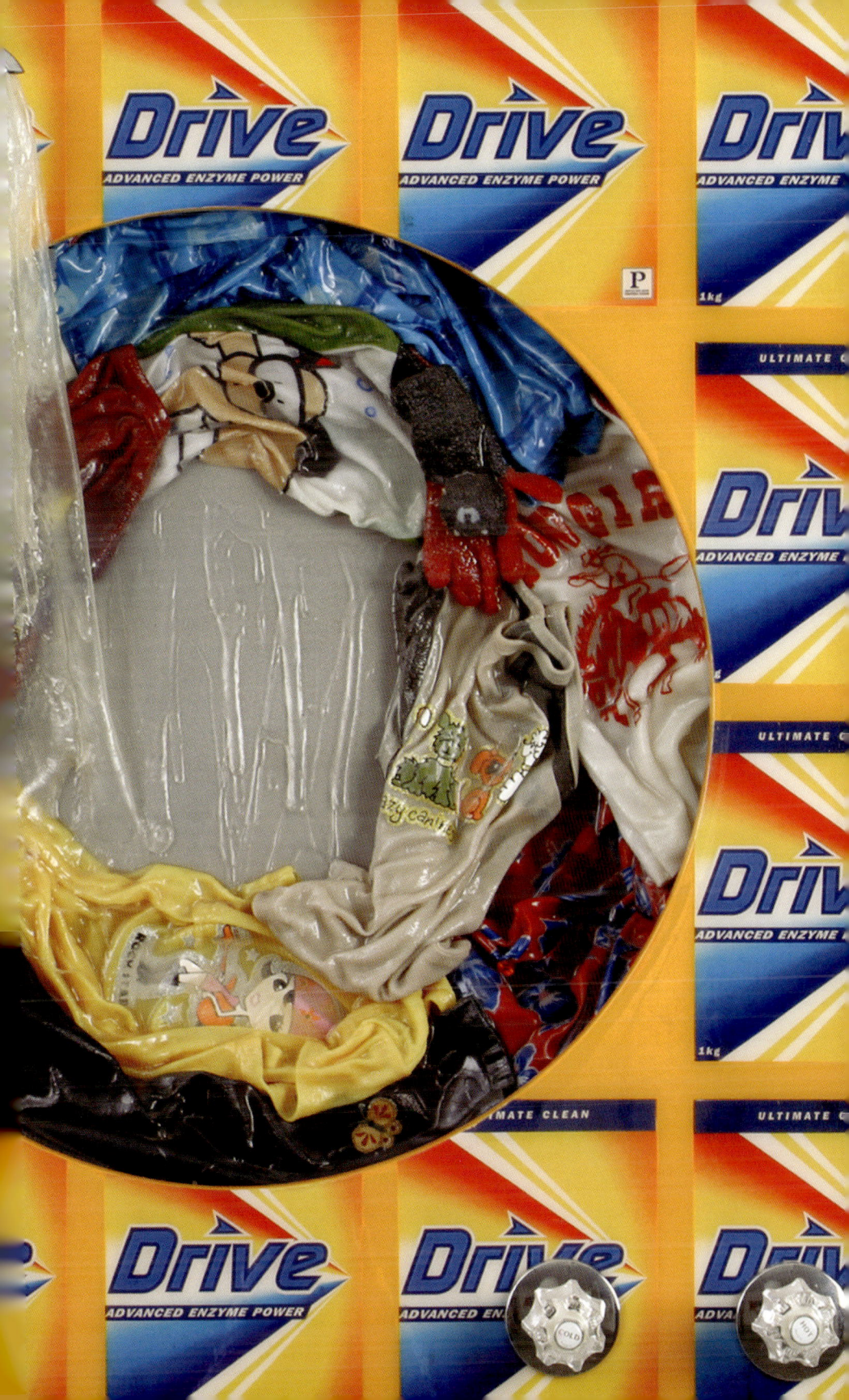

One of his works, called 'Jacaranda Time', was an easily recognisable indicator of his frame of mind at the time he painted the landscape. It depicted one of nature's most dazzling displays, where he succeeded in showing the jacaranda in all its glory as it heralded the transition from the chill of winter to the warmth of the Australian summer with a burst of colour and life that was simply spectacular.

'Autumn Trees' was another product of a settled period. It was a beautiful, peaceful landscape with golden poplars lining a pathway that almost invited you to walk down its sun-drenched corridor.

By contrast, one of his sculptures that he called 'Keep the Faith', a multi-media piece made from saw blades, metal lightning rods and taps, has definite connotations of inner turmoil and a preoccupation with his own pain and anguish.

Greg described another one of his works as an attempt to depict the conflict and confusion with which he constantly seemed to be struggling. It was a washing machine creation, called 'Drive ... Spin Out', and it offered one of the clearest insights into the enduring struggle that he waged between light and dark, highs and lows, contentment and depression.

He explained how he felt that he was constantly running on a three-speed cycle – happy and excited, or depressed and despairing, with periods of remission and calm in between. His temperament could vary as much as the temperature of the water in the machine – hot, cold, or warm.

As we came to understand these changes and their unpredictability, we learned never to be complacent. One good dose of self-doubt was all it took before the gloom would quickly descend once again on all of us. Greg would stumble, his temperament would turn cold and it often had some seriously detrimental effects.

I still recall with terrible uneasiness one such moment. Greg had nearly finished painting what I regarded as a stunning seascape. He was in the back room putting the final touches to his work. Josie and I were in the lounge room watching television. Suddenly, there was a large crash and a muttered oath, followed by another louder bang. Josie and I ran to the room to find him with a golf club in his hand glaring down at a painting that no longer bore any resemblance to the beautiful work I had admired earlier. It had been slashed to ribbons by a three iron!

At first I tried to make light of the moment by injecting what I thought was a timely vein of humour. I made a reference to the 'number three' brush and remarked that I thought he may have done better with a five wood … but my efforts did not meet with the desired result! Greg was inconsolable, he lowered his head and walked away snarling his usual self-deprecatory insults. He would vow never to paint again and go to his bedroom.

Sometimes it would be weeks before he would even look at another canvas. Sometimes he would reconsider other vocational options, like photography or professional golf, but mostly he would simply withdraw. It was not unusual for him to spend five days in bed, never venturing out of his room except for quick visits to the bathroom and an occasional foray into the kitchen. A painting that did not please him could cripple Greg emotionally for days on end.

Eventually his mood would settle, and the warmth would return to his character. This was the period I most enjoyed. Greg was balanced once again, and our friendship continued to flourish.

chapter fifteen

a tower of strength

During the times when Greg was plunged into the severest manifestations of his depression, Josie was his mainstay. I watched her handle his anguish and dejection with great skill and sensitivity. She seemed to know just the right words to say and what actions were needed. She was the one who, more often than not, would be able to restore the calm.

When Greg refused to leave his bedroom during these periods, she never became impatient. She never told Greg to 'get over it'. She knew that such comments could actually make him more depressed, and she remembered to what extremes he was tempted to go if things became unbearable for him. The vivid memory of his attempted suicide was never far from her mind.

The duration of his self-imposed withdrawals was variable to an extraordinary degree. Sometimes it was a matter of days, sometimes a matter of weeks. Josie never imposed time limits or any other restriction on his return to 'normal' life and although she never quite knew when this would occur, she was always aware that any kind of pressure whatsoever would only delay his eventual return.

a tower of strength

Greg was always the first to acknowledge that Josie's greatest contribution to his recovery from these spells was her willingness to listen and her absolute determination not to be judgmental. There were times when the two of them simply sat together in a comfortable silence, and Greg drew great comfort from her presence.

There were times, however, when he became particularly agitated, and Josie was subjected to a burst of vitriol and invective that would have daunted a less determined counsellor. She quickly learned that these were vented more from frustration than conviction, and that sometimes the mere act of letting his anguish escape in an uninhibited outburst was a partial relief in itself. Their understanding became so compatible that she sometimes intuitively knew just from his posture and his gestures exactly how he was feeling and how to respond to each situation.

She always tried to remain positive. Greg would sometimes tell her that he didn't think he would ever be able to control his destructive thoughts or overcome his anxiety which he predicted would be an inevitable part of his future. Josie would then take him back over the past few years and highlight the great progress that he had already made. She would explain to him that, like any other disease, depression could be controlled and managed by the careful use of the right medications. She would remind him of the wonderful support group he had gathered around him and that as long as he had their help then his chances of coming through his ordeal were extremely high.

One important member of that support group was Dr Westmore. One of his most timely contributions to Greg's treatment was the information and enlightenment that he provided regarding Greg's illness. When the realisation began to sink in that Greg's condition was similar to diabetes, or any one of a number of physical problems, there was a certain feeling of relief that made us all feel a little bit better. All his detractors who had been insinuating that Greg was suffering from nothing other than 'boredom with his lifestyle' or that he was 'too lazy to get off his butt', were suddenly discredited by the doctor's diagnosis.

The one thing that concerned us all about the doctor's findings was his cautionary advice that unless Greg realised the seriousness of his condition and took the appropriate measures to control it, then there could be dire, even fatal, consequences!

What the good doctor also made clear to us all was that we should not rely exclusively on the prescribed medicines to control the disease. He complimented us on the support network that we had developed to help Greg, and told us that this type of assistance was essential for Greg's continued well-being.

Josie was the epitome of the kind of support the doctor was recommending, despite the heavy toll it took on her own inner resources. There were times when she found it necessary to mask her underlying distress and concerns in order to give Greg the impression of unfaltering strength. Greg was particularly aware of Josie's demeanour during the tough times, and if she showed any sign of undue stress he would react badly. It upset him even more if he thought his behaviour was causing additional pain for Josie.

There were weeks when she would not leave his side, fearing he would try to hurt himself. This necessarily involved a great deal of her time and energy. Eventually, she had to cut back on her work as his illness made more demands on her time and financial resources. The cost of materials for his painting and sculptures was not inconsiderable, and she directed most of her income and savings to making sure that he had all he needed to keep busy at his crafts. It meant that she learned to do without many of the little extras that had been a normal part of her life.

She soon realised that there could be a number of factors that would trigger Greg's attacks. Sometimes it was dissatisfaction with one of his paintings that sent his spirits plummeting. Sometimes it was as simple as a report on the evening news. Those explicit and sometimes ugly images that are broadcast on our screens would deeply trouble him: the murders, the cruelty to animals, the assaults, and the wars. Unable to make sense of the nonsense that often permeates our world, and unable to comprehend the sufferings of so many nations, he would relapse into a deep sense of despondency.

Whilst living with Greg, I discovered him to be an extremely positive and honest person, possessing a great deal of humility. If he detected others acting jealously or observed people being the object of ridicule it would deeply upset him. Lying and snobbery were also qualities that he did not admire. The senselessness of it all would compel him to question the purpose of his own life and to wonder at the behaviour of some of his fellow human beings.

Such thoughts would invariably produce a sense of despair and despondency. Time after time Josie was there to revive his flagging spirits and to reassure him not only of his own worth but of the many outstanding individuals who made so many sacrifices and achieved so much for the sake of others.

There were times when Greg became the subject of some unkind observations from casual acquaintances. There were those who had no idea of the symptoms of depression and who tended to downplay the seriousness of his illness. There were those who suggested that painting and sculpting were not really careers at all; that they were merely 'hobbies' and that Greg should consider finding a 'real job'. Real workers didn't have time to spend at coffee shops! Real workers toiled away for forty hours every week! How could an 'airy-fairy' pursuit painting flowers and making strange statues be considered a real job?

Sometimes Josie felt herself being overwhelmed by the pressure of being expected to do so much for Greg. It threatened to take its toll on her, and she felt compelled to call on Joyce's friendship to help share the burden. Joyce was a willing listener and was always sincere in her endorsement of all that Josie was doing for Greg. On many occasions she was able to spend a little extra time at the café and provide meals for herself and Josie and Greg.

Occasionally Josie would feel that the demands on her time and emotions were so overbearing that she needed some guidance herself. At these times she would seek professional assistance and would spend time with Dr Norris or would speak with someone from various mental health organisations of Lifeline.

As she became more familiar with some of the situations and circumstances that produced stress or anxiety for Greg, she did everything she could to shield and protect him from these influences. She was careful not to overload him with too many responsibilities because she noticed that he would become worse under these conditions.

There were times when Greg felt disinclined to continue his medication. When this occurred, Josie was careful not to be overbearing or to pester Greg. Such an approach often resulted in exactly the opposite result to what was intended. Josie would simply remind Greg that she had prepared his dosage and had left it ready for him on the kitchen table. She also reminded him how important was his responsibility to himself and to those around him to do everything he could to ensure that his illness was managed and controlled.

She was tactful but persistent, gentle but firm, empathising with Greg's conflicting emotions and moods but always remaining positive and determined to do everything she could to help him. She was Greg's guardian angel, constantly tending to him and reassuring him that she would always be there for him. She never gave up, despite the enormous personal sacrifices that her devotion to him entailed. She was never too busy or too tired to respond to his cries for help.

She was a wonderful role model for me, and I learned so much from observing the way that she was able to lift Greg's spirits with her words and tender ministrations. Gradually, as I followed her example and began to practise what I had learned from her, I was encouraged and delighted at the positive response it often generated.

Both of us learned, however, that we could never rest on our laurels. We were constantly reminded of Greg's fragility, sometimes in a quite surprising and even shocking way!

chapter sixteen
nailed

One of the more shocking incidents that occurred when I was living in that household happened when Greg was working in the garage one day. He was painting, but the self-doubt had begun to surface yet again. His frustration eventually reached breaking point, and he did something totally unexpected. He took a nail gun that was resting on his workbench, placed it on the web between his right-hand thumb and index finger and pulled the trigger.

He emerged from the garage with the steel shaft of a twelve centimetre nail protruding from his left hand. It was a grotesque sight, almost obscene. I just couldn't believe it, and yet I knew it was no illusion when I felt a horrible nausea beginning to overtake me. What was even more bizarre was the calm way in which Greg was behaving. There was no screaming out in pain. There was no crying out for help. There were no obvious signs of distress on his part. He was altogether too composed. It was like watching a sequence from a horror movie!

'What happened?' I stammered after I had somehow composed myself from the shock of seeing the nail.

In a calm and unhurried voice, he informed me in an everyday conversational tone that he had put the gun to his hand and pulled the trigger. Almost as a postscript he added that it was not an accident, that it had been a deliberate action.

I was dumbfounded. The nail was firmly embedded in the soft flesh of his hand, and I knew that if I tried to extract it the bleeding could be quite heavy. I called out to Josie. She came into the room and stopped as if she had run into a brick wall. There was no point in asking Greg what had happened, she could see quite plainly the wound that he'd inflicted on himself. She took a moment to gather her thoughts and decide on an appropriate course of action.

With a composure that did her proud under the circumstances, Josie simply informed Greg that she was going to get her purse from the bedroom and that she was going to drive him down to the Mona Vale Hospital. I asked if she wanted me to accompany her to the hospital, but she excused me, seeing that I was right in the middle of exams at College.

At the Emergency ward the injury was categorised as not as serious as some others that required more urgent treatment, so Greg and Josie had to wait until their turn came. Josie refrained from asking for any further details, and Greg was obviously in no mood to discuss them. The nail protruding from his hand did produce quite a reaction in the waiting area. It was, after all, quite an unusual injury and one that not many of the outpatients had seen before.

Greg was eventually ushered into one of the cubicles and mumbled his explanation that there had been a slight accident while he was engaged in his home handyman repairs at home.

His hand was injected with a local anaesthetic and a tetanus shot, and the offending shaft was removed with a pair of surgical pliers.

The attending doctor informed Greg that what was now a dull ache would soon become much more intense and that a further injection of a painkilling drug was in order. Greg agreed and the shot was administered.

When I returned from College, Greg was lying on the couch in the living room. His left hand was now heavily bandaged. Josie mentioned that she had an urgent delivery to make to one of her clients and asked me if I would keep an eye on Greg during her short absence. I agreed, and Josie went off to make her delivery.

Greg seemed a little sheepish when I asked him to bring me up to date on what had occurred at the hospital, and began by giving me the gory description of the nail extraction, the resulting copious flow of blood from the wound and the painkilling injection.

When I decided to pursue the reasons for such an outlandish action, he slowly volunteered a few more details about what had driven him to such extraordinary lengths. He mentioned that he was seriously worried about his and Josie's financial situation. He said that all of their resources had been used up to purchase materials for his painting, and since neither of them had any regular work to rely on, their income had been seriously depleted.

Burdened by such thoughts, he had felt himself going over the edge when the latest painting on which he was working did not quite come up to his expectations. Normally this would have been cause enough to trigger an outburst, but coupled with his financial concerns it was more than enough to push him over the edge easily. When he sought to express his frustration he simply reached out and made use of the most available implements, which happened to be the tools in his workshop.

I had been concerned about the incident all day and had found it hard to concentrate at College. I was worried that there may have been permanent damage to the nerves in Greg's hand. Although the doctor had expressed the opinion that there would be no such consequences, we knew that only time would tell if this were so.

Not wishing to exhaust Greg with further conversation after his ordeal, I suggested that we might watch television while we waited for Josie to return. Greg agreed and we settled in to pass the time. We were not long into our viewing when Greg needed to go to the bathroom and rose unsteadily from the couch. I asked him if he felt okay, and he told me that he was fine.

No sooner had he reassured me that everything was all right when he staggered to the left of the doorway and crashed into the wall! I leaped to my feet and steadied him as he struggled to regain his balance. When I asked him what the matter was, he slurred an unintelligible reply. I was instantly alarmed and guided him back to the couch and encouraged him to lie down.

Greg was still mumbling and stirring restlessly while I called Josie on her mobile phone. I told her what had happened and asked her what I should do. She advised me to make sure that Greg was comfortable and to keep an eye on him until she returned. Her last instructions to me were to call her back if there were any further developments.

As the afternoon wore on, it became apparent to me that Greg was not improving. He had made one unsuccessful attempt to go to the kitchen for a drink from the refrigerator, crashing into the dining table en route and scattering the salt and pepper shakers and the sauce bottle. When I asked him to return to the lounge while I cleaned up the resultant mess, he proceeded to lurch into the bookcase, this time littering the floor with half our collection of novels, text books and medical journals. I steered him back to the couch and told him to remain there until I had finished clearing up after him.

I racked my brain to figure out what was the cause of his disorientation. I asked him if he had remembered to take his medication that morning, and I gathered not from his mumbled reply but from the discernible nod of his head that he had indeed taken his daily dosage.

Greg became more agitated when he felt I could not understand him clearly, and he struggled to pull himself up off the lounge. I advised him against further movement and told him it was important that he rest until Josie returned.

He totally ignored my suggestion and rose unsteadily to his feet. He swayed from side to side as if he were intoxicated. He pointed to the front door and indicated that he wanted to go outside. There was no way I was going to risk his walking anywhere near the busy road that went past our house, so I hurried over to the couch and gently eased him back down onto the cushions.

He suddenly relaxed and allowed me to settle him on the lounge. When

I felt reasonably sure that he had abandoned the idea of an afternoon walk, I went outside and called Joyce on my mobile phone. I was deeply worried about Greg's symptoms and asked her if she could come over to help me keep an eye on him. As I spoke with Joyce, I watched Greg through the front window rise unsteadily from the lounge and blunder around the living room.

Joyce told me that she had finished most of her food preparations for the following day, had cleaned the café and would leave a note informing her patrons that the shop had closed a little earlier than normal. She told me she would join me in about ten minutes.

When she arrived she took one look at Greg, realised that his behaviour was far from normal, and took him straight back to the hospital. He wobbled by me on the way to Joyce's car, still not sure what was happening, and looking even worse for wear.

I followed in my own car.

The medical team at the hospital soon reached the conclusion that there had been an adverse interaction between the medication that Greg was taking for his depression and the strong painkiller which had been given to him during his treatment for the hand injury. They told us that he had become delirious and had suffered an allergic reaction to the painkiller.

The doctors decided to keep Greg under observation for the next hour, and when they were confident that he had stabilised, they allowed us to take him and return home. I can only assume that Greg had experienced a period of selective amnesia, for when I queried him about some of the details of his misadventure, he couldn't remember what had happened. We all had a lot of trouble getting to sleep that night.

chapter seventeen

leaden skies

Greg's injury to his hand meant that he was unable to continue work on any of his sculptures. He also felt disinclined to paint. For his convalescence, therefore, he was relatively inactive and spent most of his time watching television and resting. It was not a good time for his fellow boarders! We began to feel sorry for ourselves and commiserate with each other over the limitations that the constant need for vigilance imposed on our lives.

The social events to which we had been invited, the television programmes that we wanted to watch, the friends that we would like to have visited, the plans that were sometimes disrupted by a call on our time and energy – all of these restrictions took their toll. There were times when one of us had to volunteer to stay in the house all day and watch Greg, lest he do something to hurt himself.

We had to be exceptionally watchful when we recognised some of the tell-tale signs that told us Greg was most likely to be feeling terribly low. He would sometimes have trouble sleeping, or lose his appetite; sometimes the tone of his voice would change, alerting us to his susceptibility to an attack. It was during these periods that Greg seemed most vulnerable and likely to be plunged back into depression. While we were constantly on the alert for any of the usual warning signs or situations that might set him off, it was also a time of great strain and disruption to our lives.

At these times the house was a decidedly unpleasant place to live. I could walk through the door then and actually feel the depression like a heavy blanket enveloping us all. The mood of the place was oppressive. I felt it eating away at my social life, impacting on my progress at College, and the anxiety it generated played havoc with my sleep.

When Greg was experiencing one of his most serious episodes, I would often return home from College and find Josie crying. Sometimes, I would be moved to tears too: tears for Greg as well as tears for myself! It was heartbreaking to see him in so much pain and yet feel so helpless. It was like a dark cloud had descended on us all when he had his depression, and there seemed no way out. I'm sure that I began to exhibit the symptoms of mild depression as well until I learned to cope with the situation.

We all wanted Greg to get better, but it was easier said than done! We would try to be positive, to build him up and we would fill his head with positive affirmations: we told him repeatedly that he had so many reasons to live; he had so much talent that it cried out to be shared; we praised his works and complimented him on an especially pleasing painting or sculpture. We urged him to spend time with his animals and to continue caring for the occasional stray or injured creature that came his way.

There were prolonged periods when we would grow increasingly frustrated and wish that we had our old lives back. We cried out for normal, happy and carefree existences. But we also craved a solution to Greg's problems and a normal, happy and carefree existence for him as well.

When this wasn't forthcoming, and when we felt overrun with the continual problems and demands we grew increasingly worn out and frustrated by the new direction our lives seemed to be taking. It was just so difficult to live in an environment where you constantly feared for someone's safety.

There were many occasions when I just wanted to pack my bags and escape. I would tell myself that wasn't how my life was supposed to be unfolding. I should've been out enjoying myself with friends, not worrying about somebody's welfare every minute of the day. How was I ever going to pass my exams when I was distracted constantly by these weird events going on around me?

If I'd known that I was going to have to live through such trying times I probably would've run as fast as my legs could carry me, and never looked back. Once I had met Greg and come to know him, however, my fate was sealed. He was a remarkable person who was suffering. He was my friend, and I couldn't turn my back on him even though I wanted to on many occasions. He was my best mate and he was in a fight for his life. I wanted to do everything I could to help him even though it was extremely difficult at times.

Even though Josie was extremely dedicated there were days when she, too, would falter. During these moments she would confess that her situation was the last thing in the world that she had planned for herself. All she had ever wanted from life was to be settled in her own house with her own garden. She loved gardens and she loved flowers. Her dream was to have her own garden filled with roses and sunflowers and irises. That was her idea of heaven!

Josie would confide these dreams to Joyce whenever the two of them had the chance to enjoy a cappuccino together at the restaurant. Each time they met in this frame of mind they would continue to elaborate on the daydreams, adding a few more fanciful details each time they discussed them. Joyce, inspired by the movie French Kiss starring Meg Ryan and Kevin Kline, imagined living among vineyards, where she could enjoy relaxing lunches, good coffee, and the occasional glass of wine with friends and family. Had I been invited to participate in these discussions I would have informed the ladies that it was always my ambition to follow my calling and make use of my qualifications to be a naturopath, and to own a small fishing boat for weekends and leisure time.

Although we would often indulge in describing these fantasies to one another, none of us had any real intention of acting on them. They were just frustrating days. We never let Greg know that we were feeling like this; he had enough troubles of his own. We all believed that if he even suspected for a minute that we felt the way we did, then he would have become even more despondent.

Gradually, we learned to cope. Through a series of graduated steps we realised that we could be there for someone without taking on the attendant problems. We learned it was imperative to safeguard our own peace of mind. We gave Greg our help and understanding but tried not to become overwhelmed with his troubles. We made every effort to help him, without completely draining our bodies of their energy reserves. When we didn't do this, we started 'burning out' and risked becoming victims ourselves. When Greg was in one of his 'holes', as we came to describe his episodes, we were providing no assistance by falling into the hole ourselves. That way, none of us would ever make it back out!

I kept reminding myself of the time when my younger sister, Tiffany, who's a scuba diving buff, explained to me how the divers' rescue system worked. The rescuer never allowed himself or herself to be exposed to the same danger as the victim; otherwise two divers would need rescuing instead of just one, with the possibility of either of them surviving extremely unlikely!

When I first moved into the house, I would end up shouldering too many of Greg's problems and taking on the role of martyr: sacrificing myself for the perceived good of Greg. I ended up exhausted and drained, and less able to cope myself.

Later, I focused on trying to be both helpful and understanding, but I soon realised how important it was to set aside some time for myself. I took the time to look after myself: I went fishing, went to watch the footy, went surfing, or went for a walk with friends. I also found it really important to talk to someone else, and had either a friend or a family member in whom I could confide. When I didn't have this type of support, then I would contact the mental health associations or Lifeline. I soon realised that a problem shared is a problem halved.

One of the more pleasant facets of Greg's 'treatment', as far as I was concerned, occurred when he would accept my challenge to eighteen holes of golf. This would have a twofold benefit: apart from the enjoyment that Greg and I shared out on the course, it would also mean that Josie could have some time to herself. It was extremely draining for her at times, and she looked forward to the respites that our golf games afforded her.

Even when I would take these steps, I still found it really hard to cope with the continued spasmodic incidences of Greg's depression and the circumstances in which I sometimes found myself. What I found particularly hurtful was the negativity that I sometimes detected, both from friends and casual acquaintances. I received comments that implied I was being unreasonable and foolish to devote so much time and effort to Greg. I was advised to move out and get on with my own life instead of saddling myself with someone who didn't seem to be showing any response at all to my efforts. I had to contend with some quite pessimistic forecasts about the end result of my association with Greg, and the gloomy prediction that I would find myself struggling when all of my good intentions came to naught.

These criticisms intensified when it became evident that I was giving money to Josie to help support Greg. Insinuations that I was being used, that Greg and Josie were taking advantage of me and my generous nature, that Greg would never get better as long as he was dependent on me for financial support only served to strengthen my resolve. I replied by expressing my firm conviction that it was far better to share our resources with the living than to leave this world with a healthy bank balance and no way of making a withdrawal! It never ceases to confound me how money issues can so often create problems within a relationship.

Some of our acquaintances were quite pessimistic about Greg's chances of survival when they learned some of the details of his attempt at suicide. They were convinced that one day he would succeed, and that all our efforts to assist him would therefore have been futile. They warned us of this likelihood and told us to prepare ourselves for the worst.

There were still others who failed to appreciate the extraordinary gift with which Greg had been blessed. From my own observation I was convinced that he had a unique talent as an artist, and that this God-given gift deserved an opportunity to be developed. Josie, Joyce and I wanted to encourage that talent, in spite of the insinuations that we were wasting our time and that Greg would never amount to anything.

It was quite a shock for me to discover that there were people who could misinterpret and even criticise our good intentions. Sometimes these expressions of disapproval came from the most unexpected quarters. I couldn't believe that a woman as selfless and as thoughtful as Josie could meet with such censure. Our only explanation for these kinds of remarks was that the people who levelled them at her had no idea of the sacrifices that were involved and the purity of her intentions.

When they accused her of interfering in Greg's life and of having ulterior motives, she would reply by informing them that her only concern was to help Greg recover and become well again. She made the most of every opportunity to spread the message that people with depression need compassion and tolerance, not disapproval and judgements.

Despite these slings and arrows, Josie in particular remained totally devoted and committed to helping Greg. For the next two years she gave him her constant and undivided attention until it seemed the worst had passed. That period, of course, was not without its difficulties and setbacks, but in the end it seemed that her persistence had paid off, and Greg was looking forward to a rewarding and fulfilling career as an artist and sculptor. She put up with his complaints about life, the suicide attempt, and the apprehension that lived with her during those years.

As Greg progressed steadily during that time, he also grew closer to Josie as he came to appreciate her dedication and commitment to his recovery. He discovered a friendship and a loving relationship that he had never known before. He has often acknowledged his great debt to her, and openly admits that if it had not been for Josie, his life would have ended long ago. He refers to her fondly as the most remarkable human being he has ever met and the best friend he could ever hope to have.

This is why I so dreaded the terrible responsibility of contacting her in the middle of her holiday on the Central Coast and letting her know that Greg had just taken one hundred sleeping tablets and was in a critical condition at the Mona Vale Hospital. His life was hanging in the balance!

chapter eighteen
the hard yards

Josie had left Church Point two days before with her car loaded with books, clothing, and natural medicines. It was the first time that she had been away from Greg in several years. A friend of hers, desperate to give up smoking, decided that a visit to a health retreat was the only way she could overcome her addiction. She was insistent that Josie go with her to give her moral support and to help her break the harmful habit before an upcoming operation.

She had left Greg happy and settled, working on his latest painting, 'Autumn Dreaming'. It was another beautiful landscape featuring all the bright colours that we associated with one of Greg's happy and relaxed periods. Josie had been so looking forward to the break and had decided to divide her time between rest and regenerative nature walks.

Shortly after I had watched the ambulance rush off with Greg's comatose body barely breathing from an oxygen cylinder, I called the hospital and asked for news. I was told it was too early yet to form an accurate diagnosis of Greg's condition, and it was suggested that I call back a little later.

When I did eventually call back the emergency staff were still running tests and taking precautions, and could not be sure if Greg would pull through. His life was in jeopardy, but they were working to try to stabilise his condition.

I thanked them for their efforts, and pleaded with them to do everything they could to save my friend.

It was time to call Josie, and it was a task I had been dreading. I dialled the number of her mobile phone.

Her happy and cheerful greeting chilled me with its friendliness and animation. For a moment I could barely begin the conversation. How do you tell someone that their closest friend could be on his death bed? How do you break that kind of news? There is absolutely no way that you can possibly soften the blow. The enormity of my task almost deprived me of speech, but I braced myself and tried to keep the terrible sadness out of my voice.

'Jose, it's me.'

'How are you,' she said excitedly.

'Not good,' I replied. 'There's been some really bad news.'

'What's happened?' she asked. The excitement in her voice was suddenly replaced by panic.

'It's Greg,' I said. 'He's taken an overdose and has been rushed to Mona Vale hospital.'

Oh no,' she said, stunned. 'Is he going to be all right?'

'I'm not sure, Jose.'

'I'll meet you at the hospital as soon as I can get back,' she said, before hanging up the phone.

My next call was to Joyce, who burst into tears as soon as she heard the news. I told her that I still had no definite word from the hospital but that I would keep her informed of any developments.

I was still in shock. I went back to Greg's bedroom and once again picked up the empty packet. The label informed me that there had been one hundred sleeping tablets in the original package. Now there were none!

I inspected the waste paper baskets in the bedroom and in the bathroom; I looked in the wash basin and the bath but there was no evidence of any pills having been disposed of. The only conclusion I could draw was that Greg had done exactly what he had told me. He had swallowed every single one of the little white pills!

Within the hour, I was on my way to see what had happened to Greg. Hospitals do absolutely nothing for me even at the best of times, but as I made my way through the entry foyer into the emergency department I had a sense of apprehension and a chill ran down my spine like I had never experienced before.

I was always aware that many people died in hospital beds, but it had never happened to anyone I knew. Could this be the first time, I thought to myself as I sat down in the waiting room. The place was quiet and dimly lit, and it reminded me in some ways of a library. But what a difference there is between a hospital and a library. In one you read books and study, in a hospital people suffer and sometimes die.

Eventually I was led into Greg's room, passing through a ward where small groups of people huddled quietly around beds of their friends or family members, talking quietly and watching me walk by. Some showed their emotions quite plainly. There was an air of sadness at one bed, where an elderly gentleman was obviously not well and struggled to fill his lungs with air in harsh, rasping breaths.

I paused for a moment outside Greg's room, collecting my thoughts before I walked in to greet him. He didn't see me enter the room. He was propped up with pillows behind his head, leaning on one elbow, and staring out the window. Surprisingly, his room was not as clinical as I had expected it to be. I could see Mona Vale beach in the distance. It was a pleasant contrast to the ward through which I had just passed, and I gazed for a moment at the sunny landscape and the people enjoying their outdoor activities.

Greg heard my footsteps and turned his head towards me. When our eyes met it was with a sense of relief as well as awkwardness. It's hard to know exactly what to say to a person who's just tried to take his own life. 'How have you been?' didn't seem like an appropriate question. Clumsily, I shook his hand and asked him what had been happening.

'I've just been having some tests,' he replied.

'What do the doctors have to say?' I asked, noticing that he was paler than usual. It was as if all the colour had been drained from his face.

'They said I'm pretty fortunate to be alive, and told me that if I hadn't arrived when I did then I would have died. They also told me that I've done some damage to my liver, but they're not sure how bad it is yet. The worse case scenario is that I might need a liver transplant.'

I wasn't sure what to say, so for a while I said nothing, just continuing to look at the desperate and almost abandoned look on his face. 'Josie will be arriving soon,' I said quickly, the prolonged silence making me feel uncomfortable.

'Good,' he said.

We chatted for a little longer. I was afraid to pursue the reasons for his extraordinary attempt at suicide, so we prattled on for a while about inconsequential things until Greg laid his head back on the pillow and wearily closed his eyes. I said nothing for a time and it wasn't long before I heard the rhythmic sound of a gentle snore beginning to develop.

Later that afternoon Josie and Joyce arrived. Since Greg was still asleep, I went to find some chairs so that we could sit around the bed and talk until he awoke.

I told the girls how worried I was about Greg's immediate future and expressed the concern that maybe he would be so disappointed at failing to carry out his plan that he would try again.

Eventually he woke up and, after greeting us all, took a moment to compose himself and then told us that he couldn't believe what he had attempted to do. Tears formed in his eyes as he recalled his desperate actions He turned towards the window and looked out at the scene below us, remarking how beautiful the ocean looked, then said that he couldn't understand how he could have tried to leave all of this behind.

Greg then began to relate the details of what had happened the previous night, saying that he went to bed feeling alone and lost. For some reason he actually felt scared. As he continued to talk to us, he began quietly to weep and I handed him a tissue from the bedside cabinet. For a while he was unable to continue his narrative, but kept remarking how he had never cried so much in his whole life before.

Eventually he took up his explanation again, and described how he kept thinking what a burden he had become to all of us. He felt that he had been nothing but a terrible disruption to all of our lives; how he had felt so inadequate having to be supported and not being able to contribute; how we had all sacrificed our own ambitions and dreams to look after him and foster his artistic career.

He told us how he had waited until I fell asleep before going to the medicine cabinet for the packet of sleeping pills. 'I felt I just had to do it,' he said. 'I wasn't fooling around this time. It wasn't a cry for help. It was a determined effort to end my own life!'

His comments made us all start to cry. No one spoke for some time. We just sat there sobbing. My mind was filled with conflicting emotions. I was crying, but at the same time I felt such a sense of relief to hear those words come from his mouth, thankful that his life had been saved. My eyes were sore. I took some more tissues and passed them to the others. I took a large handful for myself so that we could dry our tears.

Greg was staring out the window, sitting quietly as the tears continued to course down his cheeks.

'You're not a burden, Greg,' Josie said softly, 'We all love you.'

As we talked, I perceived a slow but noticeable shift in his attitude. Perhaps it was the beauty of the day outside, perhaps it was a growing appreciation of the way we all cared for him, but we soon felt that Greg was becoming quite buoyant. We began to feel a distinct sense of relief as we became aware of this change and we did not doubt him for a moment when he finally assured us that he would never attempt such a thing again. When he indicated that he wanted to return to painting as quickly as possible, we were all delighted by the announcement.

Greg's immediate concern was the condition of his damaged liver, and he asked Josie to reassure him that he would be all right. There was a slight trace of panic in his voice as he asked her if he would still be able to paint.

the hard yards

She replied that she would not know until she had spoken with the doctors who were conducting his tests.

After some time a young woman doctor approached and informed us that Greg had done some serious damage to the organ, but she would not know the full extent until she conducted further tests during the coming weeks.

Greg spent the next two days under strict medical care. Josie and I went to collect him on the day he was discharged. We packed up his things and drove him home.

His release from hospital was conditional. We would have to make sure that he rested. Josie and I would need to supervise him, and the following week he would need to go and see Dr Norris to collect the results of the tests they had run. It was a nervous wait until that time.

Even though Greg said he was feeling better, I was still worried about him.

I still recall the terrible uneasiness and anxiety I felt after Greg's return from hospital, and how a recurring nightmare continually disrupted my sleep.

In the course of the dream I walked into our bathroom and found Greg drowned in our bathtub. He had intentionally taken his own life. Frightened and upset, I lifted his naked body from the water and carried him from the room weeping. It was eerie, and the strange yellow light that was cast over his lifeless body floating in the worn tub will be forever etched in my mind.

I remember the dream was so realistic and so vivid that when I woke up I staggered to the bathroom expecting to find Greg submerged in the tub. My relief was palpable when I discovered the bathroom was empty and Greg was sleeping peacefully in his bed. I was still groggy from sleep and wanted to convince myself that he was okay, so I gently shook him until he turned over and gave me the most quizzical look.

'Are you all right?' I asked him.

'Yeah, I'm fine,' he said, glancing down at the luminous dial of his watch that showed him it was only four o'clock in the morning.

The days seemed to drag on for all of us until it was eventually time for Greg to see his doctor. I went with him and Josie to see the GP the following Monday afternoon. I thought I would let them speak with Dr Norris in private, so I went downstairs to Café Bella Cino to see Joyce.

I was deeply worried about what the results of Greg's test would be. I must have looked a little apprehensive as I walked through the front door of the café. Sensing my nervousness, Joyce decided to shut the shop early. She sent the last remaining employee home as we cleaned the tabletops. Shortly after this we pulled up two chairs and did what we normally did when life's problems became overwhelming: we made two cappuccinos and we talked.

I looked closely at the shop fittings in the café that Greg had made a few years earlier.

'Greg sure did a great job putting this place together,' I said, trying to find positives in a situation that felt hardly that. Three of his paintings hung on the wall with 'For Sale' signs beneath them.

'You can tell Greg has worked on this place,' she replied. 'It's perfect.'

Suddenly, I was overcome with a deep sense of sadness. Surrounded by reminders of the happier times Greg had spent renovating the café, I guess the events of the past week had finally caught up with me. I could no longer contain my feelings. When I began to cry, Joyce reached out and took my hand. In a world that felt so hard she gave it a soft touch. 'It will be all right,' she said.

I was grateful she did this. Never before had I been in such need of consolation.

'I hope so Joyce, I really hope so,' I said.

We couldn't improve on the silence, so we sat quietly

It was by sharing moments like these that Joyce and I grew increasingly close over the years. Strangely, in a time full of crisis, I found a friendship unlike any I had previously known. Even in the midst of our dilemma, she would remain positive. Being able to communicate with such a warm and open person made the crisis tolerable. I noticed Joyce's eyes looking at me intently as I sat at the table. They were telling me to stop worrying and they offered support. 'She only wants the best for me, for me to be happy. I am extremely lucky to have such a true friend,' I thought.

For a moment, I remembered a conversation we had the previous New Year's Eve. We had spoken about some of our hopes for the coming year. Our wishes were not too dissimilar. We hoped this year would bring with it some better times. But with Greg's recent episode landing him in hospital, it seemed our wishes had been temporarily put on hold. I made another wish as I sat at the table – I prayed that Greg would be okay.

It occurred to me then that I had probably cried more in the last two years than I had during the preceding twenty-four years of my life. I hoped there would be no additional tears with Greg's impending test results. Joyce and I would just have to sit patiently and wait for the doctors to tell us what was to be the likely aftermath of his suicide attempt.

Shortly afterwards, Greg and Josie came downstairs to tell us the results of the tests. I found it hard to contain my anxiety.

'The liver is damaged but there are signs that things are improving, and that it may well recover.'

'Is there any serious damage?' Joyce asked.

'Nothing that can be seen as life-threatening in the immediate future,' Josie replied.

I breathed a big sigh of relief when I heard the news.

'That's fantastic,' Joyce said.

I got up and began making a flat white for Josie and a hot chocolate for Greg. I thought a warm drink might be comforting at the end of a long day.

'I'm so glad things are going to be all right,' I said, as I warmed some milk for the coffee. Their worry had suddenly lifted, and the tension in my neck and back immediately eased.

'We were just talking about the renovations you did to this place,' I continued. 'They still look amazing.'

'I put all my effort into them,' Greg replied.

'When Greg puts his mind to something he certainly does put all his effort into it,' I thought, as we sat and had our drinks. When we had finished we left the café and went home for an evening meal to celebrate the good news.

chapter nineteen
resurgence

'In many ways, art enabled me to get through my depression. It became my therapy, and I used it to help brush aside my blues, literally,' Greg recalls. *'Painting helped me put back the colour in my life,'* he said.

Beautiful honey and soy aromas lingered in the air one evening as Josie, Joyce, Greg and I finished our delicious Chinese meal. I snapped the hard outer shell of my fortune cookie with my front teeth, and disentangled the hidden message. It read (in its quaint English style): 'Sometimes you have to fall into the hole to learn the wisdom.' I sat at the table thinking about the meaning of this simple statement. Perhaps Greg had learned from his horrible ordeal and would emerge a happier and more confident person?

Ever since Greg had returned home from the hospital he certainly seemed like a stronger, more determined individual. There was no doubt in my mind that he had reviewed everything that had happened in his failed attempt to end his life. I was sure that he realised that he had been given another opportunity to live and this time he was going to make the most of it. There was no way he would ever take life for granted again, he assured me.

It was almost as if the near disaster had acted as a catalyst for change in his life. He was determined to turn his life around. He knew it would

my brush with depression

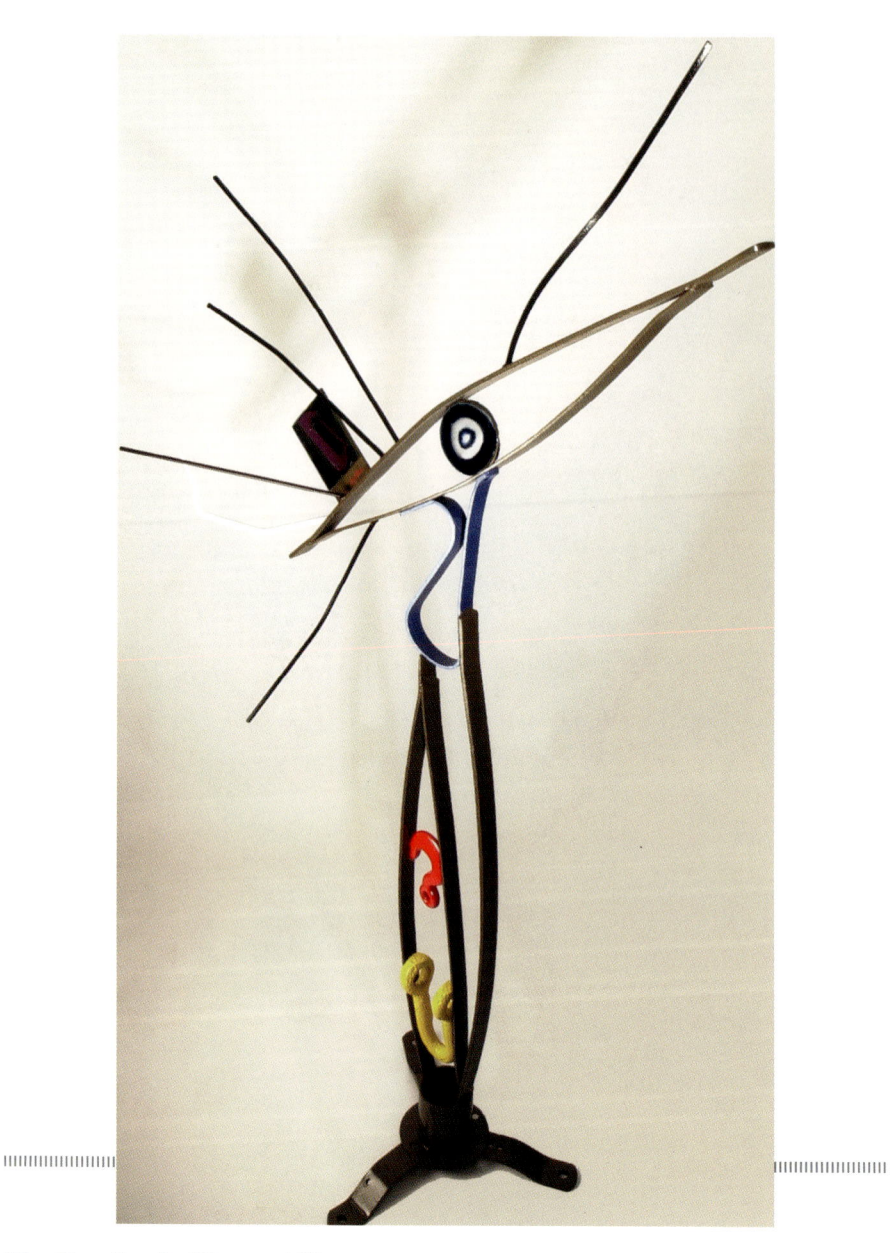

'The Question is: Who are U?'
Mirror, Steel, gemstones, 2660 x 1270 mm
This symbol of introspection seeks to portray the never-ending quest to determine our own identity and individuality.

resurgence

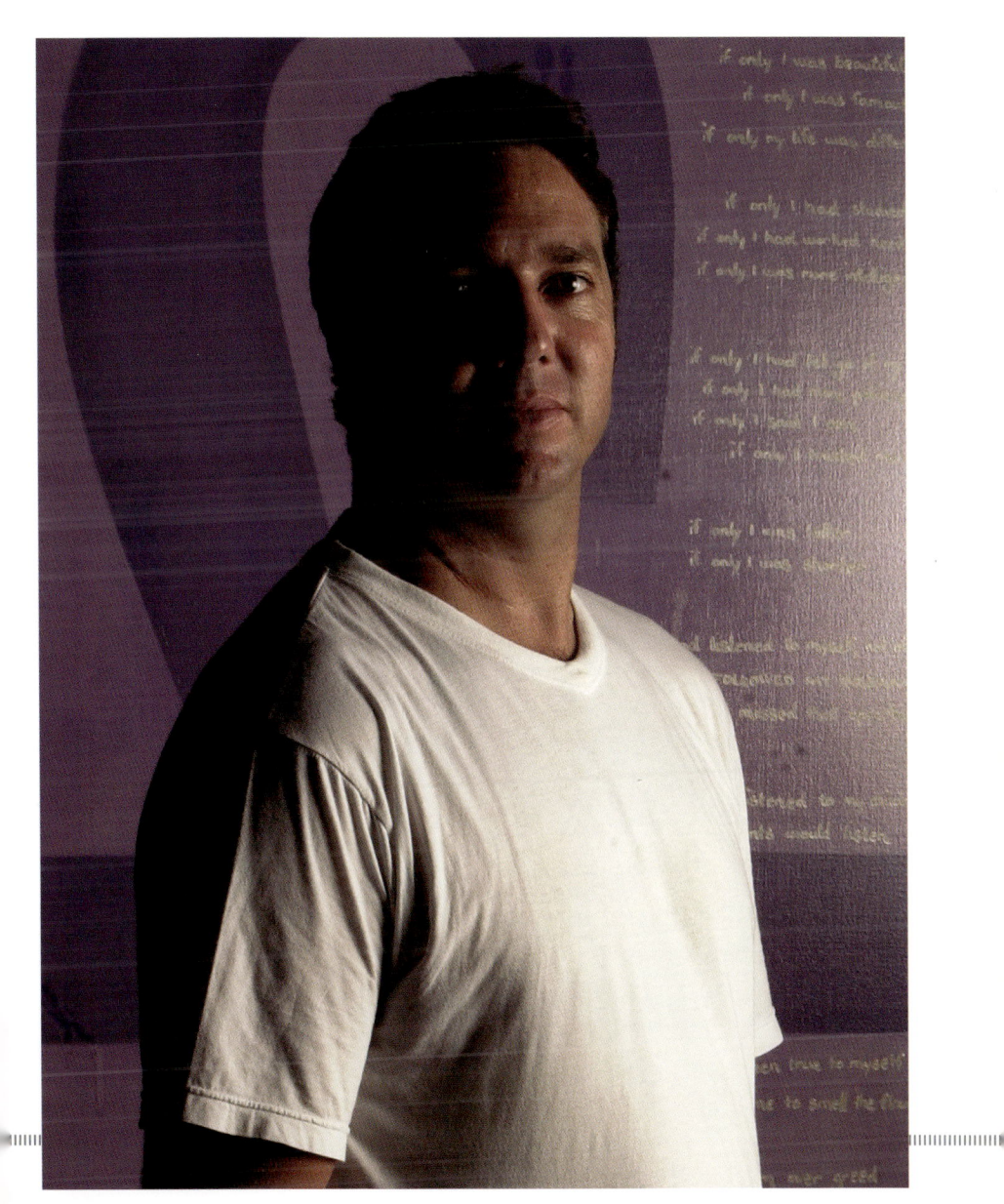

'If only…'
Oil on linen, 1220 x 910 mm
'"If only" encourages me to learn from past mistakes and regrets. My life could have been different "if only …", but analysing those errors can help me make better decisions for the future.'

greg wilson — 141

take an exceptional and courageous effort, but he remembered one of the many sayings that his grandmother had passed on to him: 'You only harvest the fruit that you plant and nurture.' He wanted desperately to rid himself of the failed crop that he had planted in the past and replace it with a harvest of optimism and hope.

He began to go back over the mistakes that he felt he had made in the past and systematically to work on eliminating those errors from his life in the future. If he became disenchanted with one of his works, he resolved to walk away from it calmly and without any of the histrionics that had sometimes resulted in the past. He vowed to be flexible and to remain positive when things didn't go his way or didn't turn out as he had planned. He even assured me that there would be no further use for the 'three iron brush'!

This self-examination and review of the past occurrences of depression became an important focal point for Greg in his attempts to nail down the causes of his outbursts. He began to see that he was more likely to have an episode of depression when he was under stress. His illness had been triggered by a number of factors: his extreme sensitivity to criticism; the trauma of his motorcycle accidents; the demands that were put on him at work; his parents' separation; his own self-doubt; and the attempted suicides.

'If only' text:

'If only I believed in myself, If only I had, If only I hadn't, If only I was beautiful, If only I was famous, If only my life was different, If only I had studied, If only I had worked harder, If only I were more intelligent, If only I had let go of my fear, If only I had more patience, If only I said I can, If only I trusted more, If only I was taller, If only I was shorter, If only I had believed in myself, not others, If only I had FOLLOWED MY DREAMS, If only I had not missed that opportunity, If only I had listened to my children, If only my parents would listen, If only I had been true to myself, If only I took the time to smell the flowers, If only I had chosen wisdom over greed, If only I had been more loving, If only I said I love you more, If only I appreciated what I had, not what I didn't, If only I thanked GOD more, If only … '

Greg also realised that it wasn't only the dramatic experiences in his life that set off the disturbing episodes. Sometimes simple triggers could cause depression. Included among these were: a fear that he couldn't express how he was feeling; a feeling of not being good enough; a fear of not achieving; of being unloved, unneeded; or a feeling of uselessness. Sometimes these simple triggers were even more harmful than some of the major traumas he had experienced.

He began to speak about these things openly and honestly. He worked hard at banishing any harmful memories that he had stored away in his mind, and any additional troubles that may have surfaced during his day-to-day activities. It didn't matter how trivial he thought it was, he would still speak about it. It was like spring-cleaning as he cleared out the clutter from his mind.

He would share any troubling emotions with Josie, Joyce or myself. He would describe his feelings and the incidents that triggered his deflated mood. Too often in the past, he had shut these thoughts away in his mind, where they would fester and continue to worsen. No longer did he shut down. He began to talk freely about his feelings and more often than not his mood would improve quite markedly.

He also realised that there were certain things in life that were beyond his control. Greg realised that he was unable to prevent wars, violence, murder, or even cruelty to animals. But what he could change was his response to these things. When confronted with these disturbing aspects of humanity, he would remain positive and do the best he could to generate peace in his own life. Instead of growing upset when he saw these things, he grew more determined to make some positive changes in his own life.

He still had to fight long and hard, but he was determined, and he had a new-found strength of purpose.

That was the major difference that I noticed when he returned home. It was this strength of mind that carried him through the difficult moments.

my brush with depression

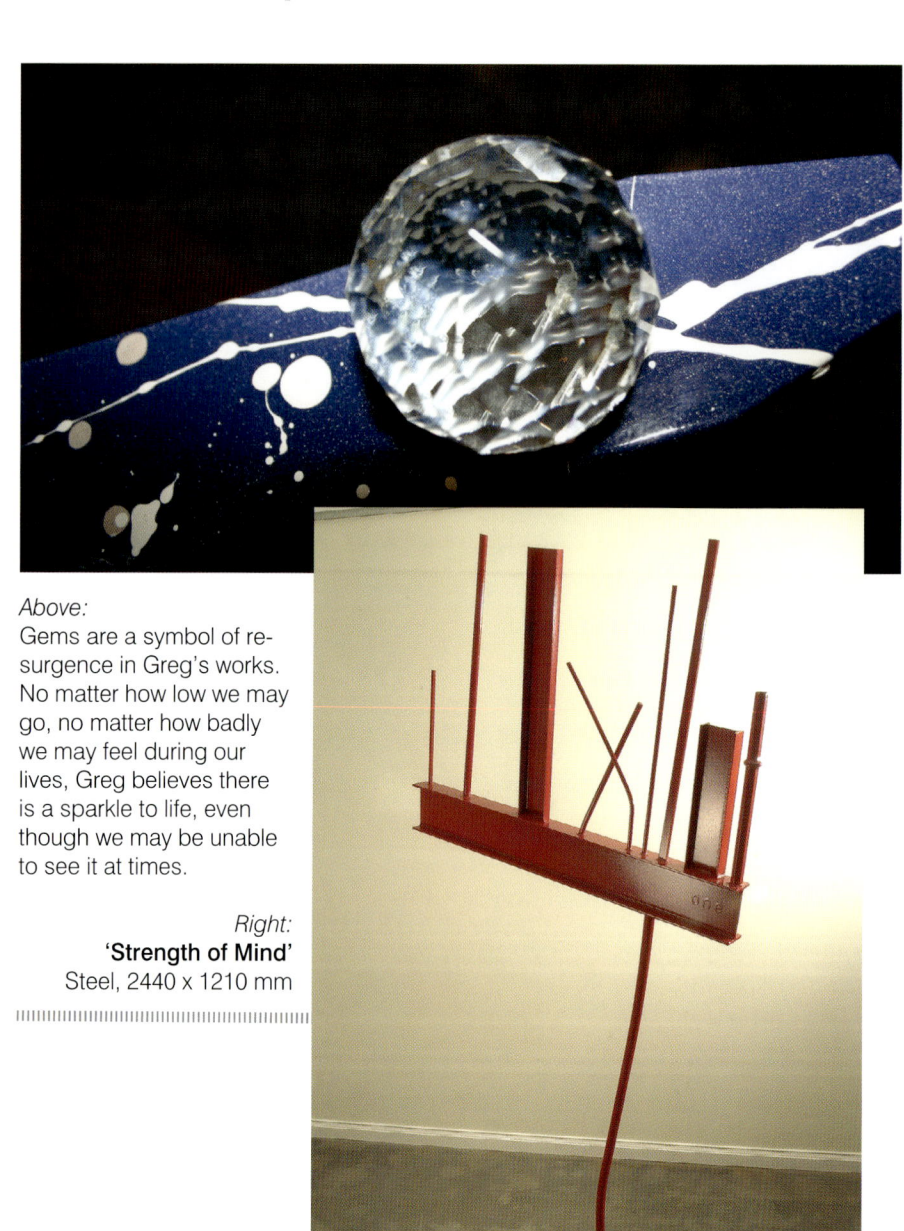

Above:
Gems are a symbol of resurgence in Greg's works. No matter how low we may go, no matter how badly we may feel during our lives, Greg believes there is a sparkle to life, even though we may be unable to see it at times.

Right:
'Strength of Mind'
Steel, 2440 x 1210 mm

144 — aaron cootes

It was this shift in his attitude that was the secret to his regaining his self-confidence. This shift also manifested itself in his work. Sculptures that had formerly seemed to focus on the macabre and sombre were now replaced by far more colourful and uplifting themes. When he completed a work that he labelled 'Strength of Mind', it was a tangible demonstration of this new-found resilience.

When I asked him to describe the thought processes that had inspired such a work, he took a moment before describing the piece quite graphically: 'At times life's pressures and complexities can seem overbearing, and our support systems appear disproportionate to the weight they have to bear. Strength of mind is then the ultimate factor in determining whether our delicately balanced lives collapse or continue to withstand these adversities. Now how's that description from a poor simple sculptor!'

It was also about this time that Greg was motivated to include some symbol of his own resurgence in his sculpture. He used small gems, or crystals, to represent the new-found spark that he felt had been re-introduced into his outlook.

We began to observe a number of welcome improvements. When problems surfaced we noticed that Greg's spirits never seemed to sink to the depths that he had previously plumbed. He would see the problem as something he could overcome. He would call upon his new-found strength of mind. 'This isn't going to beat me any more,' he would tell himself. There was a stubborn refusal to let himself be engulfed by the full force of his depression.

Despite these tenacious and determined efforts, he still had his days where he would feel his depression lurking in the shadows. While his spirits would still sink and he would become aware of many of the usual symptoms, he would fight with renewed vigour. Where in the past it could take him anything up to a week or two to return from his depths, it might now only take half a day before he was able to overcome the mood.

As Greg puzzled about the causes of his disease and how to eradicate them, he recalled the words of his doctor, who had told him that some forms of depression could be caused by genetic factors. People could inherit a predisposition in which an inadequate supply of chemicals to different areas of the brain could alter people's emotions and make them feel depressed. Greg suspected that there might have been a history of mental illness in his own family. He now understood that he could have been handed this unfortunate condition by his forebears.

His doctor had referred to this condition as clinical depression. When he explained that it was characterised by fluctuating mood swings, Greg identified immediately with the symptoms.

When Greg discussed the doctor's diagnosis with me, I realised that there was a vast difference between what most of us mean and feel when we say we are suffering from depression and the condition that afflicted Greg.

It took me sometime to reach this conclusion. One of the major reasons that I was so confused was because I used the word 'depression' to describe my own feelings of sadness or inadequacy or loneliness. That is an entirely inappropriate use of the term when compared to the mental illness that afflicted Greg and involved such severe physical symptoms.

I would have feelings of sadness in response to everyday problems, but these would normally be short-lived. Whenever I recalled how my relationship had come to an end, I was really upset. I could become withdrawn and reclusive for a while, and there were times when I would be moved to tears when I remembered the turn that my life had taken. As time passed, however, I noticed a gradual but steady improvement in my outlook.

Greg's depression was an entirely different matter. As I began to understand his condition, I realised that his depression descends on him sometimes for no apparent external reason at all. His feelings during the worst times could last for weeks or months and were far more brutal.

There was also no way that we could anticipate his attacks. There were definitely times when everything seemed to be going swimmingly for him: he may have sold a painting, he'd be surrounded by loving relationships; he'd have a great idea for one of his artworks; and yet he'd be drawn into an awful bout of wretchedness.

Even today there are times when he'll go to bed feeling on top of the world, looking forward to the morrow and enthusing about a current project, only to wake up with a glassy look in his eyes and a vacant expression on his face, and the undeniable symptoms of his illness all too apparent. At such times it is clear that there is something amiss with the supply of those vital elements to his brain.

He is totally aware of this transformation in himself, and he will sadly confide: 'It's happening again.' I really feel sorry for Greg whenever this happens. He will say to me, 'Aaron, you know I don't have any problems; my mind is clear; but I can feel the depression coming on without any apparent cause.'

It's during these times that Greg most needs my support. When Greg is feeling low it's important to be there for him, just to help him get through the mood as best he can.

I've discovered from past experience that it doesn't help to say to him: 'Hey mate, get over it and stop your acting.' Greg's condition is the result of a set of real and demoralising feelings that invade his body. I've come to understand that there's nothing that I can say or do that can improve his situation. I will always continue to extend my moral support and caring concern, but that only serves to prevent the mood from getting any worse. He just has to wait until his body recovers.

My incomplete understanding of depression prevented me from seeing the similarity between it and other physical illnesses. I failed to appreciate that just as shortness of breath was a symptom of asthma, it could not be remedied by willpower alone. The greatest mental capacity in the world will not make the asthmatic's air passages dilate and provide easier means of breathing.

The same principle was true for Greg. It didn't matter what steps he took to try to throw off his depression. When his brain's chemistry was dysfunctional he would feel terrible, and sadly there was little he or I could do to stop the ensuing despondency.

It's no good becoming frustrated with the asthmatic, saying, 'Just breath deeper and you'll feel better!' You just have to wait until they take their medication and the airways expand allowing air to the lungs.

Greg's mental illness is the same thing. It's no good becoming frustrated with the person suffering from a mental illness, telling them just to think positive thoughts and they will feel better. You just have to wait until the medication takes effect and the brain works more effectively and stabilises the mood.

Sometimes, when Greg rebounded from his periods of dejection, it seemed as if his brain had overcorrected itself and he would enjoy a period of heightened awareness and wellbeing. I have always suspected that the sense of relief that he experienced whenever he came back from his misery also heightened his feelings of jubilation and exuberance.

It was at this time that he would turn to his painting. I once watched him work on one canvas, all day and into the night, not stopping until seven o'clock the following morning. I couldn't believe my eyes when I would get up to go off to college and Greg was still sitting in front of his easel! His creativity would flourish during these highs.

One of the greatest misconceptions that I held about Greg's illness was that the depression was all in his mind. I heard other people tell Greg repeatedly that if your thoughts were positive then you wouldn't suffer from depression. Even some of the doctors whom Greg met and who had worked with depression all their lives had tried to use this kind of reasoning with him. What I learned as I watched Greg was that despite his best efforts sometimes he was simply unable to avoid the downturn in his mood.

There's no question that negative thoughts can lead to the onset of depression. There are still times, however, when Greg can fill his mind with positive thoughts and the depression still comes regardless of his positive outlook.

When I understood this, the frustration I used to feel was slowly replaced with more patience and compassion. When his downturn in mood would arrive I would remind myself that Greg had a mental illness through no fault of his own.

When I noticed Greg slipping into one of his depressed moods, I wouldn't be critical of that mood. Instead I tried to help him by lending my support or even trying to distract him. We'd play golf to try to shift his focus. But even in such an enjoyable and normally carefree environment, when others would be having the time of their lives, Greg's depression would remain. Playing golf didn't stop his feelings of despair; it just meant that he wasn't focusing on them all the time.

This condition isn't something all in his mind as some people believe. Despite his best attempts, Greg could never entirely prevent his detrimental feelings from occurring when he returned from hospital. I imagine that these moods will occur throughout his lifetime unless doctors can help find a solution to the crippling illness. Despite ongoing research, doctors still know so little about the brain. I believe the brain is the final frontier in medicine. Yet doctors were able to eradicate polio, and hopefully they will soon unravel the causes of depression and come up with new and improved medications that will help cure this disease.

Greg certainly believes he is putting the right combination of elements together to combat the illness. With his current medication, his support network and his growing conviction that he can overcome his problem, his attacks are much less frequent. There are still further improvements to be made, however, for he still has not been able to completely eliminate the occurrence of his low periods.

I can only imagine how hard it must have been for him, as he was growing up, not to have any idea what was the cause of his highs and lows, his feelings of isolation, and the unkind response that his condition sometimes provoked in others.

How much easier it would have been, for example, if the doctors could have given him the equivalent to a 'How To' booklet, guiding him in his treatment and control of the disease.

But he had to learn the hard way about his condition. People were cruel and insensitive to his problems at times. They were slow to understand yet quick to criticise.

Greg understood that there was nothing he could do to completely rid himself of these feelings. But what he discovered and learned after the attempted suicide was that he could at least manage them better. The secret to Greg's recovery was learning to cope with situations and feelings over which he had little control, and there was a number of ways he set out to achieve this.

Diet and lifestyle choices became important for Greg when he left the hospital. He noticed that when he kept his body healthy then he would feel better mentally. He tried to exercise for half an hour each day. He played golf, went for walks or lifted weights.

He had noticed that different foods would also affect his mood. Josie told him that his body was just like a car: as long as it had oil and petrol and it was regularly serviced it would perform to its highest level. Deprive a car of these things and it would eventually break down. She patiently explained to him that what was true for the car was also true for the body. When Greg was eating a nourishing, healthy diet he would function well. He would be happy and feel full of energy. If he didn't watch his diet, and ate fast food and junk, then he would become lethargic and more prone to depression. If he ate rubbish, he would feel like rubbish.

Josie encouraged Greg to eat a nourishing diet. She would make sure that he ate plenty of fibre, whole grains, oats, fish, meat, soybeans, fresh fruits and vegetables. She maintained that vitamin B rich foods also help lessen depression as they are nourishing to the brain, and that the need for B vitamins is increased by stress. Her preferred sources of Vitamin B include brown rice, fish, egg yolks, legumes, brewers yeast, liver, walnuts, beef, mushrooms, and fresh vegetables.

Greg took a little convincing to start consuming foods whose names he thought should have belonged in a foreign dictionary! But he had confidence in Josie's research and training, and the calming effect they eventually began to have on his mind as he followed her dietary recommendations gave him added enthusiasm. He also began to notice his energy levels increasing, and this gave him added resolve to continue with his programme.

As part of the diet, Josie suggested that Greg drink plenty of water. She told him that to keep the body functioning adequately it was essential to drink at least eight glasses (250 ml) per day. Finally, she recommended that Greg avoid stimulants such as coffee, tea, chocolate or excessive amounts of sugar. She also discouraged him from imbibing depressants such as alcohol. Josie had noticed that too much alcohol or caffeine in the diet made him nervous and disrupted his sleep patterns. Additionally, she made sure that he got enough rest. Greg had noticed that when he was tired, he was more prone to depression.

All of these recommendations and practices, however, were still no guarantee that the lows would not come back to trouble Greg. When they did return, however, his growing confidence and resolute determination to prevail gave him the strength to fight with all his might against his aggressor.

During such trials, he would use every means to alleviate the pressure, and part of his therapy became quite a pleasure for me when he would suggest we go for a quick round of golf or visit the café and spend time with Joyce

There was one special pilgrimage Greg would make periodically that was always guaranteed to raise his flagging spirits and inject a new sense of purpose and eagerness into his approach to his work.

He and Josie would pack the car and head south to the Shoalhaven River District, where they would visit Arthur Boyd's property, 'Bundanon'. The celebrated artist had donated the 1000-hectare property, as well as a comprehensive collection of his works, to the Australian people after his death in 1999.

All of Boyd's easels and brushes had been left untouched since his death. It was as if the room was still possessed by the pervading spirit of the great artist. Whenever Greg entered the studio he felt himself move into an almost trance-like state. He always felt so inspired, not only by the extraordinary talent that had won such worldwide recognition and acclaim, but also by the great generosity towards the public that had characterised the artist's life.

Whenever they returned home from these visits, Greg would throw himself into his work with renewed vigour and enthusiasm.

Slowly Greg became aware of a new-found self-respect. He began to make better decisions and choices and began to feel good about himself. He told himself that he was not going to act in a certain way, because that would cause him to feel depressed.

Because he made better decisions about his options his life began to run much more smoothly. As his life progressed his empathy for himself and others grew. An obvious shift in his behaviour was that he suddenly realised he didn't want to hurt either himself or those around him any more. 'I don't want to create these situations for myself or for others in my life,' he decided. 'I have had enough heartache in my life and it's time to work towards more successful choices and decisions.'

It was at this time that Greg also started working on his painting with more enthusiasm and dedication than ever before. In fact, his artwork was one of the most important elements of his recovery.

He is quick to acknowledge that it was his love for painting that started regenerating his love for life. It was the colours that he used in his paintings that started to bring him out of those trying times. It was his painting that helped him out of the darkness that consumed him.

Greg spoke about the use of vibrant colours in his work with Gillian Lord, respected journalist for the *Canberra Times*. She reported:

'Bright colours are a hallmark of Greg Wilson's paintings. So bright they make you gasp and give a flash of instant cheer. This, the artist explains, is deliberate. He's drawn to brightness because he's taunted by a world of dark and grey, the colours of depression ...'

Greg would paint all day and into the night, delighted that he had a new sense of purpose. He attacked his work with new eagerness and enthusiasm, sometimes spending up to seventy hours a week creating his artworks. His self-confidence developed to the stage where he felt it would be possible not just to control his depression through his art, but to make a comfortable and enjoyable living as well.

When he was able to start selling his work, when he saw the joy and pleasure that his paintings were bringing to others, it elevated his spirits enormously. When that realisation finally dawned, he felt as if he was really living.

resurgence

He attacked his work with a new eagerness and enthusiasm. Still, the road to becoming an established artist was not going to be easy and he knew it would take great commitment and dedication. His old destructive method of expressing his dissatisfaction with some of his work was replaced with a delightful and disarming honesty, mixed with a rather charming sense of humour.

'Hey, I feel like I'm a bit of a fraud today,' he would say. 'I'm not sure that I am good enough at the moment!' When he was so forthright in expressing his feelings it was easy for us to encourage him. Propped up by our positive reinforcement, he would resume painting again in no time

We all noticed this dramatic shift in his attitude. Joyce, Josie and I were so proud of his effort and we felt our determination to stand by him through thick and thin was vindicated. Greg told us that he would never be able to express his gratitude for the way in which we had stood by him even after his abortive effort to suicide. There was a wonderful feeling of solidarity within our little group.

Greg's determination, new-found strength of mind, his unique approach, and his ability to overcome so many obstacles would result in the creation of some spectacular works of art. Possessed by a new zest for living, he refused to confine himself to a single theme or medium – and his creativity was expressed in a wide range of paintings and sculptures.

As Greg gradually gained more confidence in himself and his artwork he decided that it was time for a new challenge. It was time to further his career and have an exciting new exhibition.

He was naturally apprehensive, but he wanted to give it another go. Greg realised that life was full of challenges, and while many chose to tackle them head-on there were others who weren't prepared to make the necessary sacrifices and effort. Greg decided that it was time to put a collection of his latest works on display through a series of major exhibitions.

chapter twenty
early exhibitions

After much deliberation we decided that Paddington, widely regarded as the art capital of New South Wales, seemed the obvious choice to further promote Greg's talent after his earlier minor exhibition.

When we were discussing the possibility of having an exhibition there, the full realisation of what we were about to do hit Greg with quite an impact. We were contemplating a step that none of us had ever really envisaged before. The novelty of the idea overcame him, and he began to entertain several thoughts of inadequacy and unpreparedness.

'Maybe I am not good enough. I'll be criticised. I can't do it!' were just some of the thoughts that raced through his mind. I was having similar doubts about my own ability as well, because I was going to help Greg arrange the exhibition and was not sure if I had the skill necessary to do so.

We sat down and talked about our uneasiness, and it was then that our mutual support network moved into top gear! Josie and I reinforced our belief in Greg, and Josie and Greg reinforced their belief in me. Soon we realised we must try, even if we weren't sure how things were going to work out. To do nothing would be far worse.

early exhibitions

Consequently, I became determined to arrange a show and make it a success. I began walking the streets talking to gallery owners and other artists. During my discussions it became clear that if the artist was talented and if you had persistence you could eventually get a space to have an exhibition. But before anything could be done it was necessary to get pictures of Greg's work so that gallery owners had some idea what to expect from the artist.

The next day I arranged for a photographer to take some professional shots of Greg's work. When this was done I put them onto a laptop computer I had recently acquired. Shortly afterwards, I began walking into galleries and showing Greg's material.

It wasn't long before my enthusiasm and belief in Greg began to pay off. The third gallery that I walked into was Global Gallery in Paddington. A talented artist greeted me inside. He was the curator of the gallery and, along with the gallery director, made the decisions on what would be exhibited. At first, he was a little reluctant to display Greg's work, as he did not know much about him. This made me slightly anxious, but I persisted, telling him of Greg's talent. After we chatted some more and he saw some of Greg's paintings he finally agreed.

I went home and told Greg that a gallery had agreed to exhibit his work. We were both ecstatic. We decided that The Many Minds of Greg Wilson was an appropriate name for the exhibition, and then began making arrangements to display his work from 17 September until 6 October 2002. It was fitting that we used this title for the show, as it seemed to capture the different frames of mind that Greg had experienced throughout his lifetime, as well as reflecting the diverse approach he took to his artwork.

Even though we had arranged to show Greg's work in a gallery, we were still a long way from realising our goal. Greg needed to replenish his supply of paints, canvas, stretcher bars and specialised brushes so that he could begin work on additional pieces for the show. We also needed to come up with some money to rent the space at Global and to pay for the transport of the paintings.

When I probed a little deeper into Greg and Josie's financial position it became clear they didn't have two dollars to rub together. They were struggling to meet the costs of day-to-day living. Much of the money they had accumulated had been spent on producing the paintings that hung on the walls.

I was a little short myself but had a good credit rating with the bank. The following Monday I met with the Commonwealth Bank manager and applied for a small loan. A few days later the bank contacted me and told me it had been granted. Subsequently, we were able to go ahead with our preparations for the show.

Soon after this, I went back to Global Gallery to arrange some of the finer details for the exhibition. I took a couple of friends with me to get their feedback on the place. The curator was committed to maintaining a high standard for the gallery. As soon as we arrived, he started outlining some procedures we needed to follow to comply with his expectations.

'You must have adequate theory to support your work,' he informed us. The curator then turned to a painting that was hanging on the wall for a current exhibition and said, 'See this painting on the wall of the three clouds.' 'Yes, I see the clouds,' I replied. 'I will give you an example of what we expect.' He then began reading a lengthy and complicated interpretation of the work along the following lines:

'The white fluffy cloud provokes the onlooker to examine the juxtaposition and binary oppositions in a world that contrasts whites and brings peace to the mind of the artist. In the cloud you will see the subconscious mind of the artist and his ability to transcend adversities and challenge the social boundaries of one's negative emotional state.'

When he had finished reading this statement, there was a lengthy silence before one of my friends, a Sydney DJ with a razor sharp wit, turned to me and then slowly back to the clouds with a slightly bemused look on her face. She then fixed the curator with a serious stare and remarked: 'Are you sure it's not pot smoke, those three big clouds?' Fortunately he had a sense of humour, and we all burst into laughter.

Shortly afterwards, Greg began to work out a theme for the show. He told me about his motivation for creating his artworks in a discussion we

early exhibitions

had when I returned home from Paddington. The fragility of life, the joy of simply being alive, a new-found awareness of the beauty of nature, as well as reflections on his near-death experience, provided the inspiration for his work. 'I want people to see and understand that my work is more than a work of art: it is a work of the heart,' he told me.

All of his works bore testimony to this, but we realised that it would be necessary for Greg to bare not only his heart, but his soul, if people were to understand the forces and elements behind some of his pieces. For this reason we chose a particular work entitled 'Shelter from the Storm', which depicted a striking contrast between a series of brightly coloured umbrellas (representing those happier times that Greg experienced) and the dark grey background that was interspersed with jagged bolts of lightning that threatened to dismantle the flimsy protection that was raised against the fierce elements. Greg explained simply that this was how he chose to represent the constant fluctuation, the constant conflict that he experienced between hope and despair.

I noticed, as Greg continued to produce his paintings for the exhibition, that he was pouring out his feelings not only on the canvases but even more noticeably in his sculptures. When he began to incorporate a number of taps into his work, he told me that they represented, better than any other item he could think of, the true fragility of life. Water was life-giving and an essential part of our existence, and the tap was a metaphor for how easily life could be turned on and off. It was a concept that had been brought home to him in stark fashion when he had crashed his motorcycle.

At the same time, he wanted to convey the clear impression that had it not been for the accident and the prolonged convalescence, he may never have chosen to pursue his artistic career. Not only did his life tap continue to function during his recovery period, but his artistic aspirations began to flow at the same time.

The significance of the tap is not always fully understood by people who have viewed his works, and often Greg felt it necessary to offer some explanation. One day a plumber who was called in to do some work for Josie saw Greg working on one of the pieces for the exhibition. It was

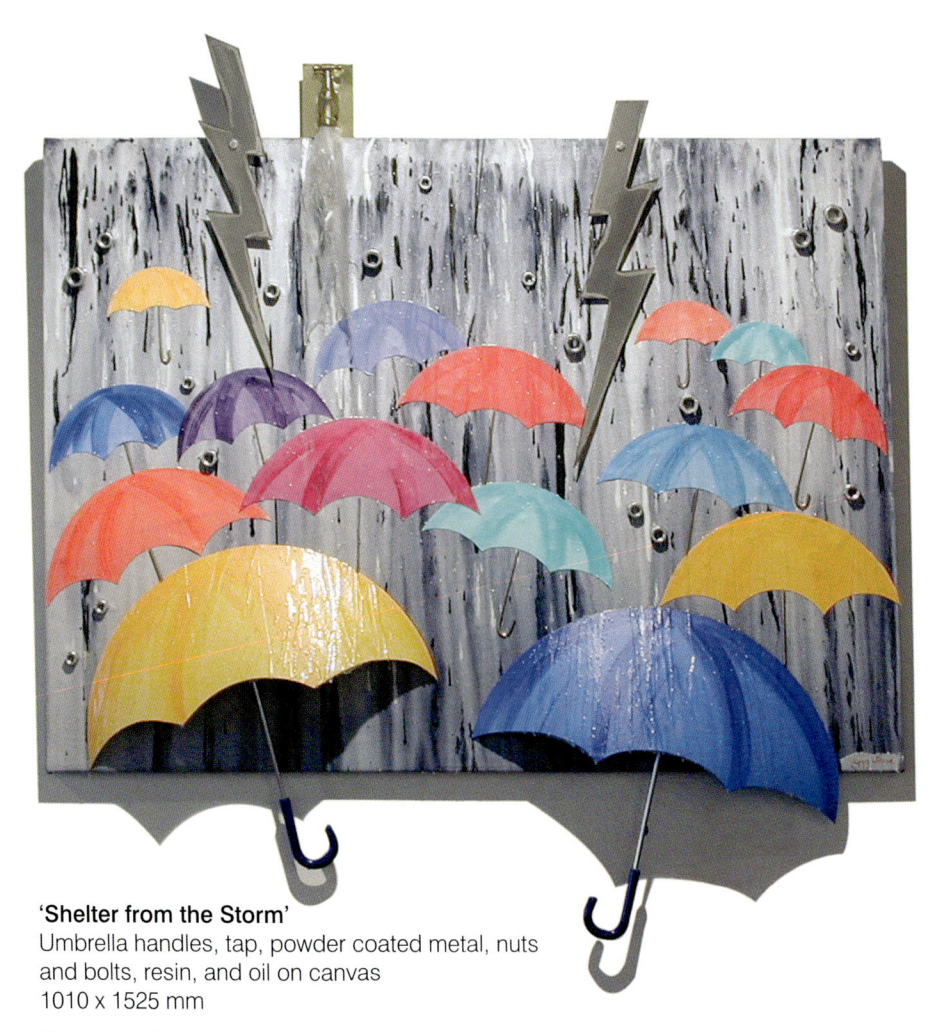

'Shelter from the Storm'
Umbrella handles, tap, powder coated metal, nuts and bolts, resin, and oil on canvas
1010 x 1525 mm

The use of the taps in Greg's work acts as a metaphor for the fragility of life, and symbolises how easily life can be turned on and off.

||||||||||||||||||||||||||||||||||||||||||||||||||||||||||||||||||||||||||||||||||||||||||||||||||||||

called 'Alone' and it, too, featured the taps. The bearded gentleman, in his late forties, remarked: 'That's a strange subject for a piece of art. I work with taps all day, and I don't find them particularly artistic. They're just accessories to me!' Josie, who happened to be within earshot, approached him and asked: 'What do you see when you look at the piece?' 'It's just a tap,' he replied.

early exhibitions

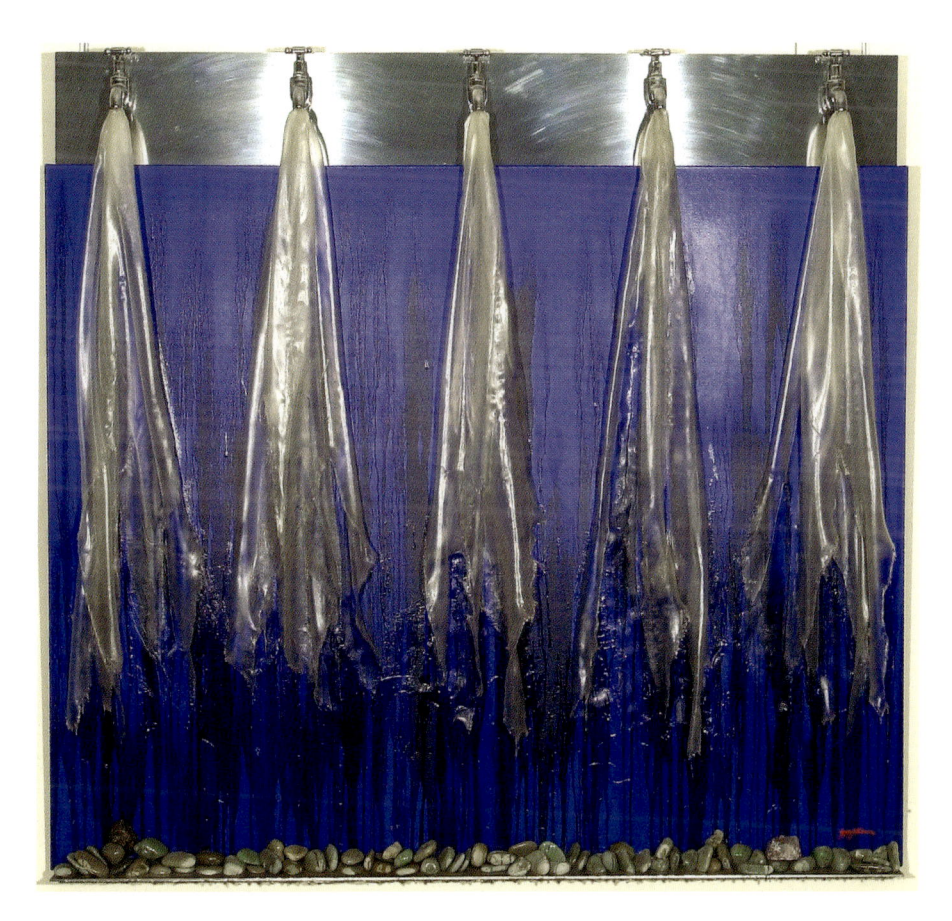

'Catharsis'
Clear powder coated aluminium, chrome taps, resin, rocks, gemstones, oil on canvas,
1425 x 1550 mm
There are times when we need to be immersed in life's regenerative waters and rediscover the lustre of our own existence.

'Well,' she said, 'the artist has a different interpretation of the work. To Greg this work has great poetry and meaning.' She related the meaning to the plumber. Then she explained a little bit about Greg's background, and how he had gone through the torment of depression. Later, she directed the plumber's attention to the gutter at the base of the painting. 'Greg uses the gutter as a metaphor for being down and out in life, something he can relate to because of his experiences.'

She also pointed out to him a number of shiny gems positioned in the gutter. 'Even when Greg hit the gutter, and he's been there a few times, the spark of life was never extinguished,' Josie said. 'It's also significant that despite all of Greg's experiences his spirit never gave up in the struggle for survival and his creative urges continued to flow undiminished.'

'You see his work through the eyes of a plumber, but you are not seeing it through the eyes of an artist,' Josie said.

'You're right,' he exclaimed. 'Now I see what he means. That's really incredible when you understand where the guy is coming from. I never though about taps in that way, but that puts a whole different light on what I now see. They could be a real talking point for my customers,' he said. 'I'd like to buy that for my office!'

Another innovation that Greg continued to use, and one from which I took a great deal of comfort, was the inclusion of a glowing crystal in his pieces. One of them first appeared in his work 'Catharsis', and is now something he includes quite regularly. He puts a gem into each of his sculptures to represent the idea that life is precious, that life does sparkle, even though we may be unable to recognise it at times.

'Blue taps' was another work that we chose for the exhibition, and even though it featured the lightning and flowing water, it again depicted a number of saw blades, sharp cutting instruments, that recalled for Greg the severe lacerations he received during his accident, lacerations that required major surgery and which left his neck, legs and arms badly scarred.

Roads are also a recurring element of Greg's work, and I was

early exhibitions

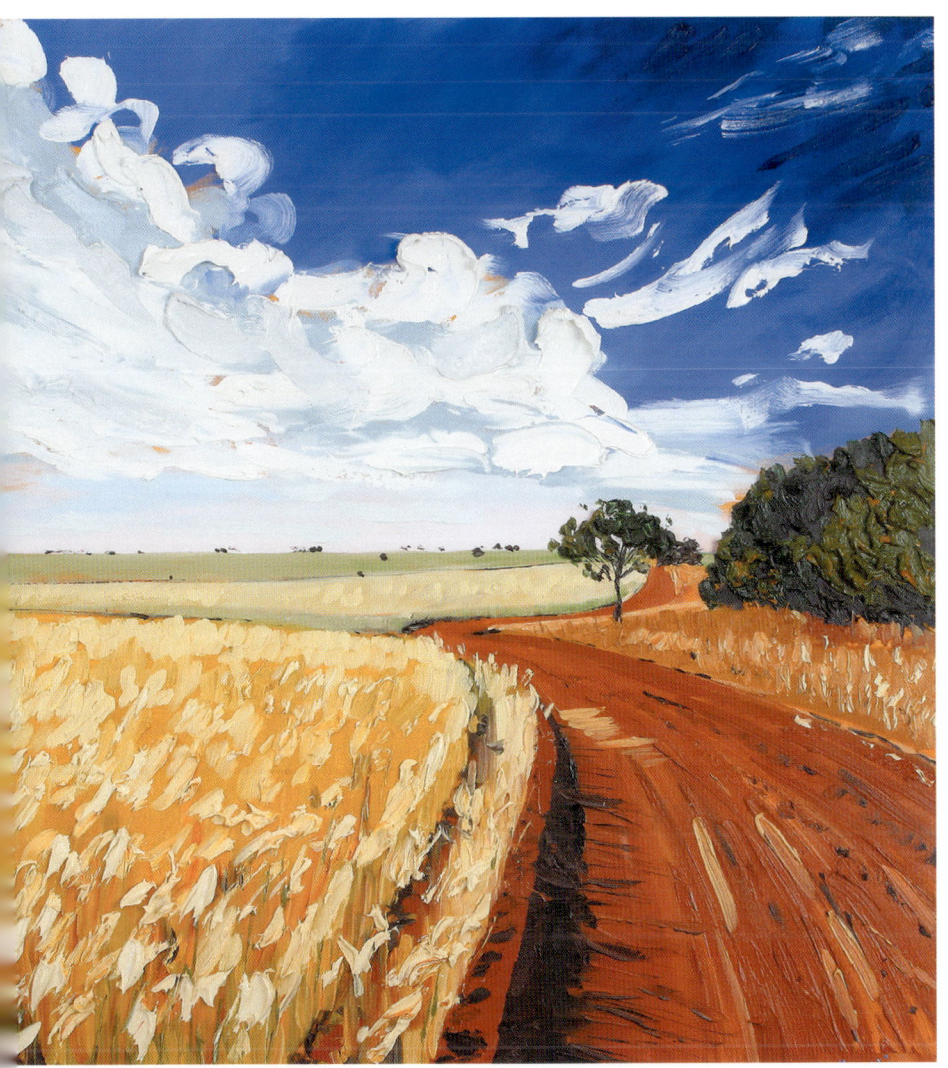

'Track through the Field'
Oil on Canvas, 920 x 1210 mm
The Australian wheat field is the source of our daily bread.

particularly impressed when he produced a painting that he called 'Track Through The Field'. The roads, he told me, represent the ever-present choice we have of determining our own destiny, of deciding on the path we take with our lives.

my brush with depression

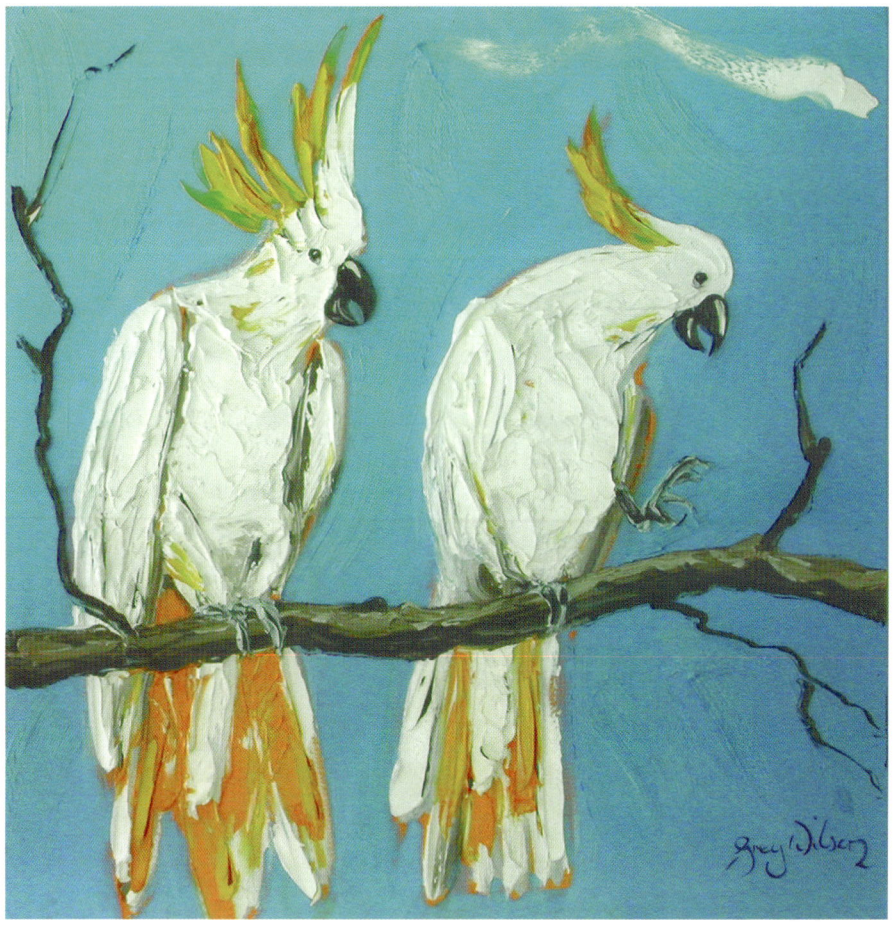

'Two Cockatoos'
Oil on canvas
910 x 910 mm

He also painted a number of beach scenes for the exhibition. 'Australians, in the main, are coastal dwellers, and much of our leisure time is spent enjoying the beach and the ocean. They are our summer playgrounds,' he said. The inspiration for these works was drawn from our own wonderful Northern Beaches of Sydney.

Greg was not about to let an opportunity go by to portray the brilliant wild life of our countryside, and he included a selection of some of his

early exhibitions

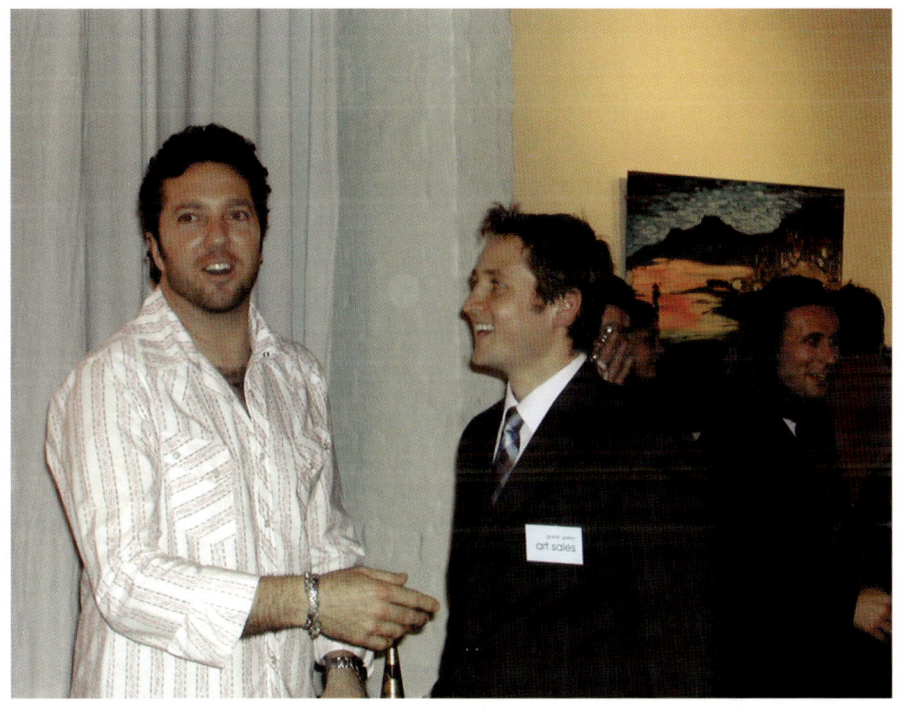

Greg and I during the Paddington exhibition, 17 September 2002. 'What an amazing turnout.' Greg said to me. 'It only goes to show that with hard work, perseverance, and great friends like you, it can happen. I couldn't have done it without you, thanks mate.'

favourite animals and some of our most colourful fauna.

As strange as it may seem, Greg thinks it was spending so much time in hospital and on his own that had a lot to do with the development of his imagination. He recalls how desperately he wanted to go outside the hospital grounds, to walk on the grass, smell the flowers and stroll among the trees – activities that he had previously taken so much for granted.

During his recovery, he would try and relieve the boredom by using his imagination to transport himself to far more pleasant surroundings. He would picture himself walking along the beach or being back in nature. He focused on colour and form, and although he may not have realised it at the time, these imaginary journeys and the vivid colours he was able to conjure up in his mind were to provide the inspiration for his later artistic endeavours. He was able to recall a lot of these images for the landscapes he prepared for the exhibition.

It was not long before we had finalised our preparations for the display, and soon the opening night rolled around. Even though we remained positive, Greg, Josie and I were decidedly nervous. Many of our doubts resurfaced. Was this the right thing to do? Would it work? Would anyone turn up? Once again, we sat and encouraged each other. Our nervousness only began to ease as a steady stream of people started arriving at the gallery.

To our relief, the night turned out to be a huge success. Not only did a large number of people attend but Greg sold many paintings as well. After the evening was over, a happy gallery director invited Greg to extend the exhibition for two more weeks and asked him if he would like to display his work there again.

It was lucky that we were able to overcome our fears and took a chance with the Paddington show. Had we not, then his work would not have made such an impact on Robert Miletic, the director of sales at the Park Hyatt Hotel in Sydney. A visitor to the Paddington exhibit, he became an admirer of Greg's work and, after seeing the show, was keen to organise a solo exhibit at the hotel so that clients could meet the artist and view a collection of his works.

Two months later on Wednesday 11 December Greg held his next exhibition in the boardroom library of the Park Hyatt, Sydney. The Opera House and harbour provided a stunning backdrop for Greg's paintings. It was a unique experience for himself and the Hyatt. Greg had never displayed his work in a hotel, and never before had an artist been invited to have a solo exhibition there.

Robert was even more enthusiastic about the exhibition when he learned Greg wanted to use the opening night to promote and support a charity that helped those with depression. It was becoming increasingly important for Greg to do so. His life experience had left him with a strong empathy for those with mental illness.

It was Greg's concern for others, whom he felt didn't recognise the

early exhibitions

signs of depression, that prompted him to get in touch with the Mental Health Association of NSW Incorporated to see if he could lend a hand. I went with him to Sydney to meet Gillian Church, one of the key members of the organisation. We were impressed with the principals and the staff of the establishment. Their philosophy was outlined in a brief statement: they acted as a non-government, non-profit and voluntary organisation working to advocate, inform and promote good mental health for all members of our community. It didn't take us long to realise that Gillian Church was, and continues to be, a remarkable director and a wonderful human being who works tirelessly trying to meet these goals.

With the help of the Park Hyatt, Gillian and the Mental Health Association of NSW Incorporated, we decided to use the opening night to raise the awareness of mental health and generate some money for the organisation. When news of Greg's personal crusade to help those with depression became more widely known, it attracted the involvement of some wonderful people.

Janice Walker, who was a friend of Josie's, came around for lunch one Sunday and learned about our endeavours to raise money for the Mental Health Association NSW Incorporated. She wanted to help us generate as much interest in the evening as possible. As well as being Josie's friend, she was also an employee of Channel Ten. She began wondering if there was anyone at the television station who might be interested in helping us on the night.

Janice told us that Jessica Rowe, the Evening News reader, might help, since she was a really caring person and her mother had lived with episodes of mental illness. She had a great empathy for the cause of mental health, and would be a wonderful choice if we could persuade her to come.

When Janice returned to work she e-mailed Jessica to see if she would be interested in speaking at the dinner, or attending the night for the Mental Health Association of NSW Incorporated.

Janice got the reply a short time later. Unfortunately, Jessica's extremely busy schedule meant that she had a prior engagement. What followed next was quite unexpected and deeply appreciated. In the e-mail

Jessica volunteered to do a short speech on video so the Hyatt could play it on the evening. We were thrilled about her participating in this way.

We met up with her when we went to collect the tape. I have to say that she is a remarkable woman, and an extraordinary person, deeply committed to helping those with mental illness. Jessica is one of those people who easily earns the admiration and respect of those with whom she speaks. A kind-hearted and generous individual, she is quick to get behind causes related to mental illness. She gives freely of her time, and has been a big support to Greg.

We knew that with the help of so many wonderful people the night could only be a huge success. Robert's thoughtful and professional traits, combined with his exceptional customer service and organisational skills, helped create what we still regard as one of the best shows of Greg's career.

At Robert's suggestion, the Park Hyatt generously donated a night in the luxurious Presidential Suite, worth thousands of dollars, as a lucky door prize to help generate more money for the Mental Health Association NSW Incorporated. It was a generous contribution by the management. Robert and Greg have since become firm friends and we meet with him regularly. Jessica and Greg delivered talks that held the audience enthralled. They had both experienced first hand the devastating effects that depression can have on people's lives.

early exhibitions

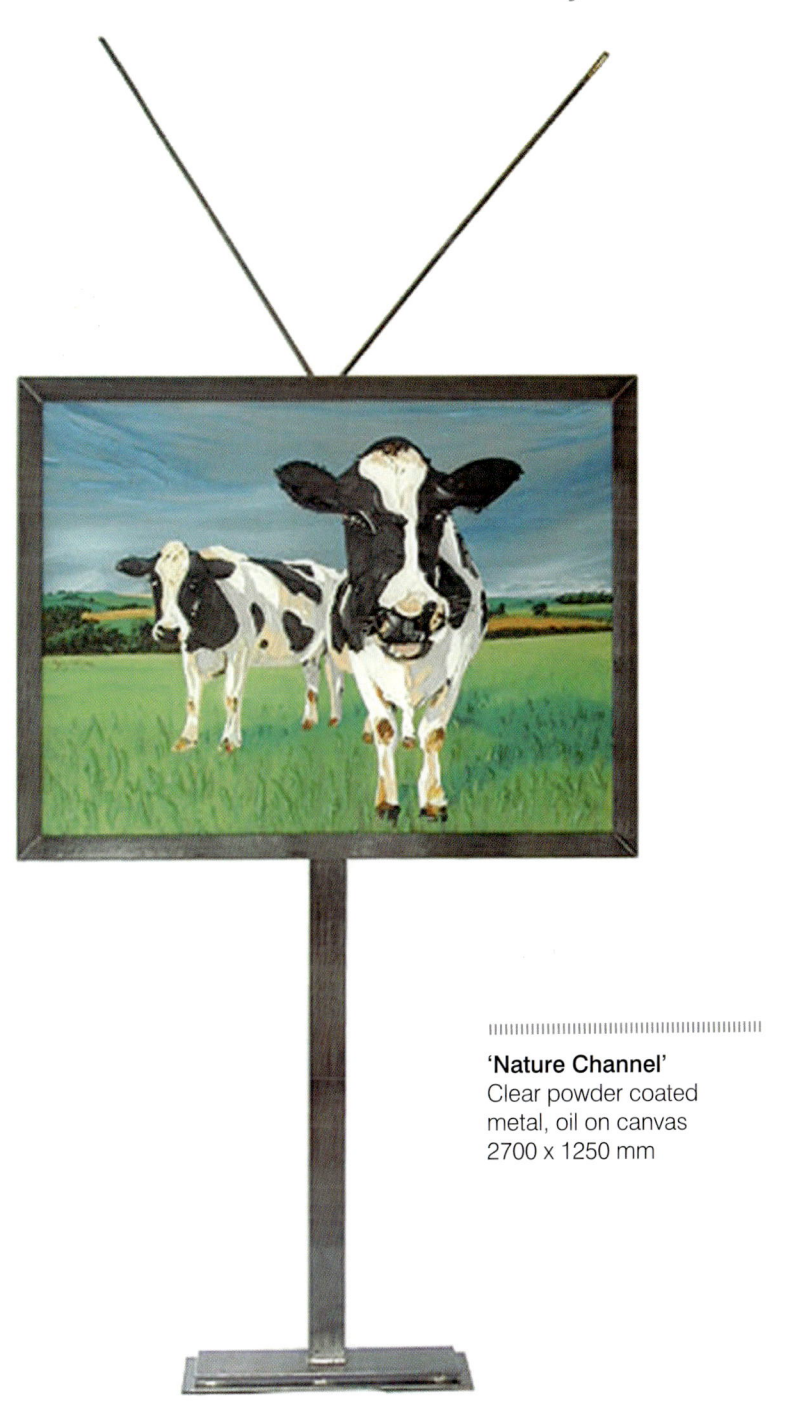

'Nature Channel'
Clear powder coated
metal, oil on canvas
2700 x 1250 mm

greg wilson

chapter twenty-one
trials and tribulations

Although Greg was really enjoying his new role as an artist, his desire to be a painter and sculptor brought with it a unique set of challenges that almost led him back into his depression. He had to work hard to make sure that the uncertainties and self-doubt in the early part of his artistic career did not lead him back into his despair.

Even though he sometimes doubted his ability he persisted with his dream. Depression always seemed to catch up with him whenever he felt that he hadn't taken advantage of the opportunities that life placed in his path. Underachievement was something that left him feeling quite empty.

He learned that failure was not just a lack of success. Failure for him was not trying; failure was not taking the chance; failure was not following one's heart and chasing one's dreams. Whenever he had given his all and tried his hardest, then he was proud of his attempts, even when things didn't quite work out as expected. He would then tell himself that maybe it wasn't the right time; that he could always make another all-out effort when he felt the time was opportune.

He acknowledges that, although his artwork points to a study of art, he is largely self-taught, although his decision not to study formally sometimes met with criticism at his earliest shows.

trials and tribulations

'How can you call yourself an artist when you haven't studied?' he was asked on one occasion. At first he found such remarks extremely hurtful and for a time he thought there may have been some substance to the subtle criticisms. He would become dejected and disheartened, but eventually decided to put his trust in his own feelings of self-worth and have faith in his natural ability.

The next time someone questioned his credentials, Greg asked if having a degree or having completed some kind of extended apprenticeship would make his art appear differently. Do we ask the creator of life where he studied or how many degrees he has? When it was evident that no reply was forthcoming, Greg told his would-be critic that the important thing about his paintings was not where he had studied, but how hard he had tried to express his thoughts and feelings and observations on canvas.

There were occasions when he felt tempted to retaliate to remarks that had negative overtones, but would resort to a ploy that he'd used as a young boy to lighten the moment. He would recall a saying that he had learned in kindergarten and repeat it until his uneasiness had passed: 'Sticks and stones will break my bones, but names will never hurt me!' He was also mindful that any prolonged preoccupation with criticism could well bring on another bout of depression.

He often recalls that when he started painting, nobody believed in him except his three closest friends. Fortunately, the faith that they had in his ability was all the encouragement he needed and helped him disregard the disparaging remarks and cynicism of his detractors.

Not surprisingly, he observed, the strongest criticism seemed to come from the least accomplished of his acquaintances!

These lessons taught Greg to surround himself with positive people, and to take heart from the positive feedback they provided. On one occasion he was approached by an accomplished artist who attended one of his early exhibitions. She told Greg that she saw something special and quite unique in his work, and that he could take his place with many of the fine artists that she had met. Her words gave him an enormous lift and strengthened his resolve to continue with his chosen vocation.

He set about collecting a whole range of books on art and the technical

my brush with depression

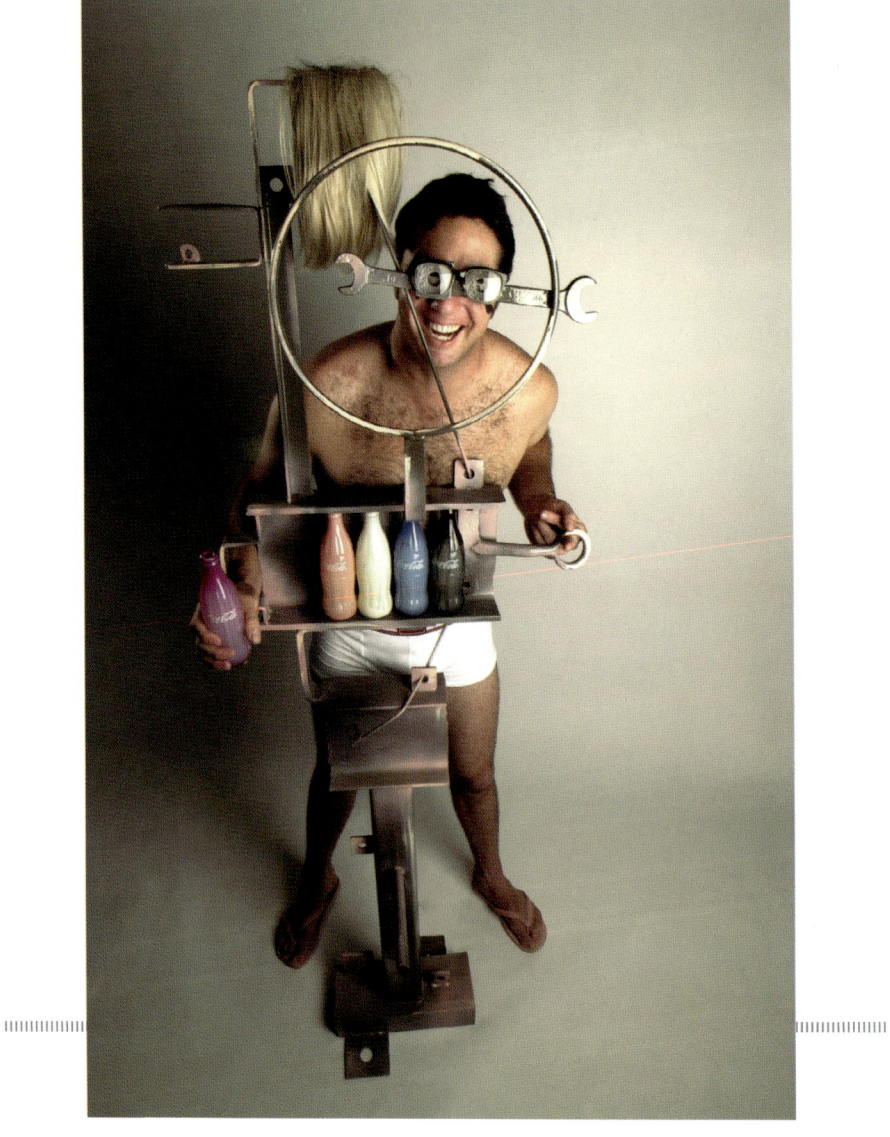

'The artist series – Andy Warhol'
Metal, wig, coke bottles, spanner, glasses
1950 x 650 x 330 mm
When photographer/friend Ian Hamilton and Greg attempted a photographic session during a heat wave, Greg tried to mimic the eccentricities of Andy Warhol, the inspiration for this particular work in progress.

trials and tribulations

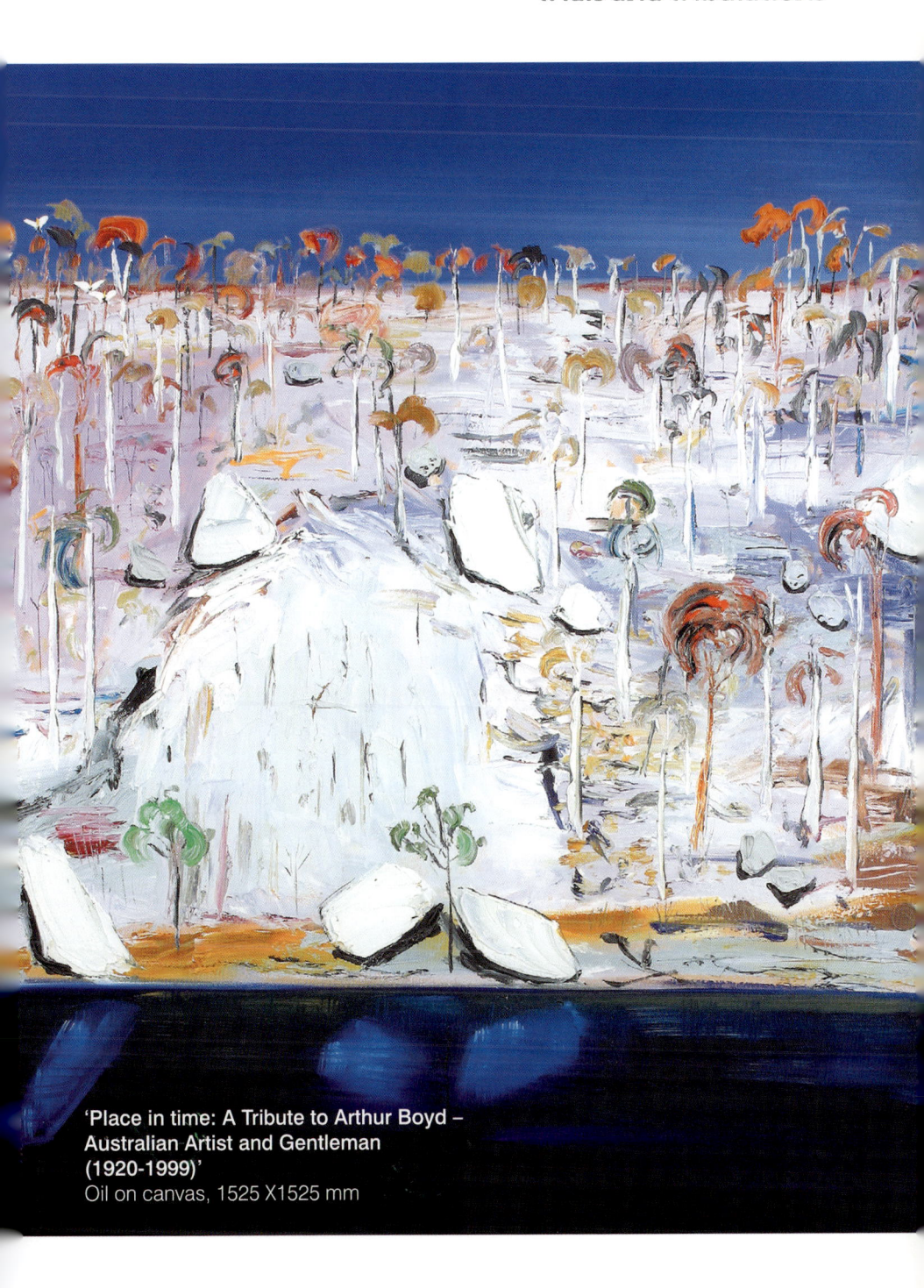

'Place in time: A Tribute to Arthur Boyd –
Australian Artist and Gentleman
(1920-1999)'
Oil on canvas, 1525 X1525 mm

greg wilson

aspects of painting. He studied the masters, Monet, Van Gogh, Picasso and Warhol and developed a particular affinity with the works of the Australian Masters, Whiteley and Boyd. Day after day and night after night he applied himself to his trade, more determined than ever to become a better painter.

He was soon being well rewarded for his efforts. One gentleman who had attended the Paddington exhibition subsequently dubbed him the 'Rebel of the Art World,' because his artwork 'resisted definition'. This tag stuck, acknowledging Greg's diversity. Somebody else called him a 'master of all,' describing his talent as 'varied and excitingly imaginative'. He couldn't believe that one person could paint, use wood, fibreglass, metal, cement, glass, even plaster in his artworks so effectively. What was initially regarded by some as a possible drawback is now something that persuades people to purchase Greg's work.

I remember with great satisfaction the time another visiting artist came to inspect Greg's work. The elderly gentleman wandered around the gallery slowly and purposefully for some time before introducing himself to Josie. He explained to her that he had been all around Australia many times visiting galleries and he continued: 'I know Arthur Boyd's work exceptionally well. This painting hanging on the wall that Greg has created as a tribute to him is outstanding. In all my years looking at galleries I have not seen anyone recreate his style of work so effectively.'

'How old is Greg?' he asked.

'Thirty-three,' Josie replied.

'You tell him from me to persevere with his painting. He has a huge future ahead of him if he stays with it. The boy has got it,' he said, smiling. 'You can tell that his soul is truly in his work!'

Greg was delighted. It made the endless hours of study and analysis all worthwhile and vindicated his individual approach to his art. What he depicted on canvas was truly an extension of his heart and soul.

chapter twenty-two
finding the promised land

In late 2002, Josie, Greg and I went to the Hunter Valley, a tourist area in New South Wales, for some rest and relaxation. Greg's favourite pastime was playing golf at the Cypress Lakes Resort and Country Club, and we had gone up to test our skills against the course. It tested me, more than it did Greg, who plays to a six handicap.

While we were enjoying our weekend escape, we went for a drive and came across a new development called the Hunter Valley Gardens that was due to open the following year. It was situated in Pokolbin, the commercial centre of one of Australia's premium wine producing districts. Nestled at the foothills of the Brokenback mountain range and set in the heart of the Hunter Valley vineyards, the twenty-five hectares of spectacular international display gardens were a showpiece, unlike anything I had seen before. I could not even begin to imagine how splendid they would look when they were completed.

As we walked through the partially completed village that was part of the development, we noticed there were a number of the boutique specialty shops that were available for lease. The village was quite spectacular in its own right. The small buildings, with a French country feel, were set among beautifully landscaped gardens complete with picnic facilities, restaurants, a rotunda, and a beautiful chapel.

my brush with depression

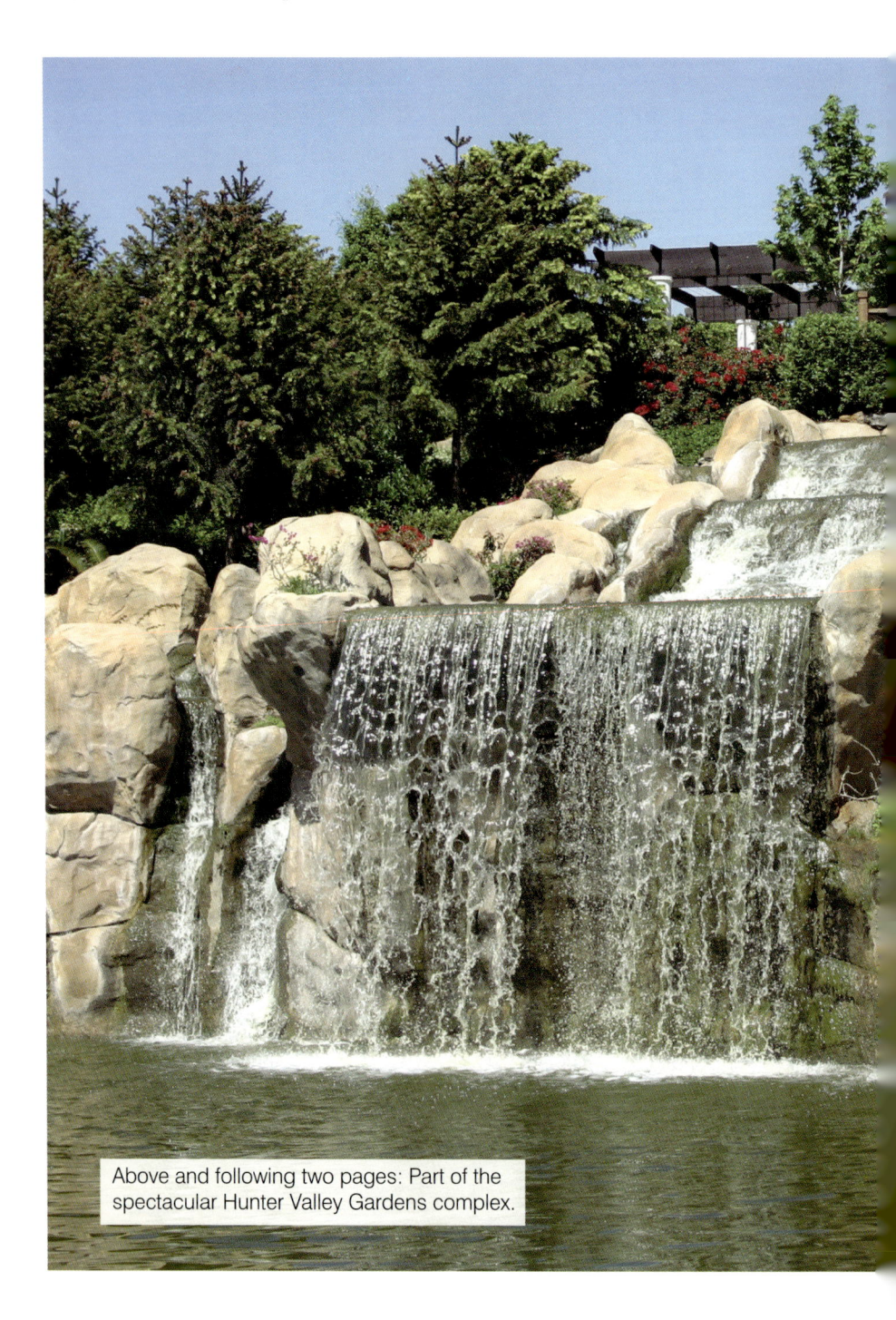

Above and following two pages: Part of the spectacular Hunter Valley Gardens complex.

finding the promised land

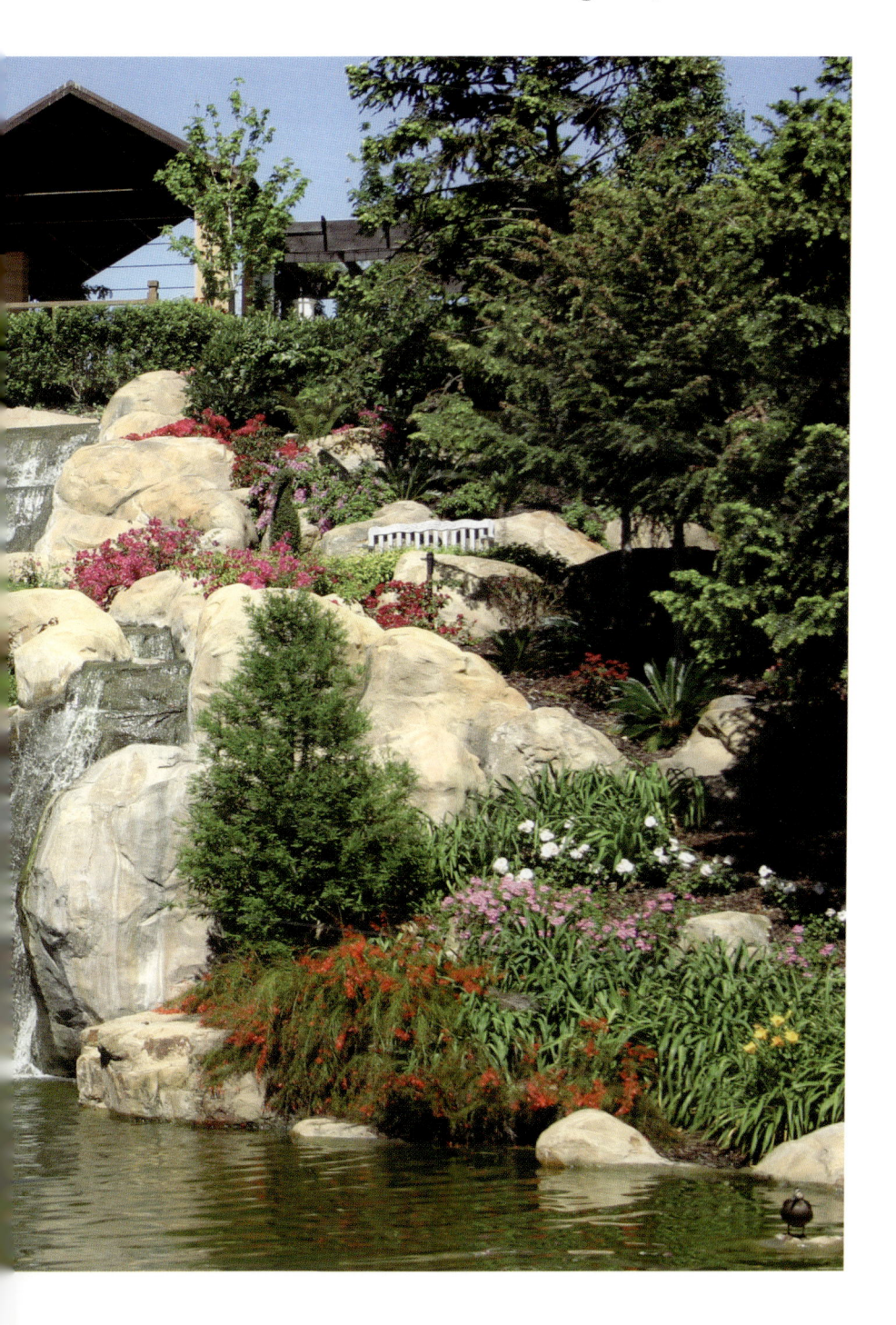

my brush with depression

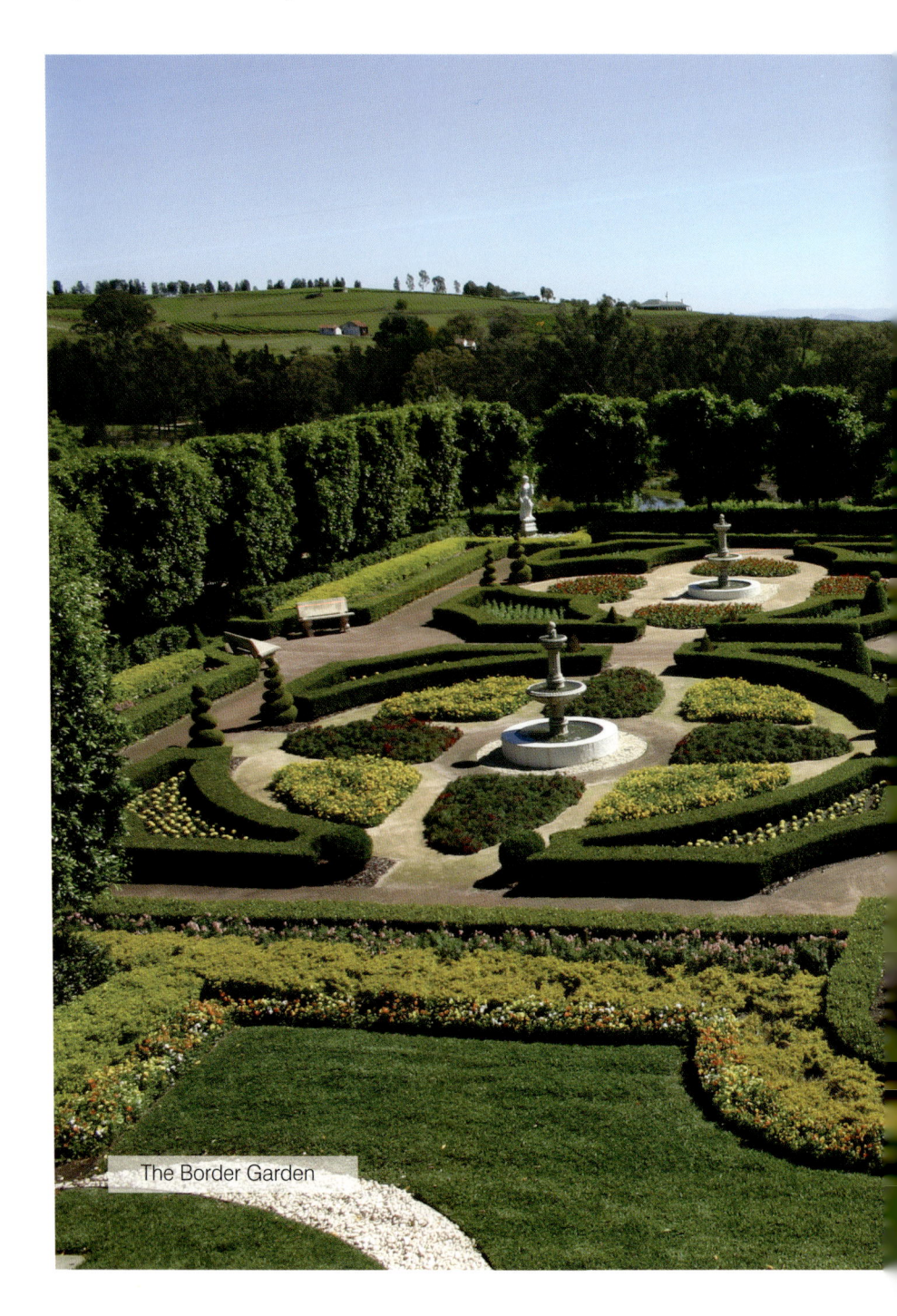

The Border Garden

finding the promised land

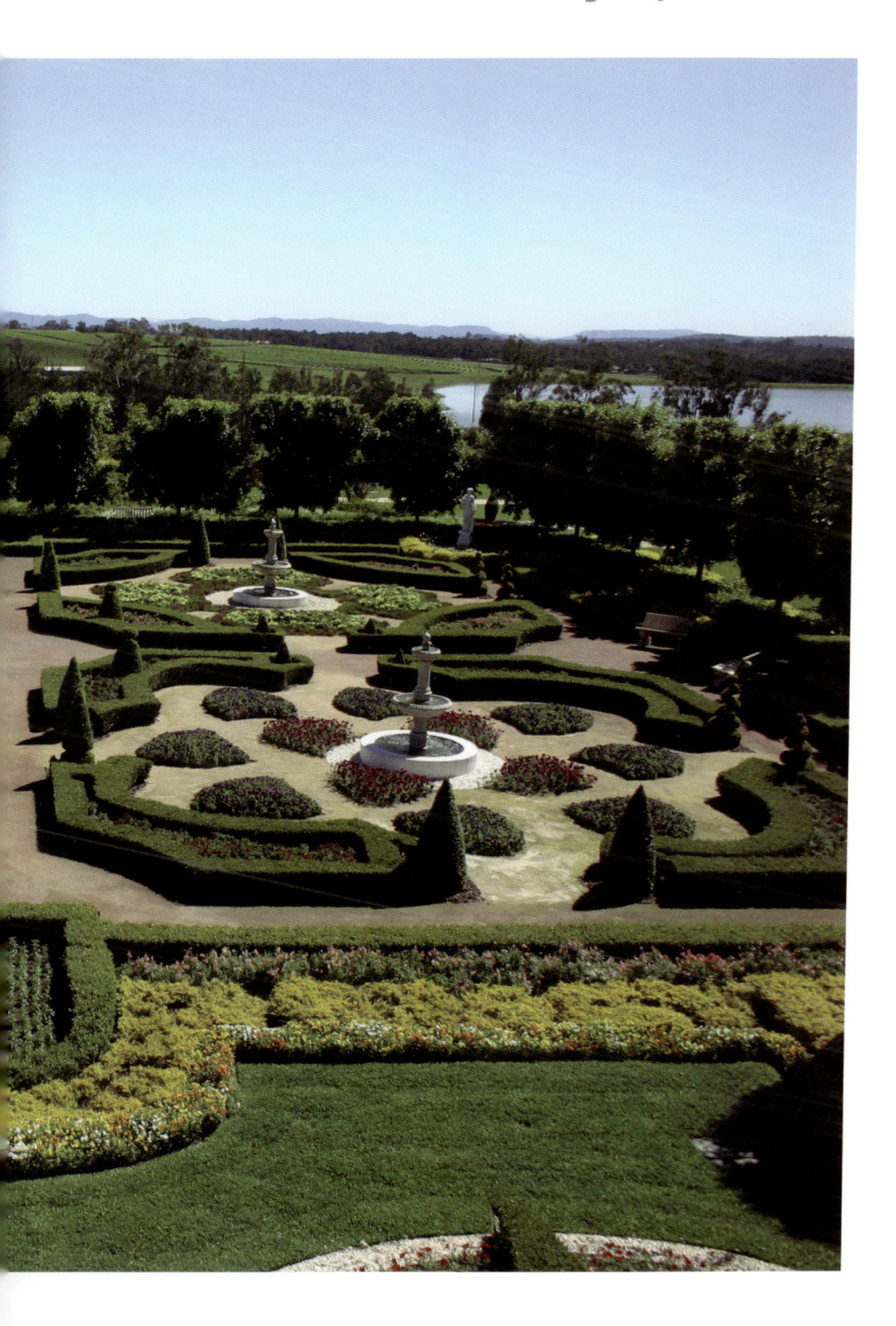

my brush with depression

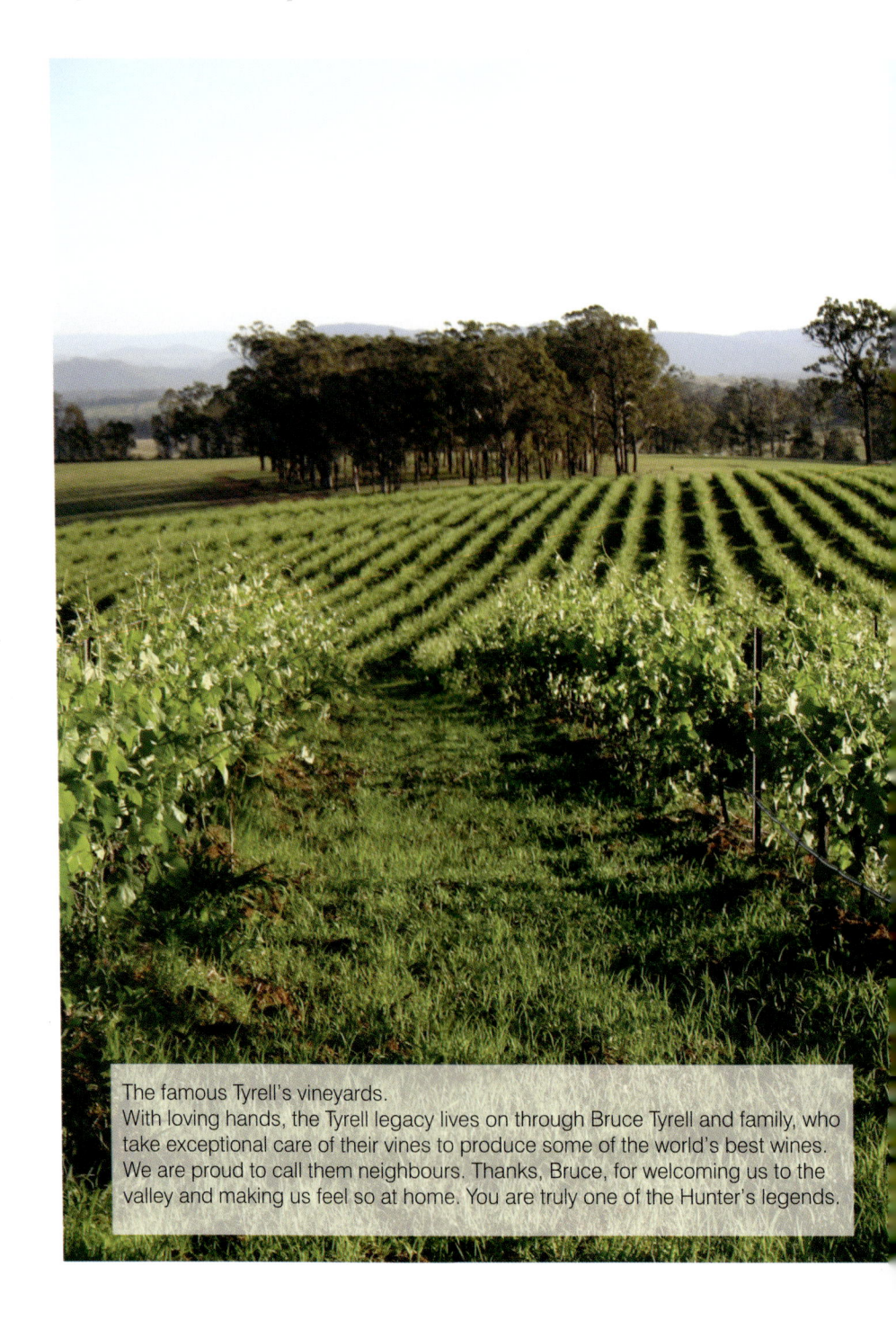

The famous Tyrell's vineyards.
With loving hands, the Tyrell legacy lives on through Bruce Tyrell and family, who take exceptional care of their vines to produce some of the world's best wines. We are proud to call them neighbours. Thanks, Bruce, for welcoming us to the valley and making us feel so at home. You are truly one of the Hunter's legends.

finding the promised land

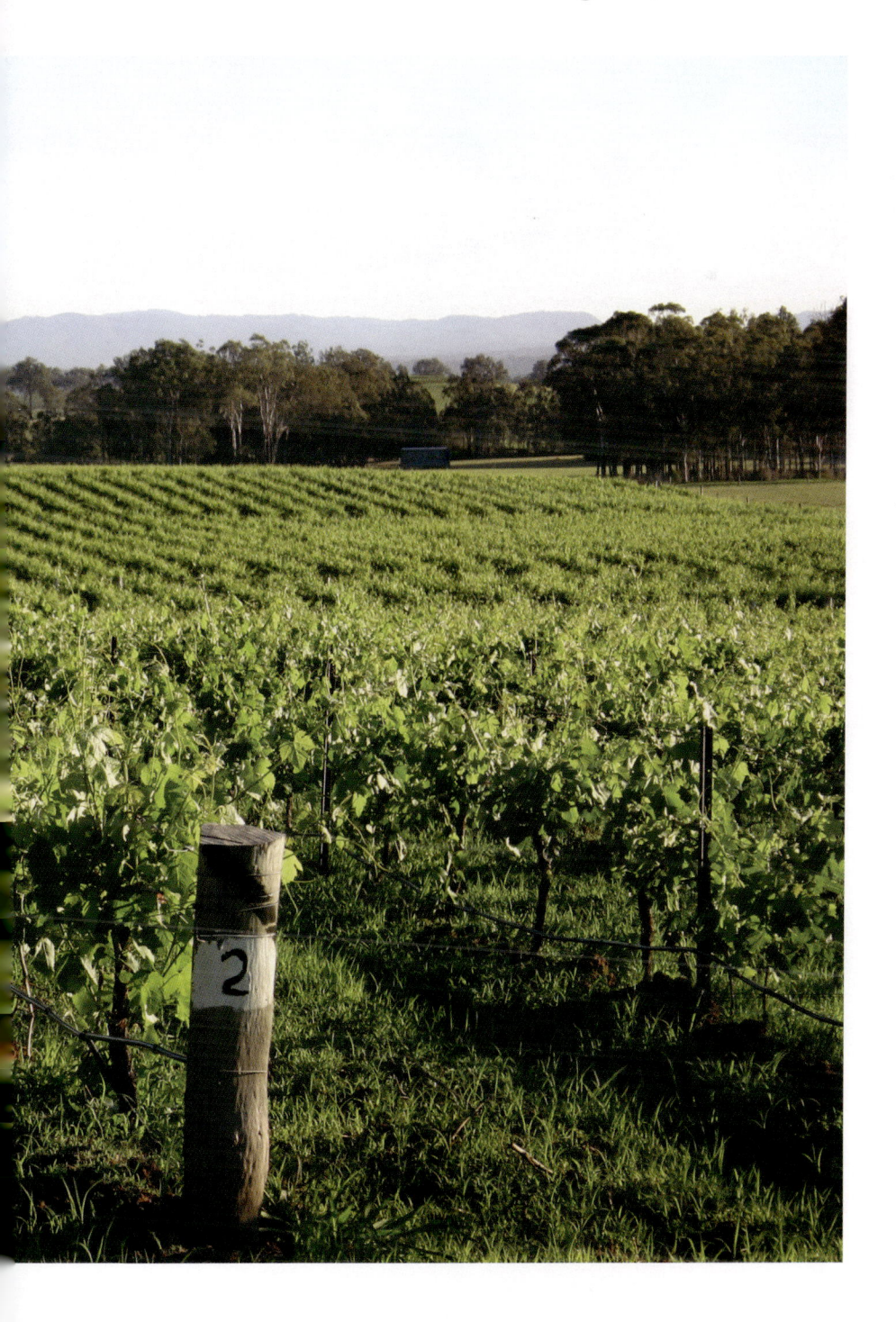

We stopped to watch a group of happy and smiling tourists, laden with their recent purchases, emerge from one of the shops when a wonderful idea occurred to Josie and me almost simultaneously. This would be an outstanding site for Greg to have a gallery. We discussed the idea excitedly over a cup of coffee in the village square. The more we thought about it the more animated we became. We could barely contain our enthusiasm and decided to make immediate enquiries about leasing one of the shops.

It wasn't long before we had singled out the General Manager of the project, David Mulham, who was most encouraging, and who offered to take us on a tour of the gardens. Even though there was still much work to be done on some areas of the landscaping, all of the completed sections were breathtaking. David walked us past a 10-metre waterfall, through the twelve feature gardens, and told us that eventually there would be more than eight thousand roses on display.

The tour heightened our sense of anticipation, and we could hardly wait to become part of this delightful community. We truly believed that we could establish a successful business in these beautiful surroundings, and we were convinced that we would love the other outstanding attractions of the valley.

Not only would we be surrounded by the gardens, the mountains, the vineyards and four championship golf courses, but we would have access to some of the world's best-known entertainers who performed regularly at the wineries.

We enquired about the cost of renting the premises and learned it was quite substantial. In order for us to go ahead with the venture, we would have to draw on all our resources. Joyce sold her business; Greg and Josie agreed to put in all the money they had, and I began making arrangements to sell an investment property that I had in Sydney. As well as this, we needed to borrow additional funds from the bank.

It was quite a risk we were taking, and we knew that we would have to live quite simply in order to achieve our desired goal. We all liked being with one another and thought that it would be a great lifestyle.

We approached David with our proposal, hopeful that we would meet

finding the promised land

the strict Gardens criteria for tenancy. Then we waited. A few days later he rang us and gave us the good news: we were accepted as tenants.

This meant that we needed to move to the area and Josie and Joyce began searching on weekends to see if there were any places that would be suitable. After some extensive consulting with real estate agents and searching over the Internet, Josie, Joyce, Greg and I finally found a property that we all loved in the Pokolbin area. It was forty acres of partly cleared land, part bushland, and part grape vines. A large barn and workshed that had been used for manufacturing furniture were the only buildings on the property, but they offered great potential, not only as a dwelling but as a studio and workplace for Greg as well.

We put in an offer to buy the place and the contract was exchanged a short time later.

Widespread bushfires caused some anxious moments for us all before we moved to the area. Ironically, I had asked the former owner of the property if they had ever experienced any serious bush fires or was there any risk from fires given that our residence was so close to the bush.

He assured me that there hadn't been any fires there since the great inferno in the late 1960s, and that the prospect of any serious threats was extremely unlikely.

I couldn't believe it when we returned home and I turned on the TV at Church Point and discovered a high-ranking fireman reporting on the news that there was a widespread outbreak of fires across New South Wales, the worst since the late 1960s. When they gave an overview of the location of the fires throughout the state, Pokolbin was listed.

When we rang the gardens to enquire about the seriousness of the threat, David told us that he could see the fire from his office window, and that the advancing flames were headed for our property in the distance. He later confided that he thought there was a real chance that our property was going to be endangered, and for a while he believed our home was going to be burnt to the ground.

It took twelve fire engines, thirty firefighters, and a helicopter to stop the blaze.

'Escape'
Oil on linen, 1525 x 1225 mm

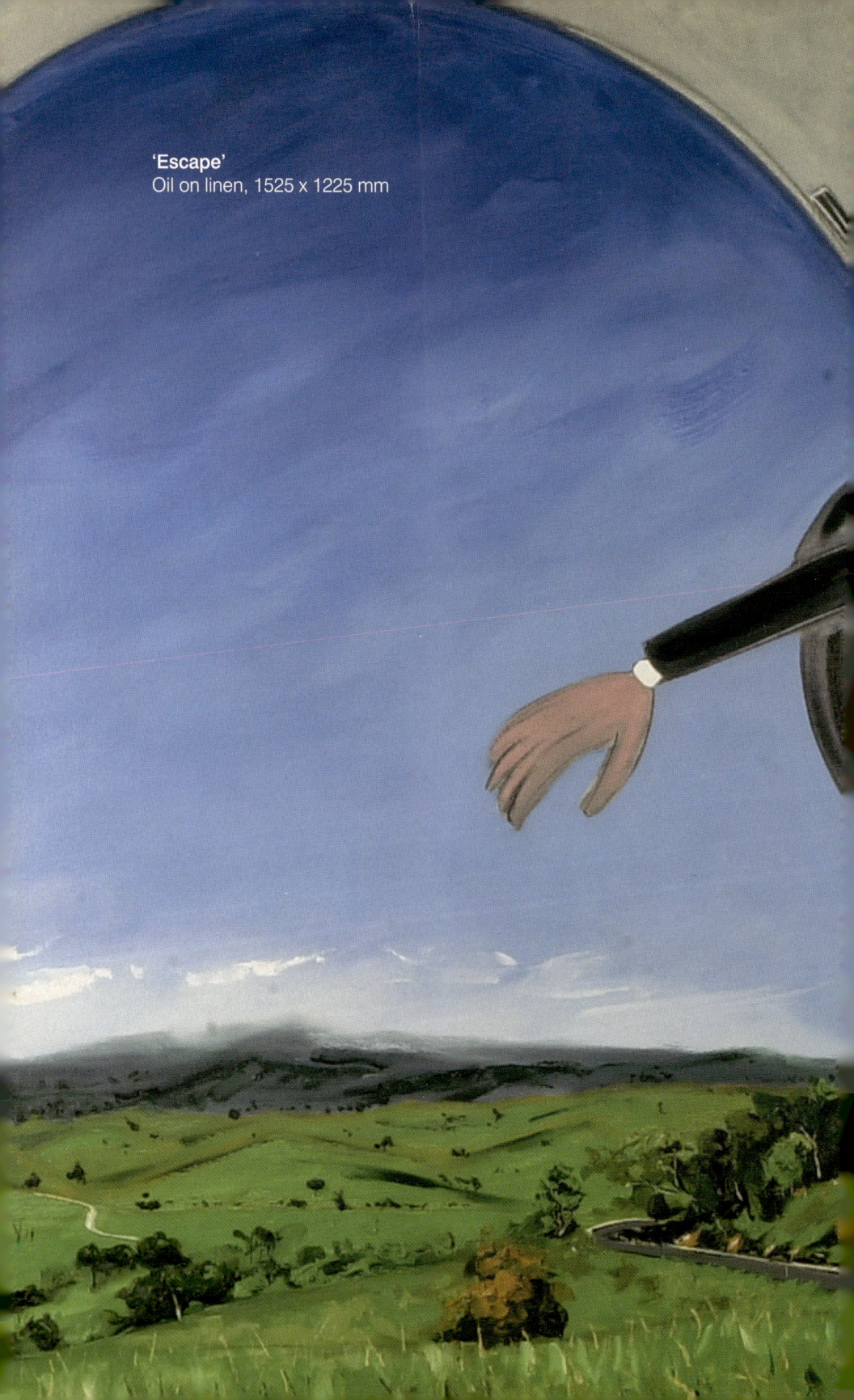

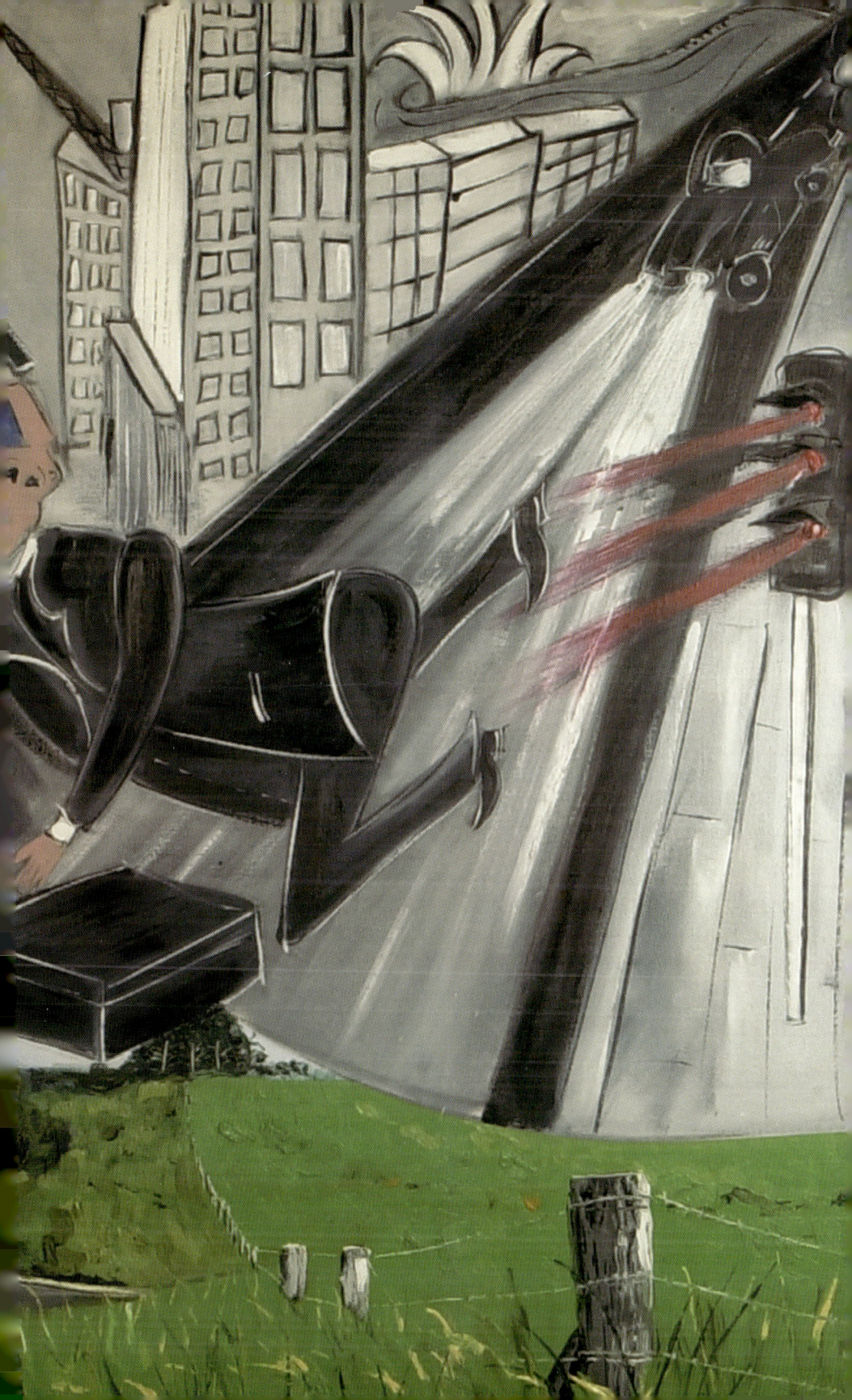

Fortunately for us, our settlement was delayed for a week. Otherwise we would have been evacuated from the property on the day we were due to take up residence.

When the fires had been extinguished, we made plans to move from our home at Church Point. We loaded up a small truck that I had borrowed from Dad, and made the two-hour journey north from Sydney. I had to do ten tiring trips before all our possessions had been relocated.

I was delighted but exhausted when I headed back to Sydney for the final time to return Dad's truck. I started to relax when I reached the freeway, and even though it was already four in the morning, I thought I'd be back in Pokolbin for breakfast. I was almost savouring the smell of freshly cooked bacon and fresh farm eggs when the truck lights suddenly went out and I was left negotiating a tricky bend in complete darkness! The alternator had failed and left me without dashboard lights, headlights or tail-lights. Fortunately I was able to avoid hitting any guard rails and was just coming to a halt when a huge semi-trailer careened past, going like a bat out of hell!

When my shattered nerves eventually settled I called roadside assistance and tried to catch up on a little sleep while I waited for the mechanic. I made it back to Pokolbin in time for morning tea, but was so tired I simply stretched out on the sofa and fell fast asleep!

In the meantime, the rest of our gang of pioneers went about putting the place into shape. Joyce was a little dismayed when she saw the kitchen, and after the deluxe equipment she had enjoyed using at the café she found the four-burner barbecue just a little primitive. There was no kitchen bench, and she had to make do initially with a dressing table as the only place to prepare our food.

Growing up in the city, Greg never really imagined himself leaving. However, when he first started visiting the country with Josie it made him feel more at peace. He realised that the scenery was beautiful, and that he would love to live in the Hunter region. The countryside made Greg feel more peaceful. When Greg lived in the city he felt trapped in a never-ending competitive environment where it was all about looks

finding the promised land

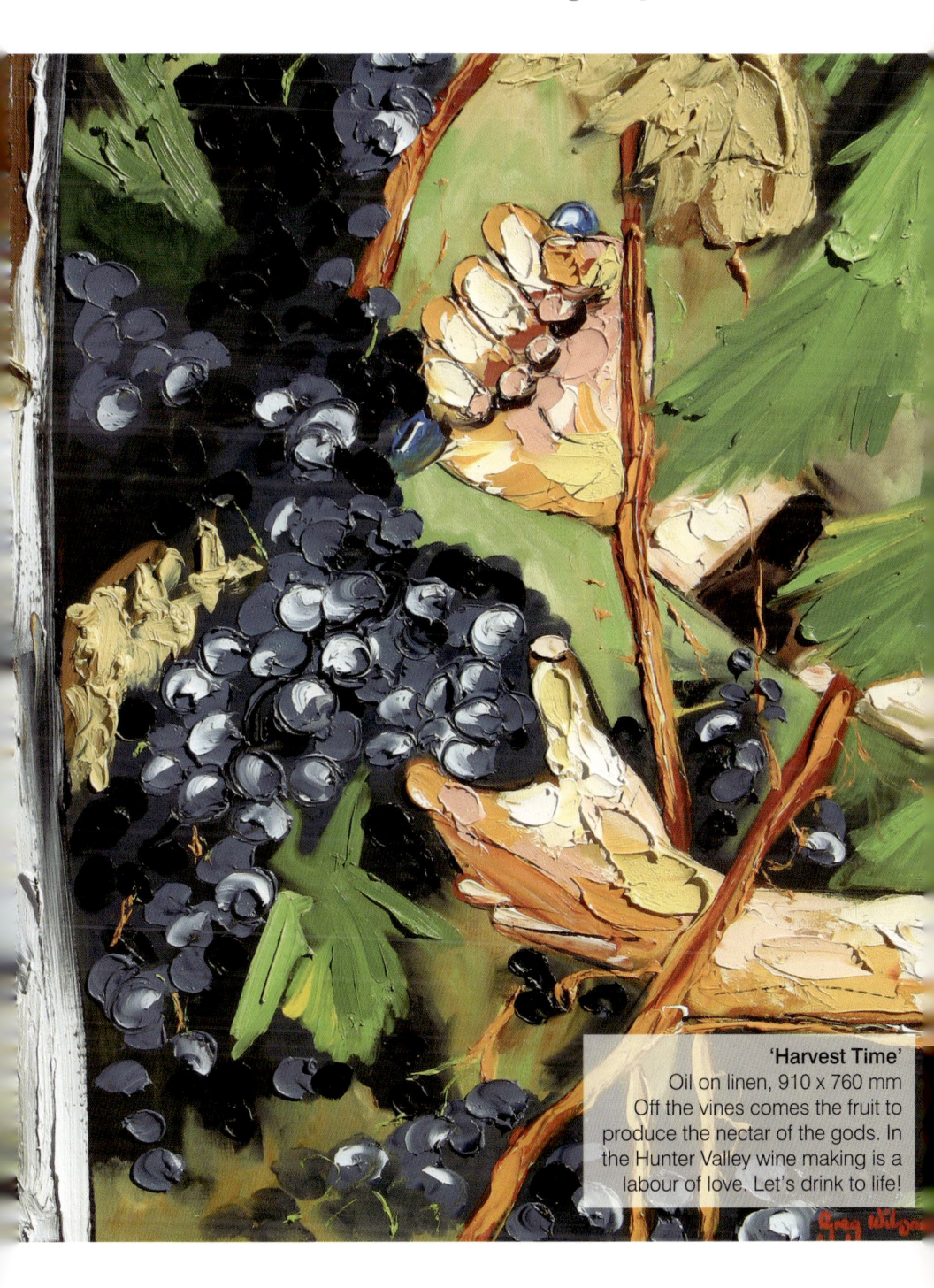

'Harvest Time'
Oil on linen, 910 x 760 mm
Off the vines comes the fruit to produce the nectar of the gods. In the Hunter Valley wine making is a labour of love. Let's drink to life!

my brush with depression

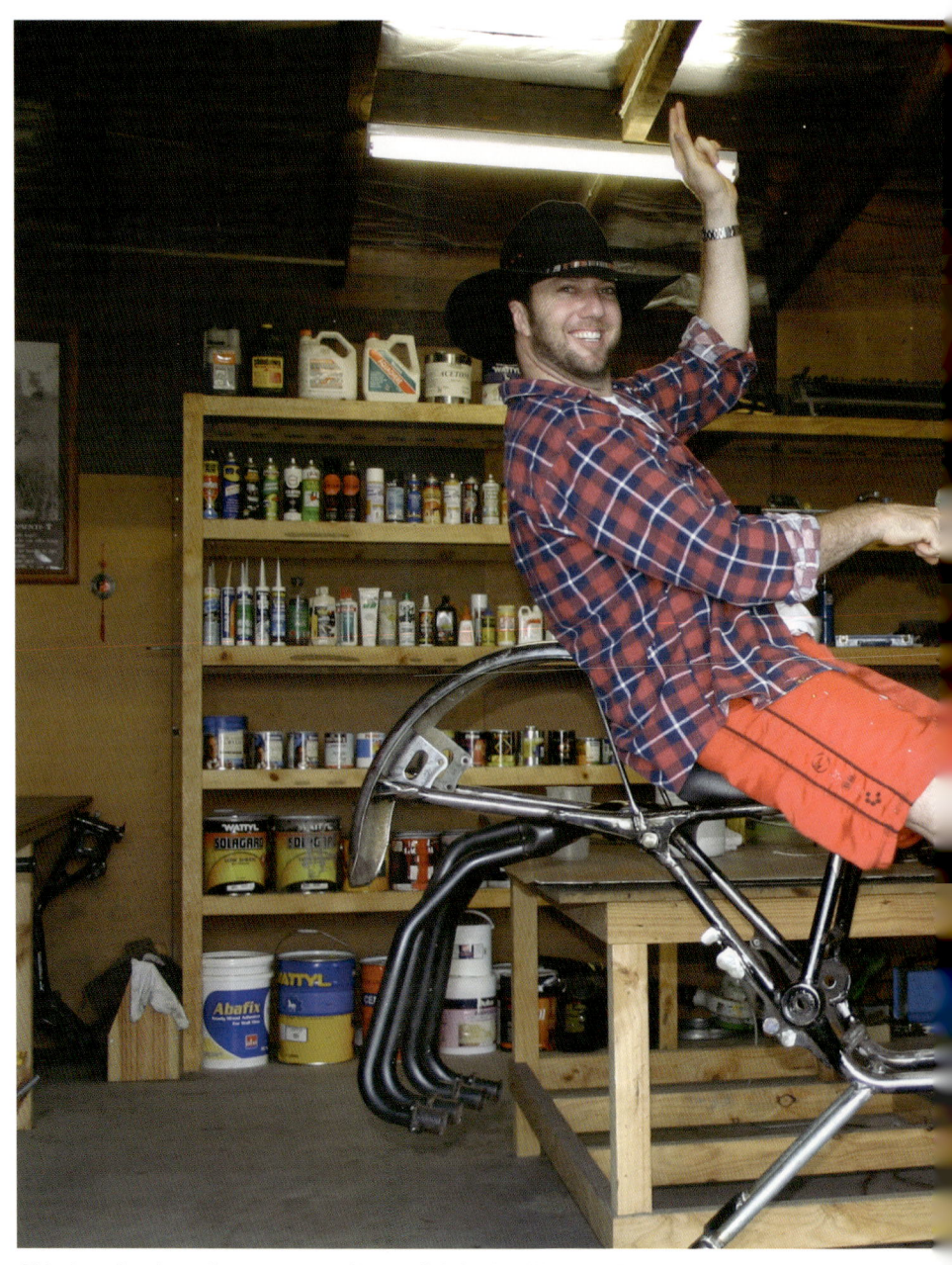

Ride 'em Cowboy. Greg on one of his unfinished quirky creations – a horse-powered motorcycle.

finding the promised land

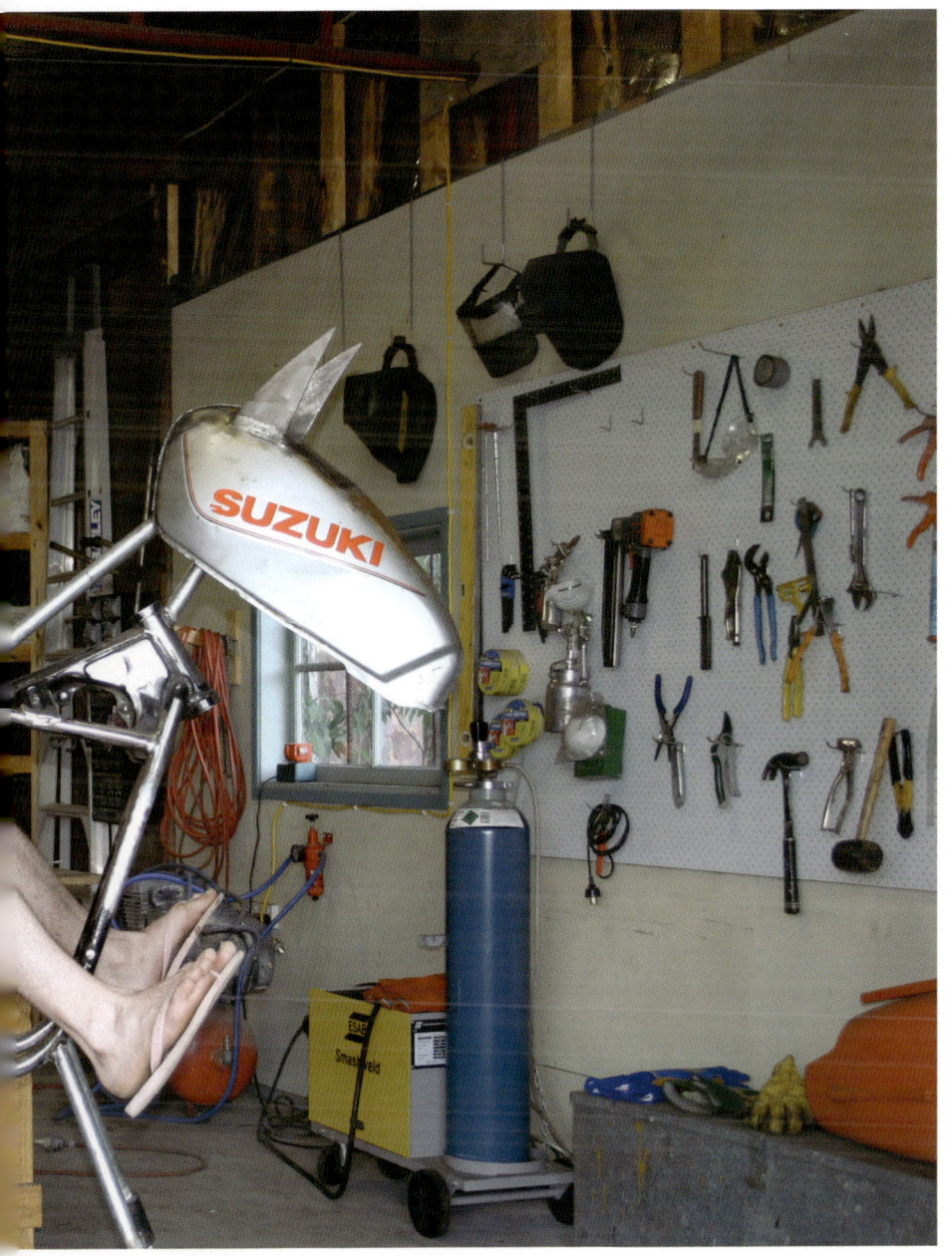

'It's a much slower pace nowadays than it used to be in my wild youth. But what a great feeling to take each day as it comes, living the simple life in the country. I've happily traded in my motorcycle leathers for a cowboy hat, and my motorbike for a safer two-door ute!' – Greg

greg wilson

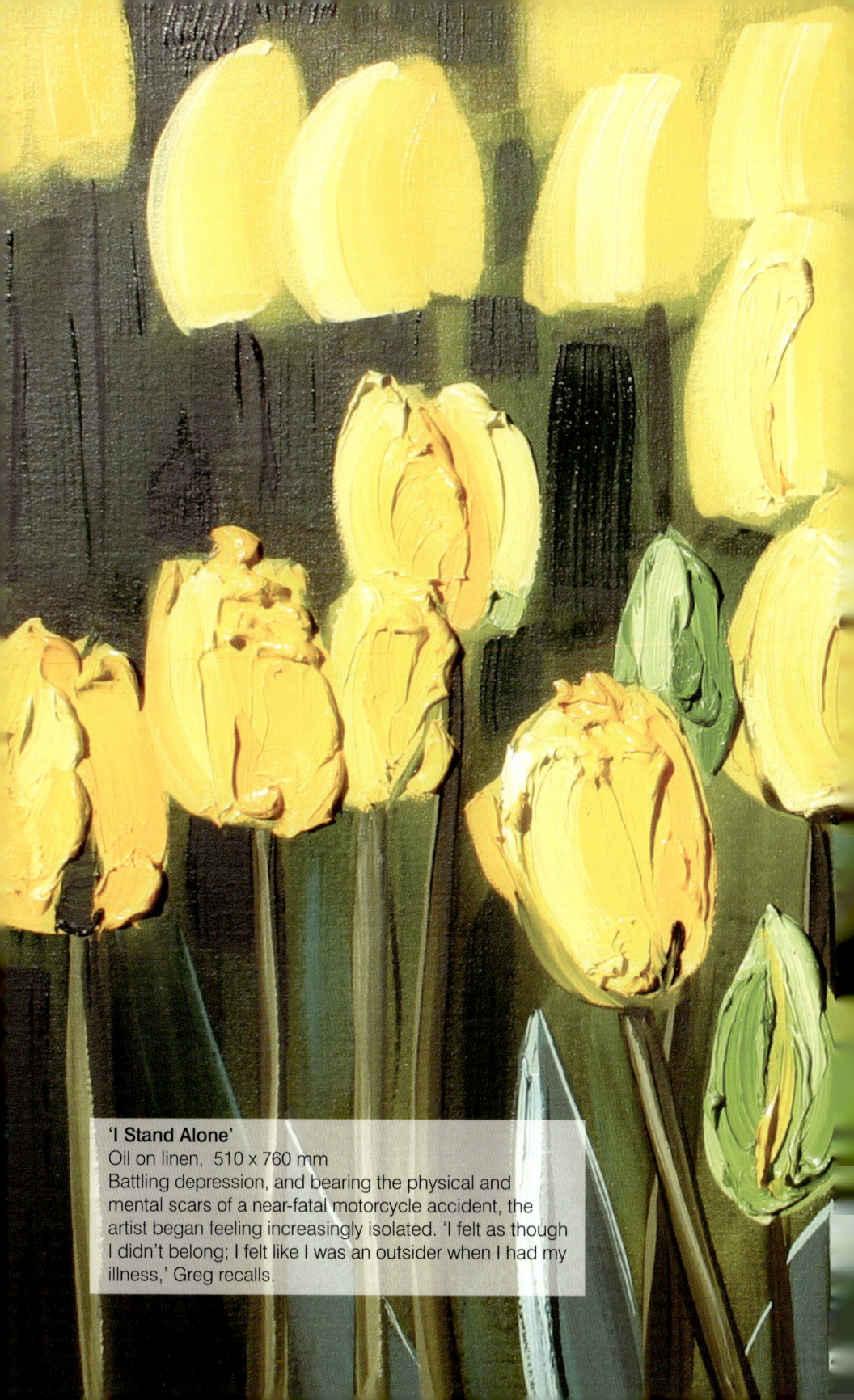

'I Stand Alone'
Oil on linen, 510 x 760 mm
Battling depression, and bearing the physical and mental scars of a near-fatal motorcycle accident, the artist began feeling increasingly isolated. 'I felt as though I didn't belong; I felt like I was an outsider when I had my illness,' Greg recalls.

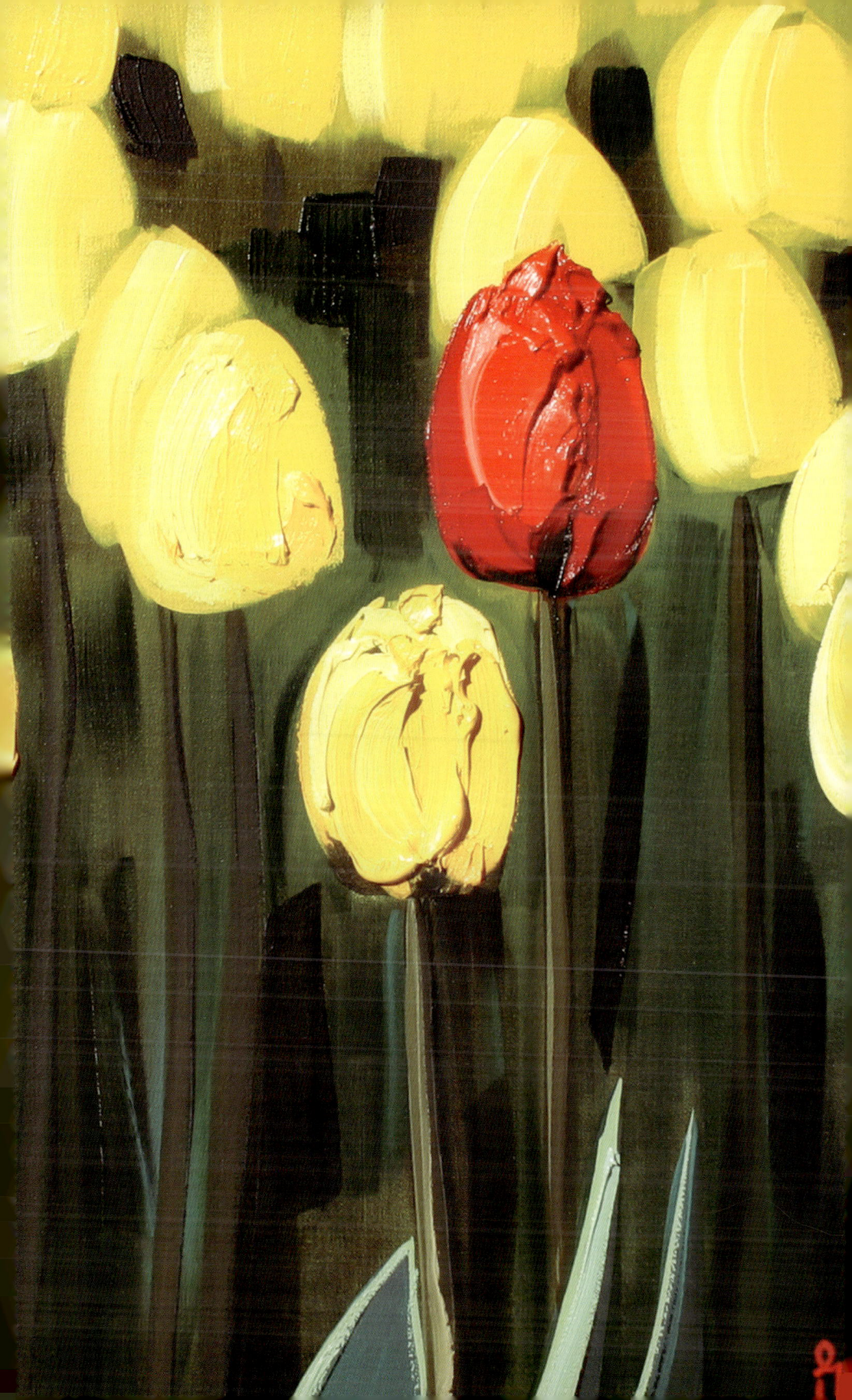

my brush with depression

and fashion, what car you drove, where you lived. When he went into the mountains he found that all the shackles and chains came off. It was extremely calming.

He did a painting, shortly after our arrival, which he titled: 'Escape'. The accompanying description of the work beautifully captured the essence of Greg's feelings. 'Who has not felt the call of the Australian countryside – its serenity and peace – in stark contrast to the pressures and frantic pace of city life?'

The local townsfolk provided quite a contrast also to his city associates, and their laid-back attitude appealed to Greg enormously. He took great delight in relating an incident that happened when he went down to the village hardware store to replenish his supply of paints. The young girl behind the counter, who had served him a few weeks previously, was a little surprised when he returned, and she remarked: 'You're still painting, then?' When Greg explained to her that painting was his profession, she exclaimed: 'That's good! Maybe you could paint my house for me!' We remind Greg of this offer whenever he has a slow period!

'Home'
Oil on Canvas, 1525 x 1525 mm
'Heavenly landscapes surround me on my property and provide ideal inspiration for my work. I see a work of art everywhere I look in the Hunter Valley.'

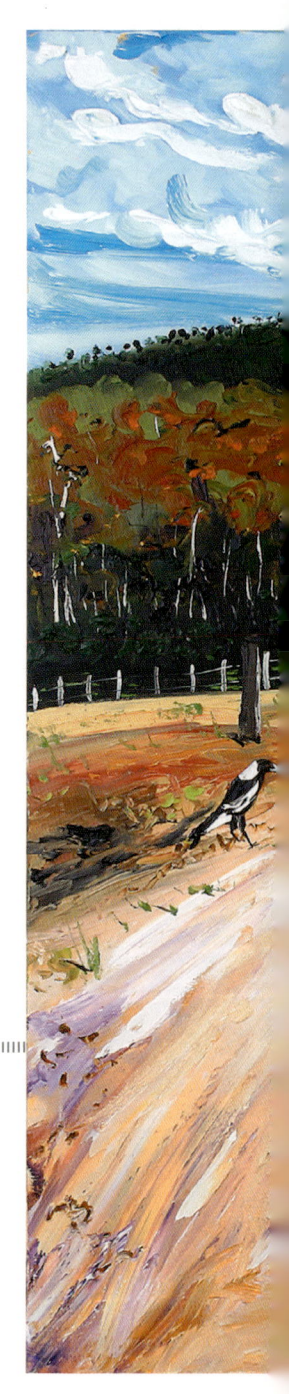

finding the promised land

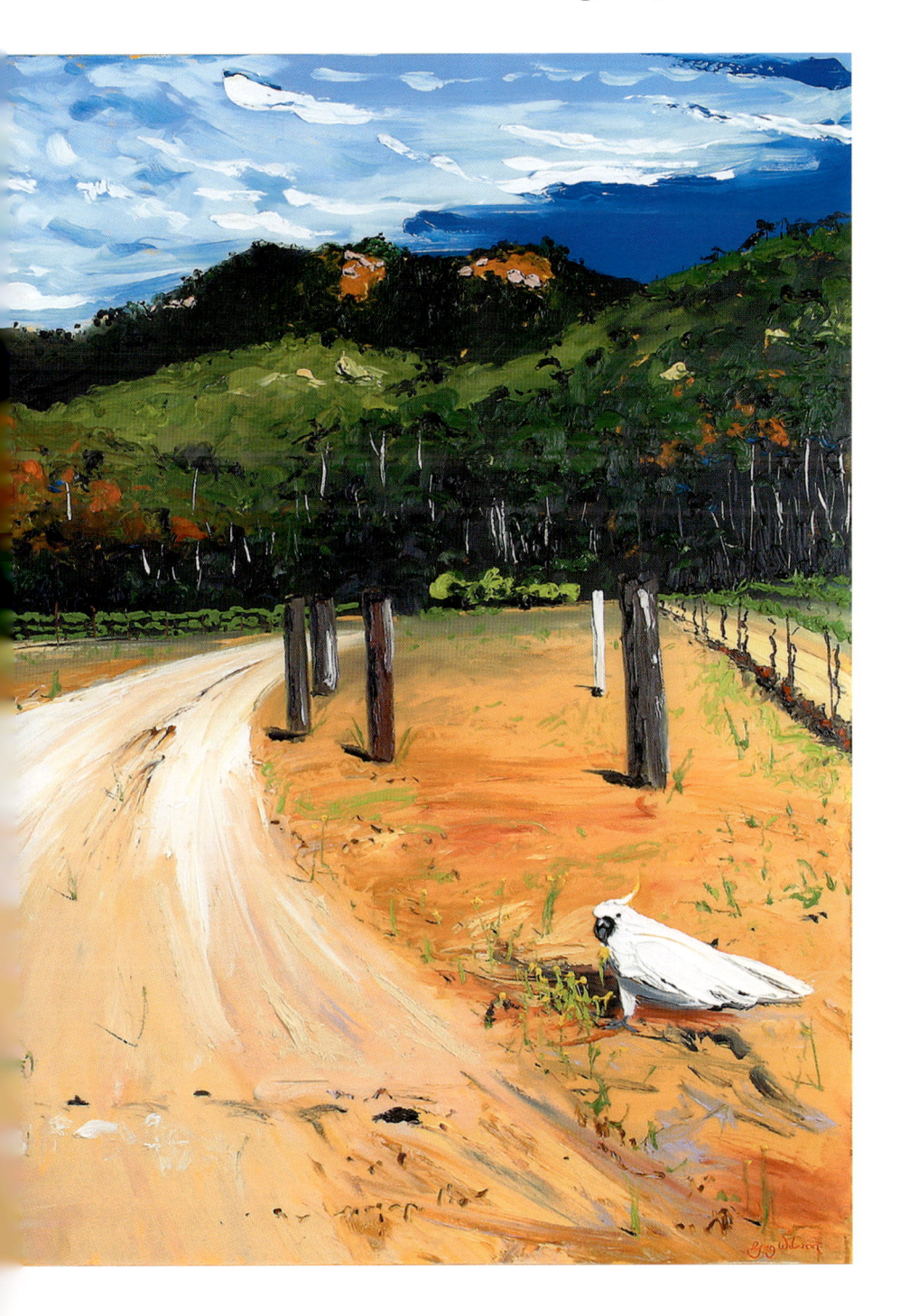

greg wilson — 191

Josie loved the country lifestyle, although a number of incidents caused her a few anxious moments during the settling in period. Before we had a chance to renovate the old barn that eventually was to become our main residence, she had to visit our quaint old outhouse at one o'clock in the morning. As she attended to her needs, she had a sudden shock when she perceived two eyes peering at her in the moonlight. She sat frozen to the spot, conjuring up all sorts of ideas about strange country yokels roaming the neighbourhood. It was only when the eyes moved away and she was able to discern the outline of one of the local foxes that she began breathing again!

Greg was totally occupied for the following week, calling on his carpentry skills to begin the first of our renovations: an indoor shower and toilet!

I fell in love with the place, although it took me some time to adjust to being so far from the surf. I had always found the ocean a source of great relaxation and serenity, a place where I could get away from all the cares that had surrounded us with Greg's illness. However, I soon found there were plenty of other places in the valley that afforded me the same peace and calmness.

Some of our 'city-slicker' friends took great delight in calling us their country cousins. They loved reminding us of how the town received its name. Pokolbin was named by a German settler who had arrived at the height of summer when the temperatures had soared. He promptly called the place Pokolbin, which translates from the German as 'hell-hole'! It was not unusual for our telephone calls from friends in the city to commence with: 'How's life in the hell-hole?'

Nothing, however, could have been more inappropriate to describe our slice of heaven! There was so much to do and see when we first arrived, and we divided our time between fixing up the rudimentary accommodation on the property and visiting the local wineries and gardens.

Shopping in the village was a social event, and we were delighted to be readily accepted as members of the local community. People would go out of their way to greet you and spend time chatting, offering to

finding the promised land

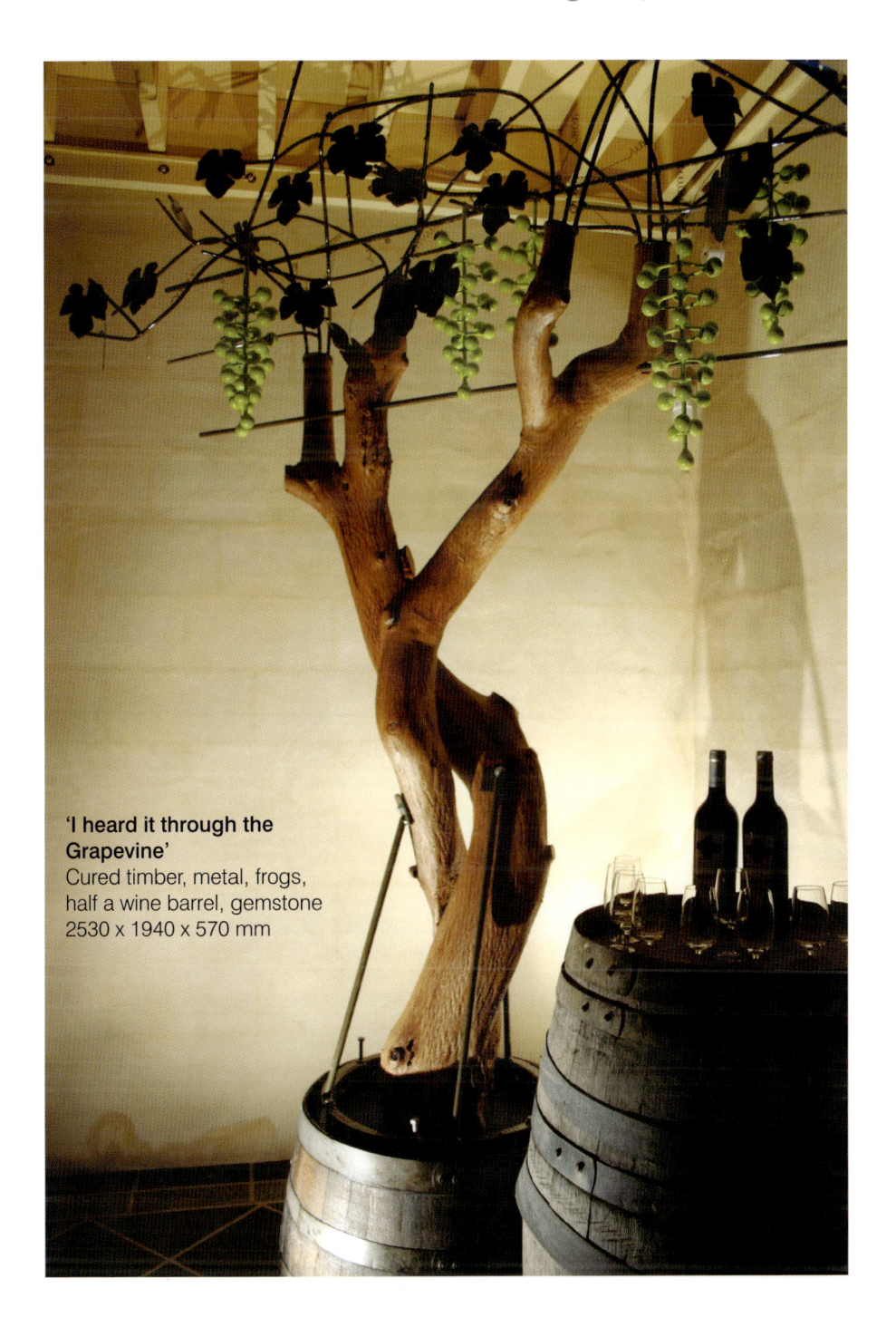

'I heard it through the Grapevine'
Cured timber, metal, frogs, half a wine barrel, gemstone
2530 x 1940 x 570 mm

greg wilson — 193

my brush with depression

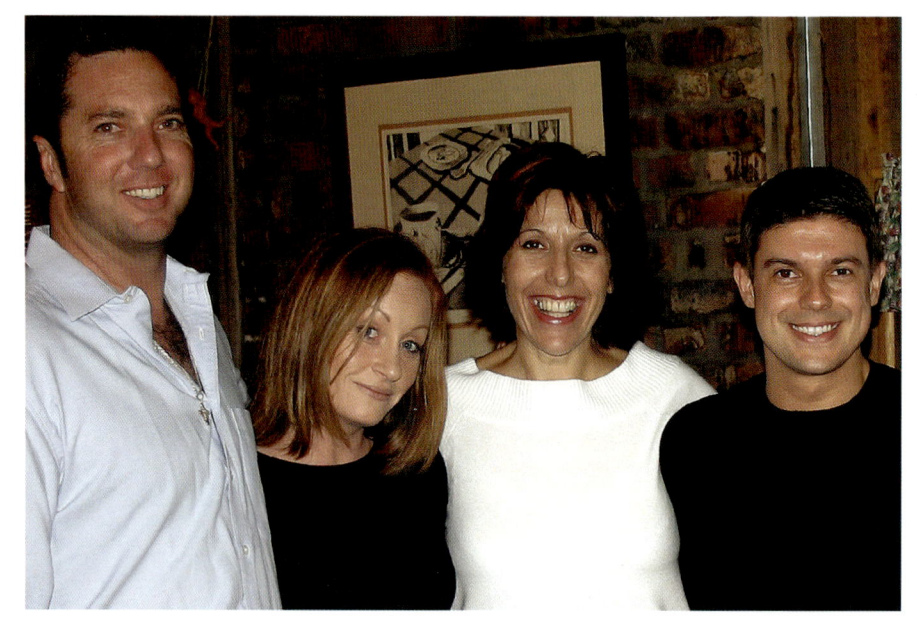

Greg (left) with close friends, Simone Miletic, Joyce Biviano and Robert Miletic.

help in any way they could, and inviting you to lunch, dinner, or a visit to their vineyards.

I came up the driveway one afternoon to notice Greg's old cowboy hat moving slowly along the grapevines. It was only when I stopped the car that I heard the sound of the old Victa motor mower. The previous owner had used a tractor and slasher to mow between the vines, but we had no such luxury available. It was quite amusing to see Greg labouring along with a carefree smile on his face, even though it appeared that he would have to spend a few weeks to complete the job!

During the next few months, we also prepared the new gallery. Greg did most of the work himself, painting the walls, making the skirting boards, grinding and sealing a concrete floor, and I helped where I could. Furniture wasn't a problem, either. I called on the family connections and soon two stylish red lounges, with a truckload of dining and bedding, arrived from John Cootes Furniture.

finding the promised land

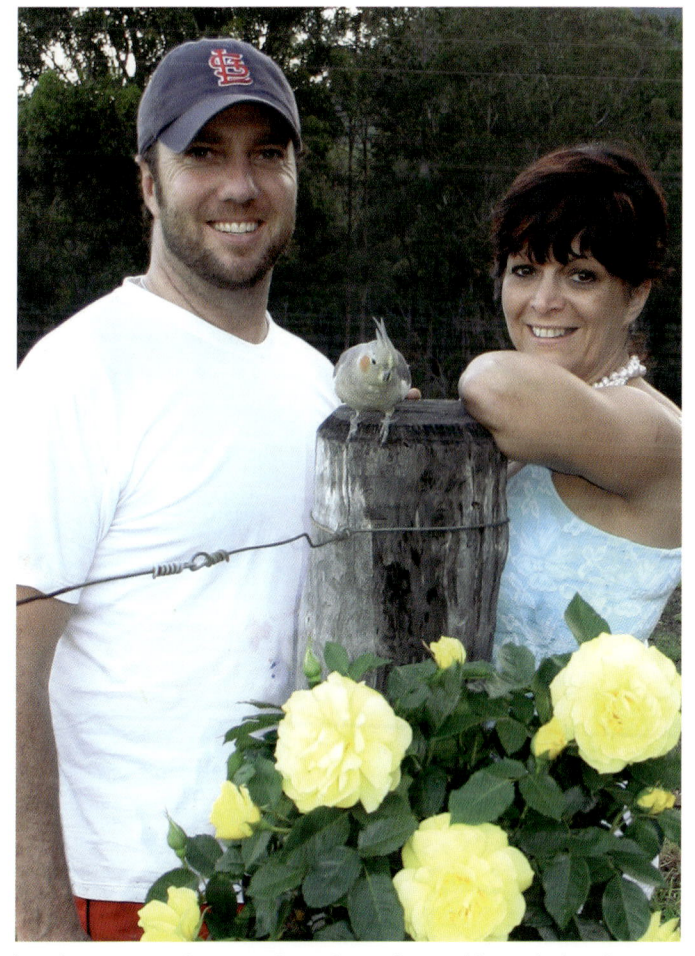

Jess is never too far away from the action and loves being the centre of attention. She doesn't like to miss out on a photo opportunity and is seen here with Greg and Josie.

As well as working on fitting out the gallery, Greg was eager to prepare as many paintings and sculptures as he could to ensure that the collection was varied and comprehensive. He threw himself into his work with a will, and produced an impressive number of works in a relatively short time. His enthusiasm almost brought him undone, however, when he was working on a sculpture representing his concept of the solar system.

He had been using a welder extensively during a morning session and inadvertently grasped a metal bar that had become extremely hot. A searing pain scorched the palm of his hand, and he dropped the welder onto the floor. He was so anxious to complete the work, however, that he went straight to the first aid cabinet, applied a rough bandage to his left hand and continued with the sculpture. Things only got worse, though, when the loose end of the bandage later became entangled in the spinning blade of an angle grinder. The machine slammed into his wrist, slashing an artery and causing blood to spurt from the wound.

Frantically, he called Joyce at the gallery. She raced back to the property, helped stem the flow of blood, and rushed him to the Cessnock hospital. The attending doctor stitched up the wound and gave Greg a tetanus booster. He told him to return home and rest, as he had lost quite a large amount of blood.

Greg rested for an hour and was back at his workbench as soon as he felt that his dizziness had passed. His keenness was an encouraging sign for all of us, not only because it meant he was back doing something he loved, but that the chances of his having a lapse into depression at such a positive time was highly unlikely.

It was at this time that Greg decided to acknowledge his new-found freedom in the countryside by including a small, discreetly placed, bird somewhere in his paintings or above his signature. For him it was an acknowledgement of his mental freedom and his peace of mind.

It was with this vibrant sense of optimism that we had settled into our home at Pokolbin, and the same spirit persisted when we opened our gallery in February of 2002.

chapter twenty-three
the greg wilson gallery

'Art is not what you see, but what you make others see.'
— Edgar Degas

The gallery looked most impressive for the opening. Greg wanted to use the event as a means of drawing attention to the mental health cause. After the highly favourable impact that Jessica Rowe's contribution had made at the Park Hyatt in Sydney, he hoped that she might be interested in helping us further.

When she accepted our invitation to open the gallery, it was my designated task to pick her up from Sydney. As I was leaving the Hunter Valley, I bumped into a couple of tradesmen from the gardens. They appeared quite envious when they learned I was to spend two hours chauffeuring Jessica, an extremely attractive woman with a dazzling smile. Three hours later I picked her up from her home in Sydney and had begun driving to the gallery. It was a strange trip back. On the way along the F3 motorway I heard the blast of a horn. I thought it was some admirers of Jess and looked up expecting to see some hormone-crazed teenagers. Instead it was my father, now sitting in the outside lane, casting furtive and quizzical glances in our direction.

I had been really busy with preparations for the gallery opening and had not been in contact to tell him that I was picking Jessica up. The look on his face, when he saw my passenger, caused me to burst into spontaneous laughter. He glanced over a few times, and I was worried he was going to have an accident before he waved goodbye.

We arrived a few minutes before the opening. Already in attendance was the Mayor, John Clarence of Cessnock, who had accepted our invitation to welcome Greg to the Hunter Valley and Gillian Church, the Director of the Mental Health Association of New South Wales Incorporated.

It was a special moment for all of us when Jessica got up to speak and officially open the Greg Wilson Gallery on 15 February 2003. She held her audience spellbound, not only because of her polished delivery, which she had honed by presenting the evening news nightly on Channel Ten, but also because she spoke with such conviction and passion about mental health issues.

She explained how depression had already impacted upon her life. She was only ten years old when her mother was diagnosed with the disease. She described the heartache and anguish that her mother's behaviour had visited upon the family. Particularly vivid was the way she told how her mother had a maniacal preoccupation with cleanliness, and how she sometimes worked throughout the night vacuuming and

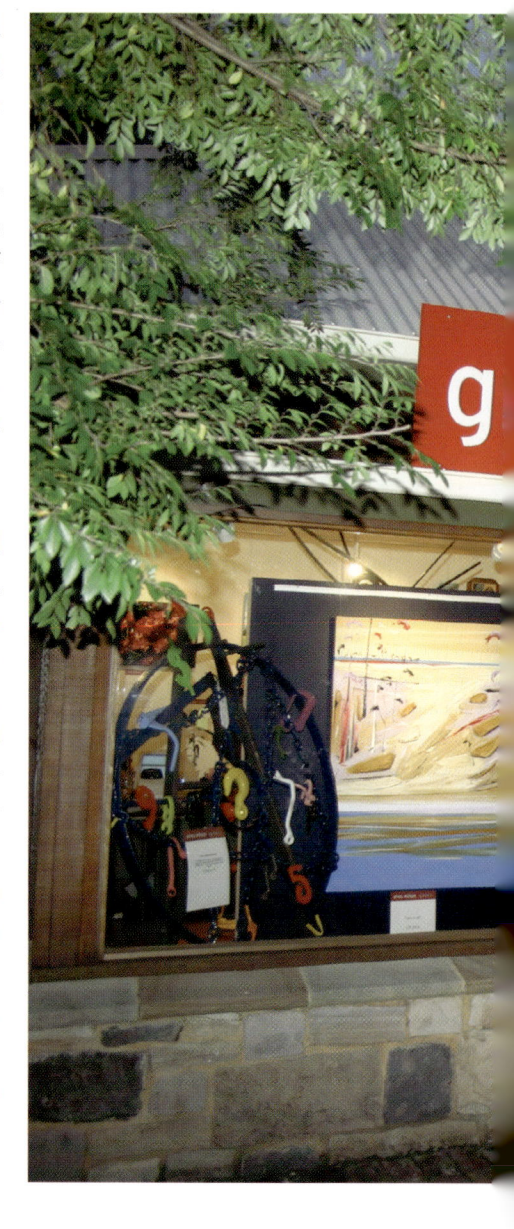

the greg wilson gallery

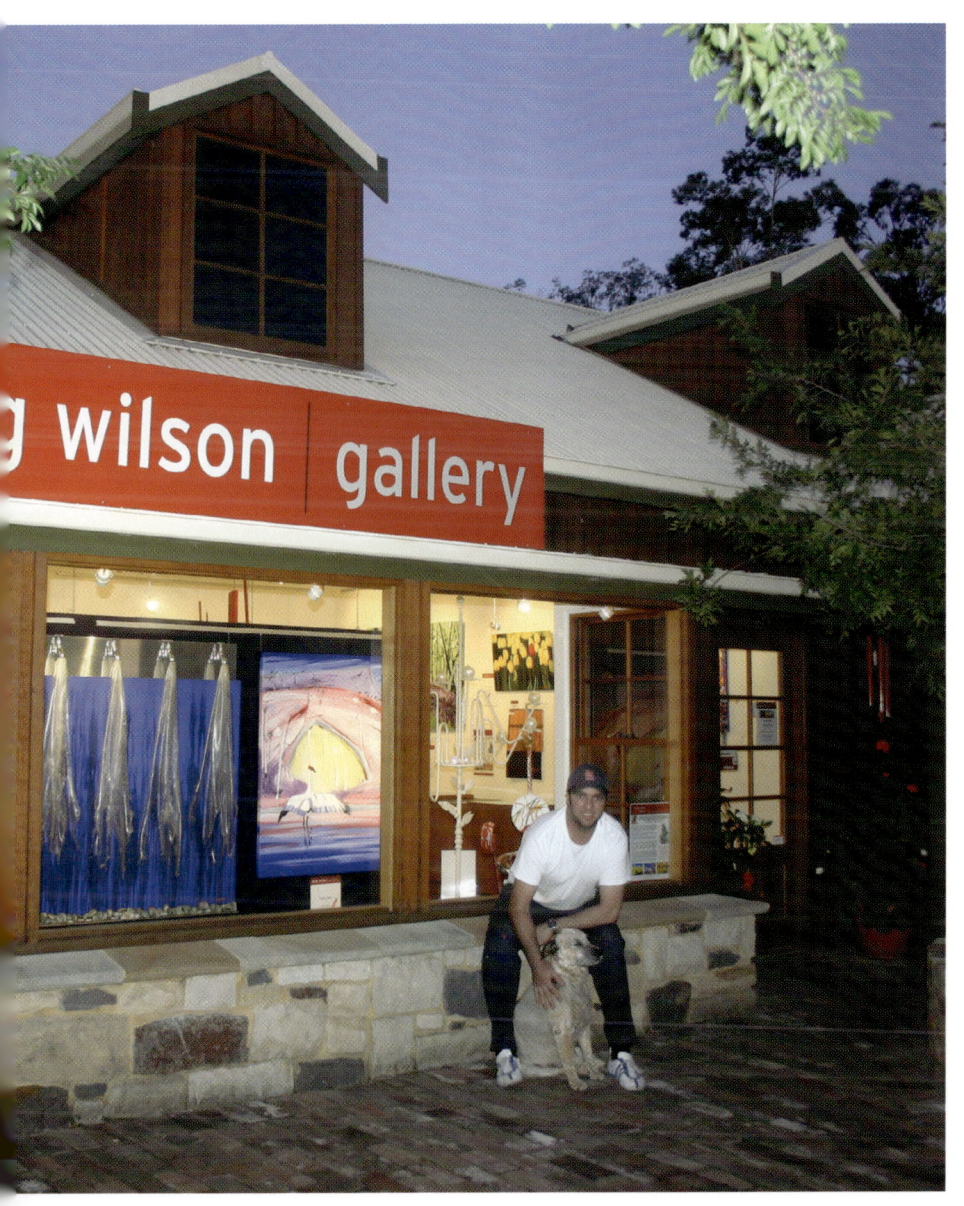

Dusk at the Greg Wilson Gallery. Greg and Jackson sit and contemplate the next move.

my brush with depression

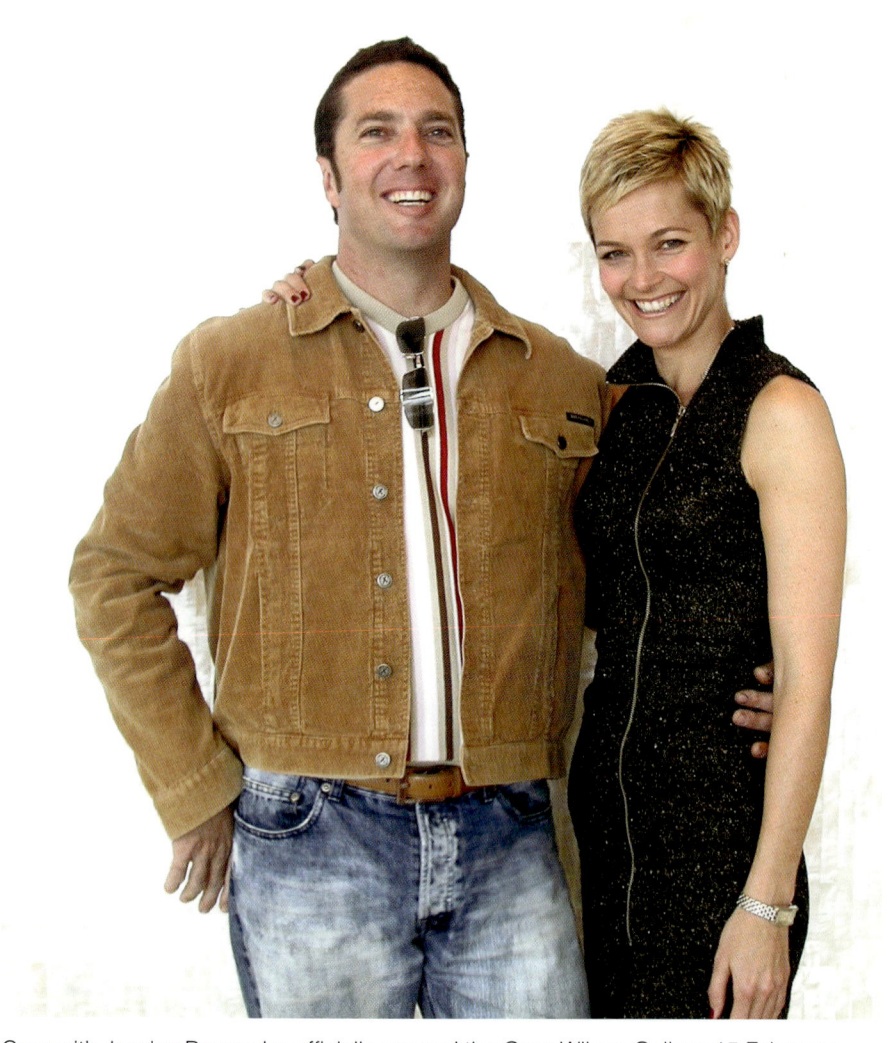

Greg with Jessica Rowe who officially opened the Greg Wilson Gallery, 15 February 2003. Jessica is an extraordinary person, deeply committed to helping those with depression. She gives freely of her time and has been a big support to Greg. Thanks Jessica, you're an angel!

scrubbing their house almost in a frenzy; how her mother would lose her appetite, could not sleep, and could not tolerate the sound of music or traffic.

I listened in fascination as Jessica described what I saw as the

200 — aaron cootes

the greg wilson gallery

extraordinary similarities between the suffering of Greg and her own mother. Particularly chilling was the way she described the time when her mother confessed that she had actually contemplated taking her own life on a number of occasions. It brought back a host of evocative memories to Josie, Joyce and me.

Jessica paid tribute to Greg for providing such a readily accessible 'sanctuary' for anyone who wished to discuss depression or gain inspiration from his story. She also commended him for establishing his art school for children in the area and the assistance he gave to the Mental Health Association of New South Wales Incorporated by donating a percentage of his sales to their programmes.

She completed her presentation by thanking us for the opportunity to shed a little more light on the subject of depression and to dispel some of the myths that surrounded it. She expressed the hope that Greg's continued crusade to combat the effects of the disease would help remove the stigma that some people still associate with it. She complimented Greg on the outstanding calibre of his artwork, predicted a bright future for the gallery, and then declared our pride and joy officially open!

Her address was met with lengthy applause and hearty congratulations. After being interviewed by representatives from the Newcastle media, she joined other guests for a celebratory glass of champagne and further discussion on her own outstanding career. Her parting words to Greg before I chauffeured her back to Sydney were most encouraging. She told us that she knew good things were going to happen because of our presence in the valley and that Greg would bring a lot of relief and consolation to many sufferers of depression.

That confidence was well founded. The attendant publicity and the widespread media coverage had an immediate flow-on effect, and we were surprised at the number of visitors to the gallery who were prepared to discuss mental health issues that they had previously regarded as taboo. Their openness and candour were refreshing and encouraging. Greg was called upon frequently to offer words of encouragement or advice to people who came to discuss their problems with him.

A Newcastle woman came to visit the Hunter Valley Gardens shortly

my brush with depression

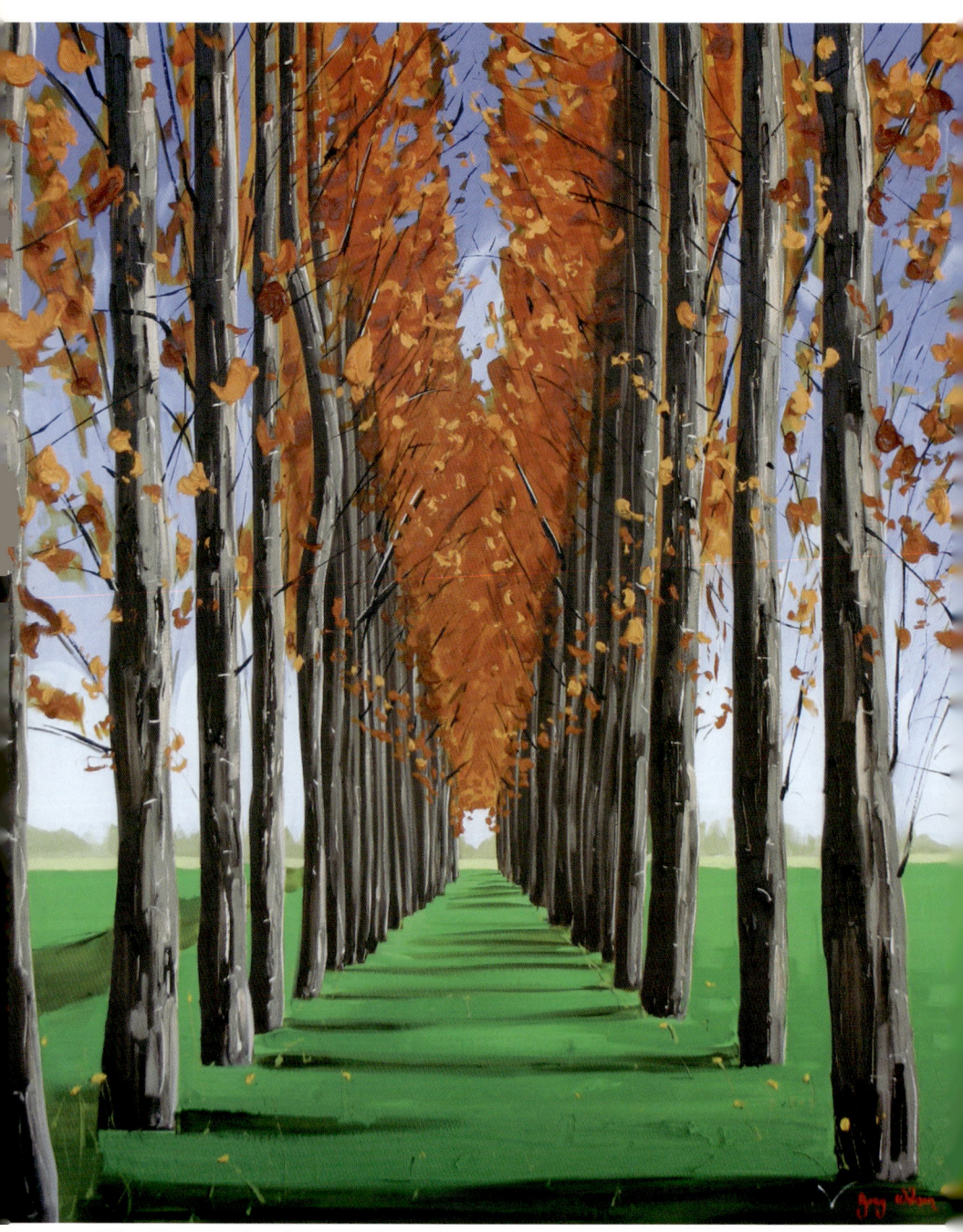

'Way Home', Oil on linen, 1210 x 1010 mm

the greg wilson gallery

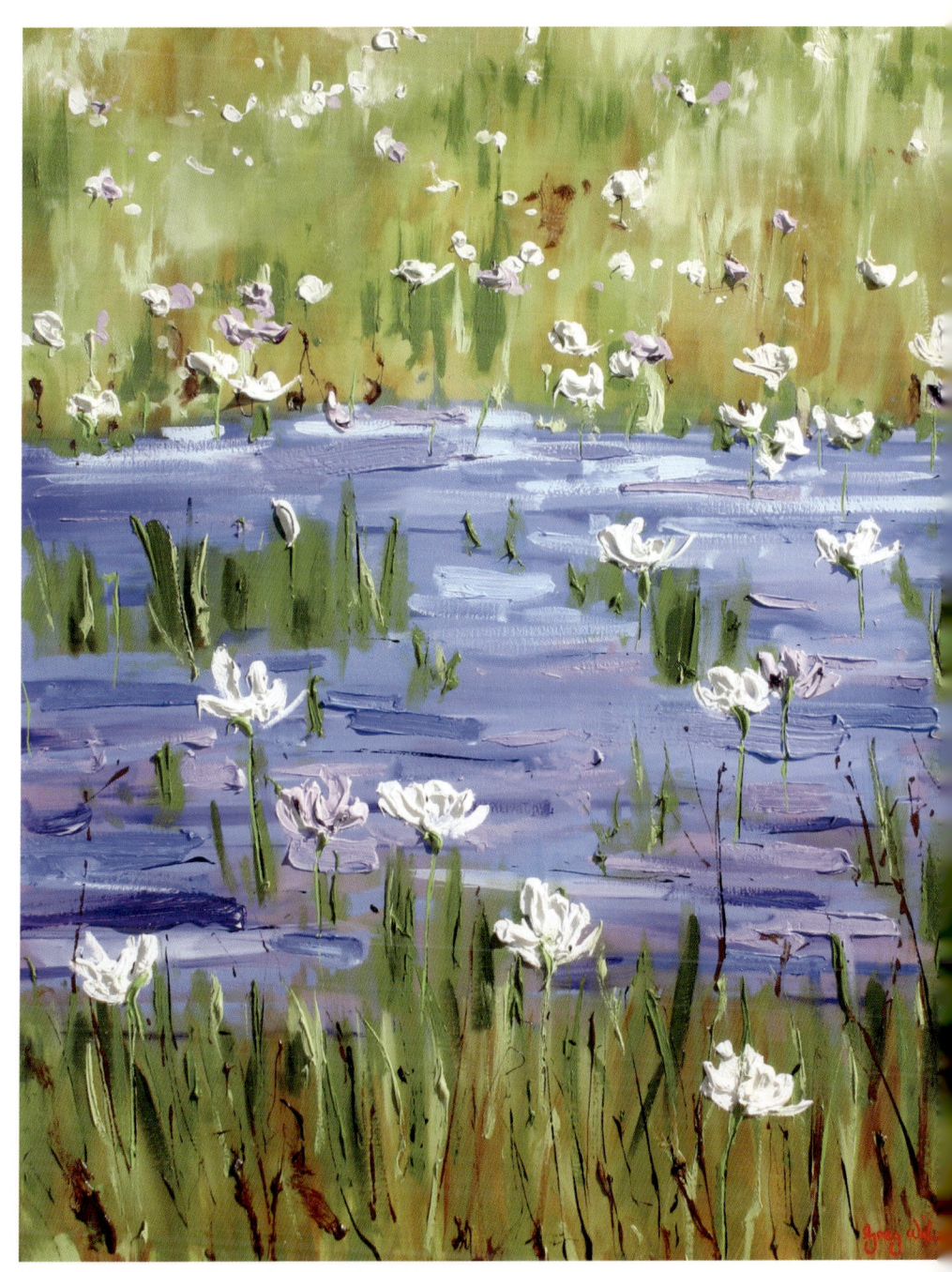

'Touch of Colour', Oil on linen, 1010 x 760 mm

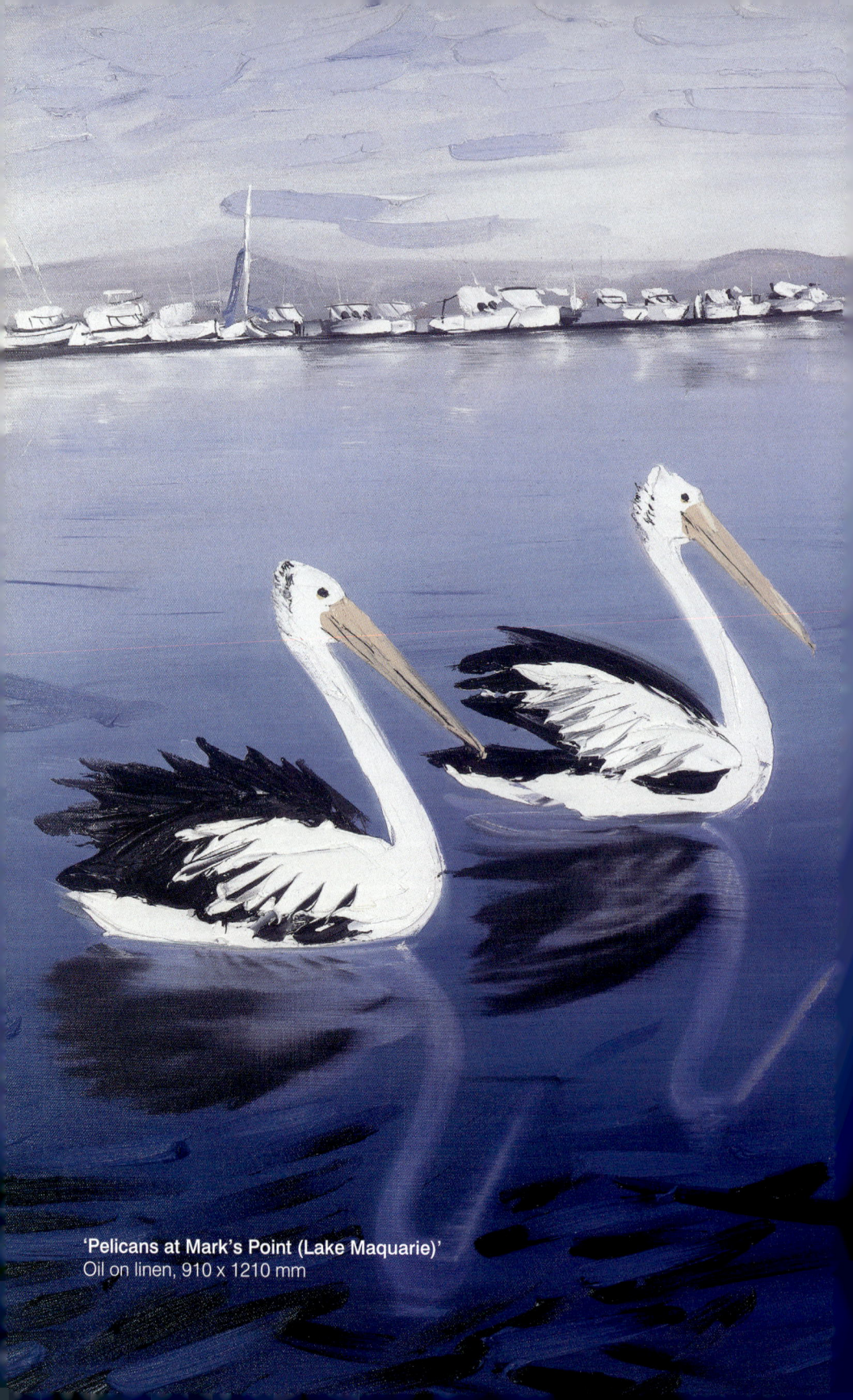

'Pelicans at Mark's Point (Lake Maquarie)'
Oil on linen, 910 x 1210 mm

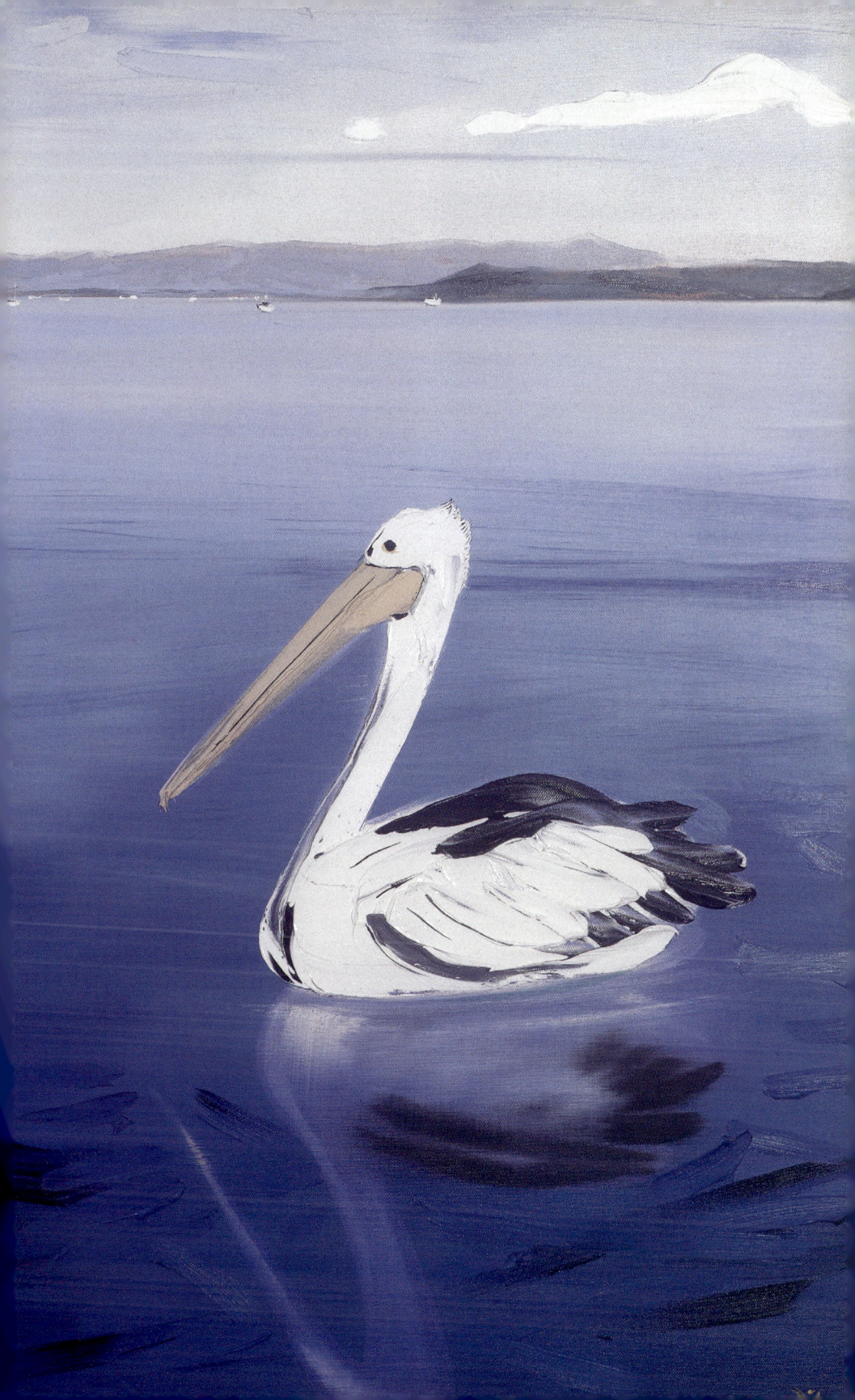

my brush with depression

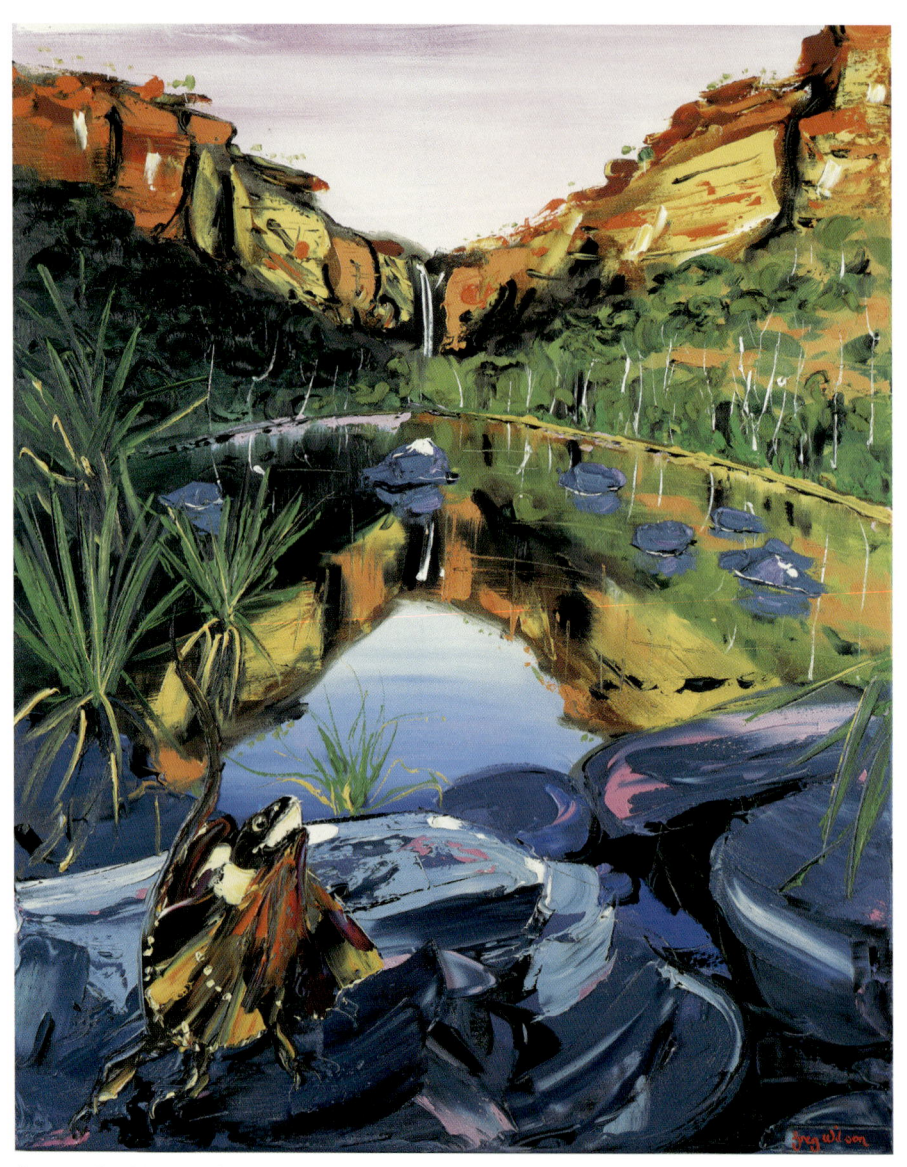

'Lenny the Lizard'. Oil on linen, 1010 x 760 mm
Australia is host to a large and varied lizard population. When Greg noticed one of the reptiles basking in the sun on the middle of the road, he was determined to stop an approaching tourist bus, which he feared would run over the helpless creature. The artist was amused when Japanese visitors began taking photos of him holding the animal by the tail. He was unable to contain his laughter when he was affectionately referred to as the 'Crocodile Hunter' in broken English. This painting reminds him of the funny incident.

the greg wilson gallery

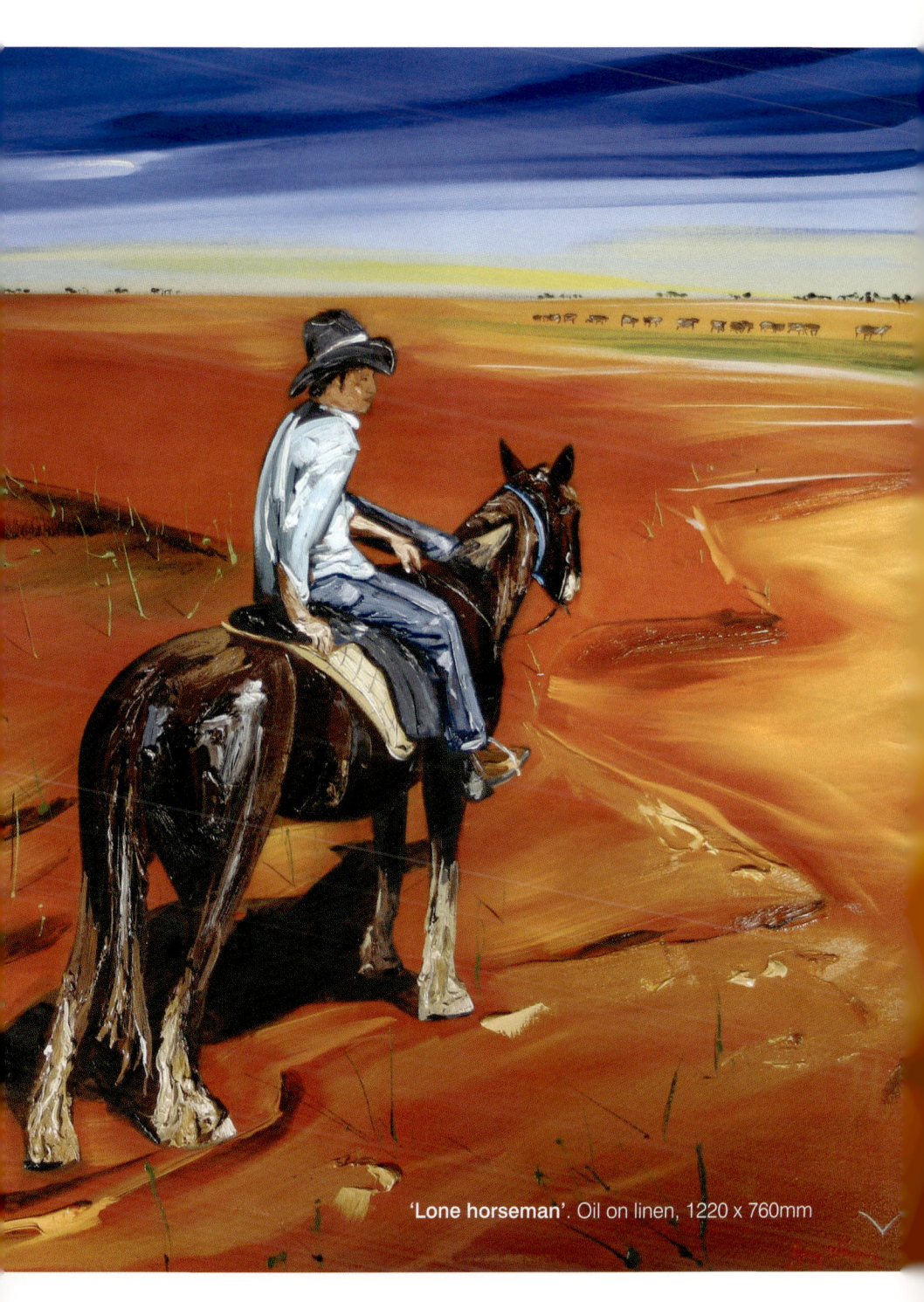

'**Lone horseman**'. Oil on linen, 1220 x 760mm

greg wilson — 207

'Bright Days', Oil on linen, 1010 x 1210 mm

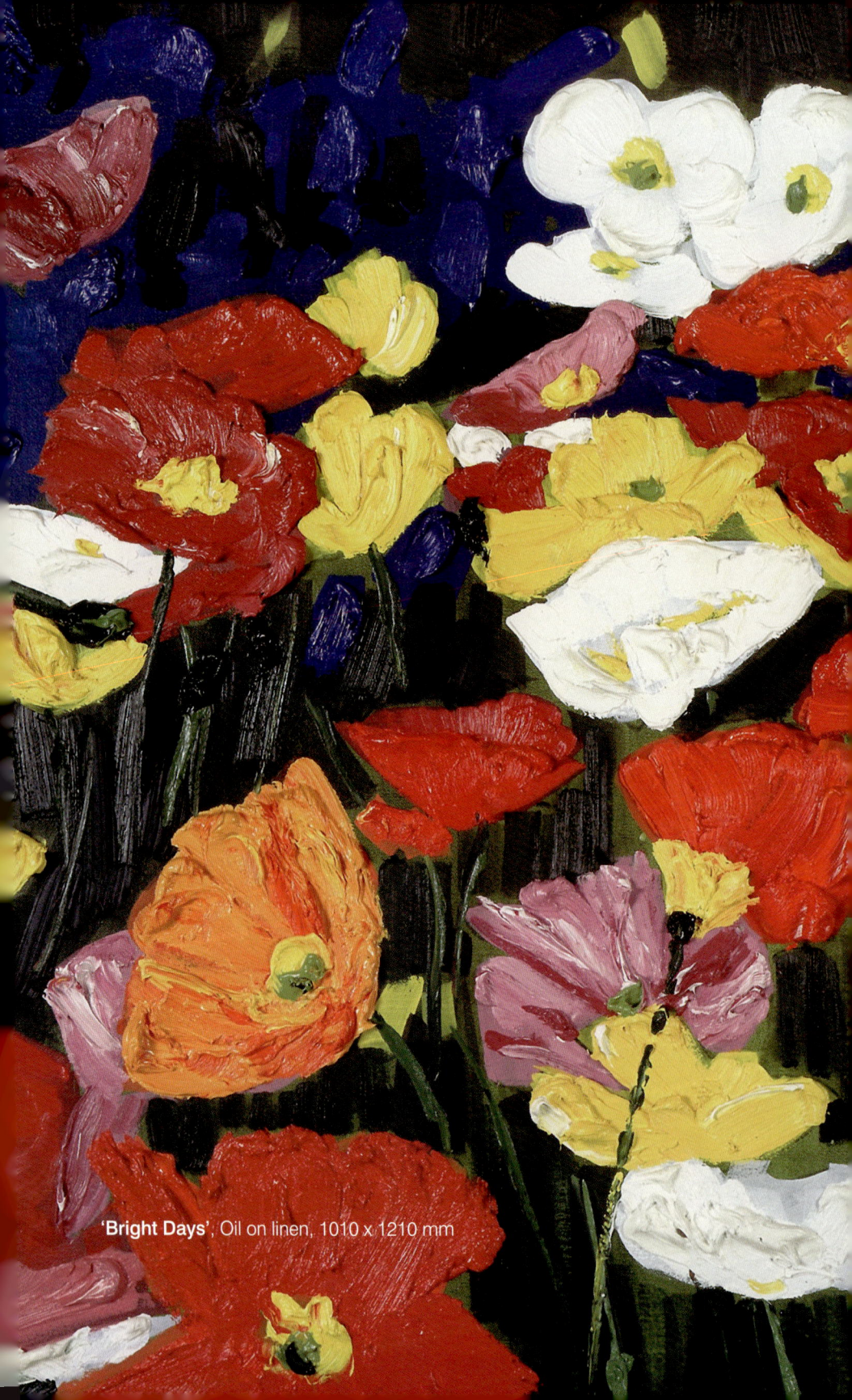

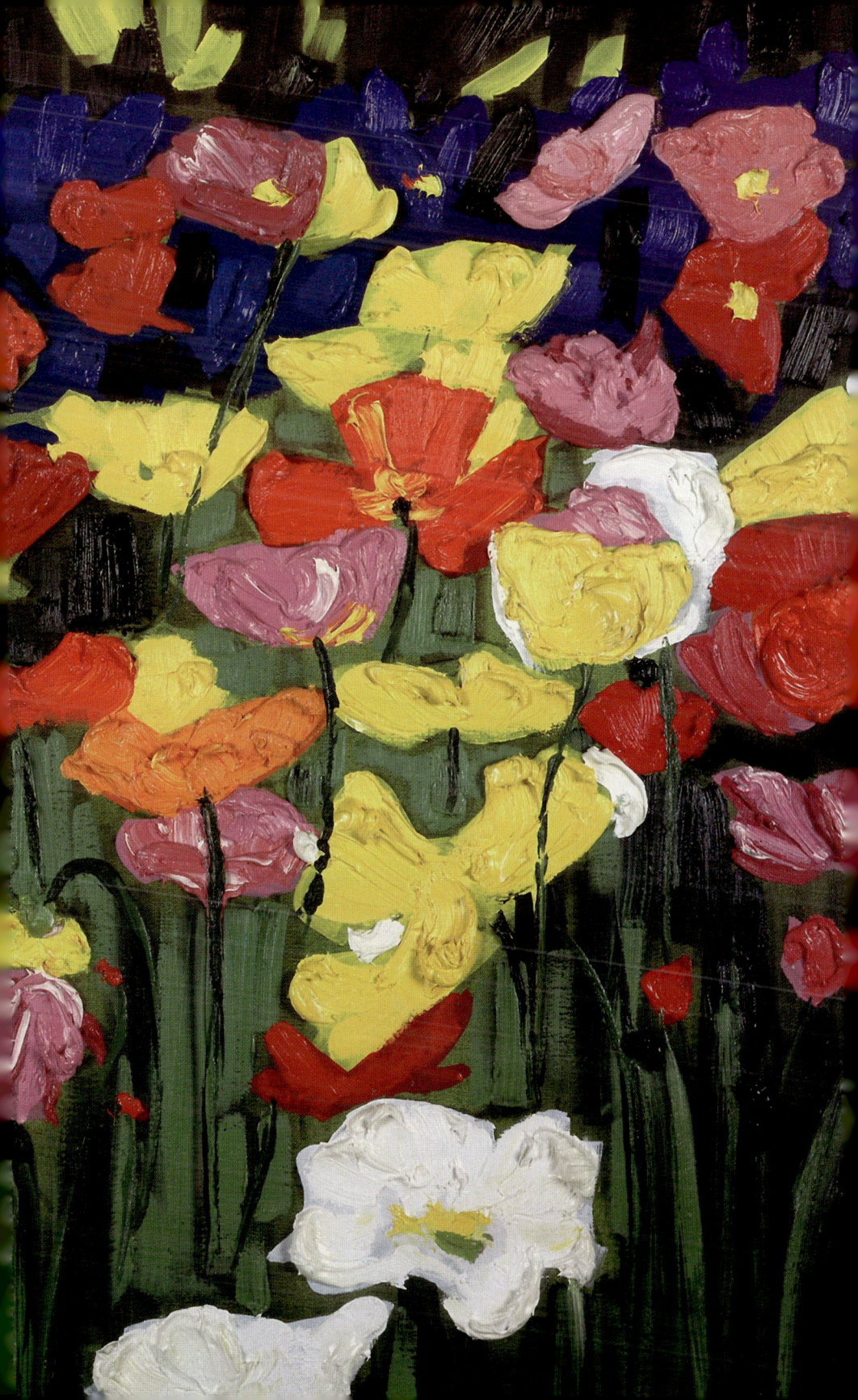

my brush with depression

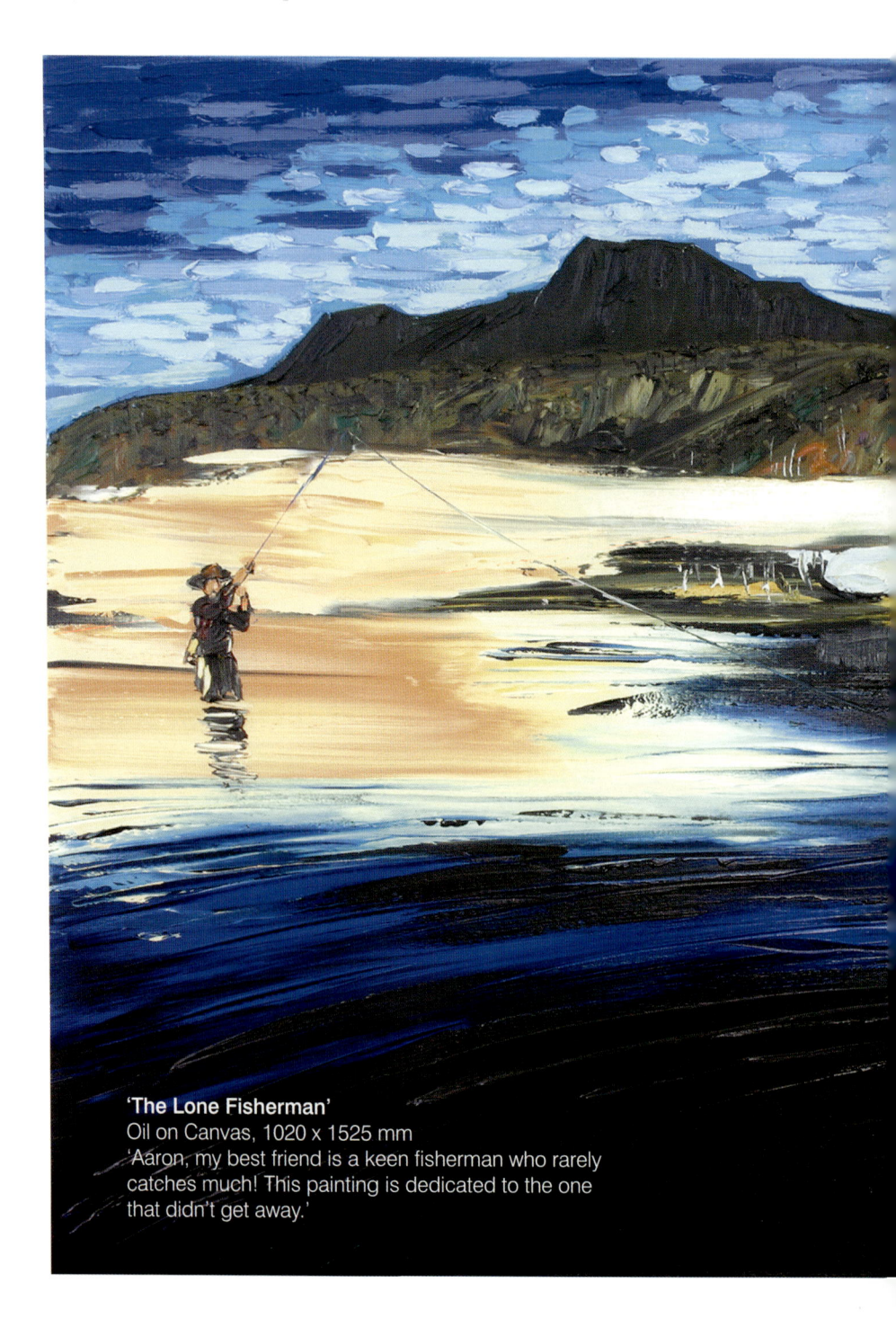

'The Lone Fisherman'
Oil on Canvas, 1020 x 1525 mm
'Aaron, my best friend is a keen fisherman who rarely catches much! This painting is dedicated to the one that didn't get away.'

the greg wilson gallery

greg wilson — 211

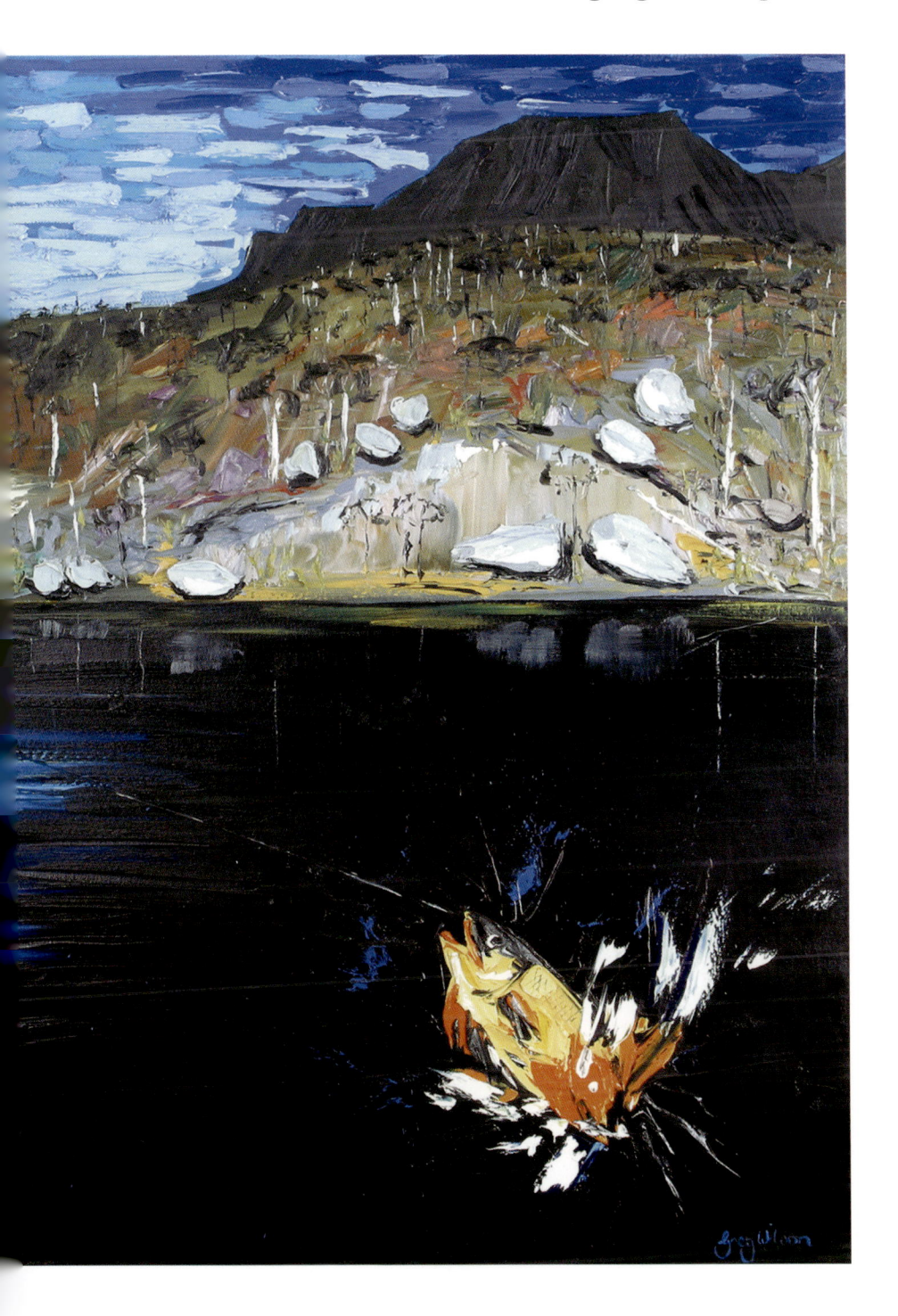

my brush with depression

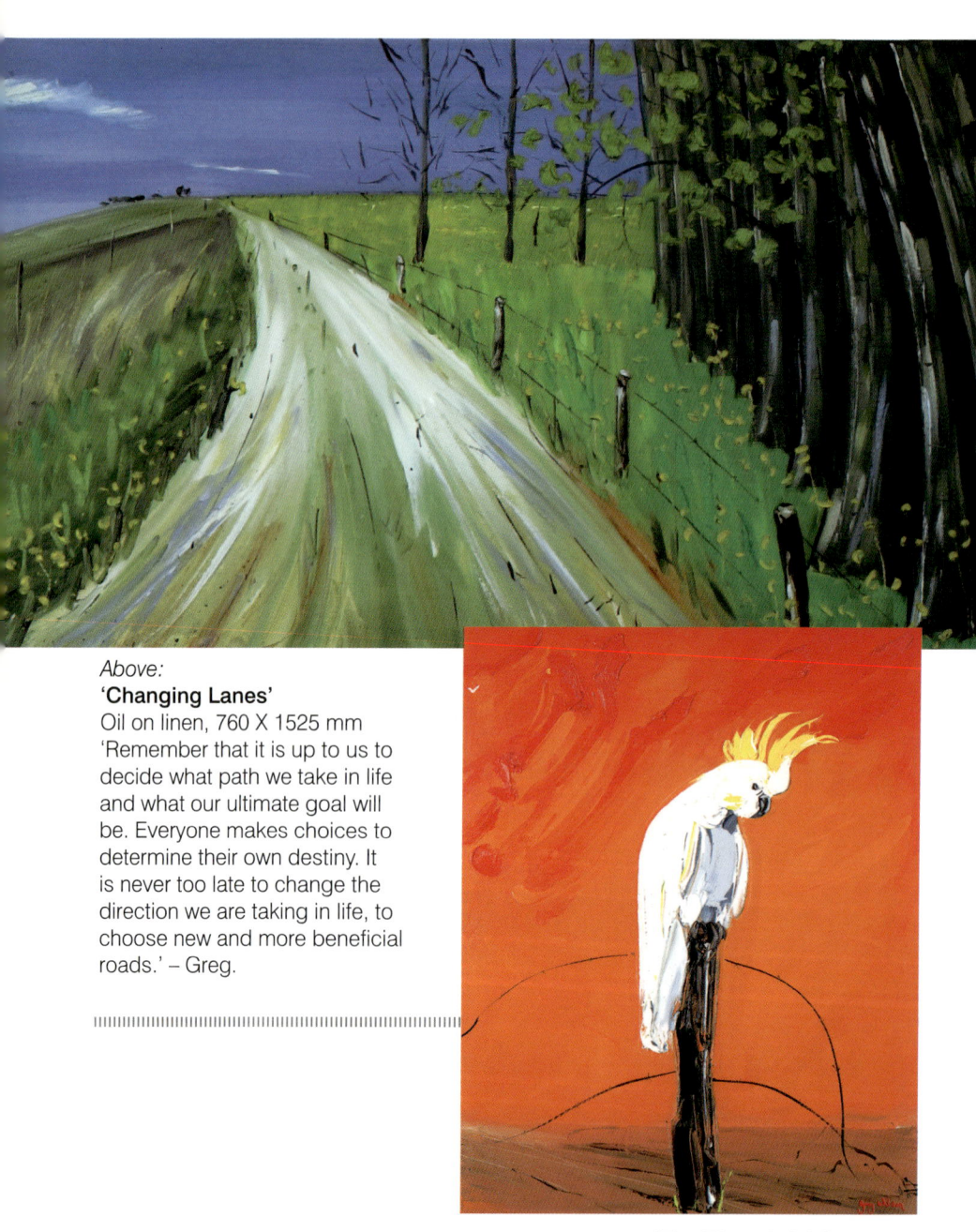

Above:
'Changing Lanes'
Oil on linen, 760 X 1525 mm
'Remember that it is up to us to decide what path we take in life and what our ultimate goal will be. Everyone makes choices to determine their own destiny. It is never too late to change the direction we are taking in life, to choose new and more beneficial roads.' – Greg.

'The Thoughtful Cockatoo'
Oil on linen, 760 X 610 mm

after the gallery had opened, and noticed the colourful selection of artworks in the gallery as she walked through the village. She called in to have a closer look, and was soon reading Greg's profile from the brochure that we display on the wall. When she finished reading she began looking closely at each of the works.

Josie noticed that as she stood in front of a striking landscape called 'Vibrant Day' she appeared to be wiping tears from her eyes with a tissue she had taken discreetly from her handbag. Josie thought there might be more to what she saw than a woman observing a beautiful painting – although she knew that Greg's art did sometimes provoke such a response – and quietly asked if there was something the matter or if she could help in any way.

The woman replied by confiding that she had a 17-year-old daughter who had recently shocked her by disclosing that she had entertained thoughts of suicide during a particularly severe attack of depression. Seeing Greg's paintings and appreciating that something so beautiful could come from someone who had suffered so much was quite moving for her.

The mother confessed that she did not know how to discuss depression with her daughter and had always shied away from the subject whenever it looked like being introduced into their conversations. She asked if there was any way we could help her. We were able to reassure her that she was doing the most important thing for her daughter by offering her love and support, but it was just as vital that she encourage her daughter to discuss her feelings openly and without any embarrassment. Greg told her that any talk of suicide should always be taken seriously and usually represented a desperate cry for help.

He suggested that she arrange for someone to be constantly with her daughter during the darkest moments of her depression and that she seek professional assistance as soon as possible.

The mother thanked us sincerely for our advice and time and told us that she felt much better equipped to broach the subject with her daughter.

The same woman contacted us shortly afterwards and told us her daughter had burst into tears of relief when she learned what had transpired at the gallery. Both mother and daughter had then engaged in one of the most open and candid conversations they had ever shared. In the middle of the exchange the daughter had embraced her mother and told her that she had been feeling so alone and so confused recently that she had once again been planning to terminate her life, this time with an overdose of sleeping tablets. She promised to abandon all such desperate measures in future, now that she felt she could confide in her mother.

Such stories were a constant source of encouragement for us, especially for Greg. Suicide is the most difficult consequence of depression for us to accept. It involves so much pain and suffering for everyone involved, victim and friends, both before and after the event. Oftentimes there is a huge burden of guilt left with the family or friends.

I can remember the self-reproach I inflicted upon myself after Greg's attempt to take his life. I berated myself that I had not been observant enough to detect the ominous signs; I had not been receptive enough when he may have wished to discuss his concerns with me; or I had not been patient enough to spend the time with him and perhaps allay his fears. I felt overcome with a dreadful sense of guilt for a long time after the terrible experience!

It was only on further deliberation that I realised that Greg had done everything he possibly could to conceal his real intentions from all of us. In some cases, this reluctance to discuss the problem is the reason there is no intervention at all. He admitted that outwardly he tried to convince us that he was getting better, while inwardly he was in turmoil.

Using the knowledge gained from these previous incidents really gives Greg a great sense of satisfaction. These experiences continually motivate him to help others. Yet sometimes it has been others who have both motivated and inspired Greg. One of them came from a most unlikely and unexpected source!

chapter twenty-four
an unforgettable encounter

One of the most remarkable moments in the gallery was the time Frank Ancona came to visit. Nothing could have prepared me for what was about to happen on that day, and the memories will be forever imprinted in my mind.

I remember the morning clearly. I was working on my computer at the back of the gallery when Josie called to me from the front room. 'Aaron, come out here. There's someone that I'd like you to meet.'

I strolled out into the front area of the gallery and saw a tall gentleman with broad shoulders waiting expectantly. He introduced himself with a strong American accent and told me that his name was Frank Ancona. His face was wreathed in a beaming smile, and I liked him immediately. Something about him told me that he was a warm and genuine human being, and as our conversation progressed I felt that my initial assessment had been correct. After we had exchanged hellos and observed the normal courtesies he explained that he was a visitor from New York on a brief holiday to Australia. He had come to the Hunter Valley to visit the Gardens and to sample some of the local wines. He had noticed the gallery and decided to drop in for a quick look at some of the art.

I offered to make him a cup of coffee while he inspected some of Greg's work, and as I was boiling the water I noticed that he had stopped in front of a recent work that Greg had completed. It was a sculpture that he had designed in the aftermath of September 11, 2001. It was meant to represent the ground zero site in New York, and the work was titled 'Come to Light'. A short caption beneath the piece read: 'The flame of liberty and hope continues to burn brightly, even in the face of the greatest adversity.'

Frank stood transfixed in front of the work and there came over his face a look of such sadness that I felt reluctant to disturb his quiet reflection. Eventually, however, I asked him if everything was okay. He turned slowly towards me and told me in a faltering voice that he had been a part of that terrible event and that he would never forget the horror and tragedy of what had been the worst day of his life. He told me that he had been a New York firefighter.

Like most Australians, I had seen the dreadful scenes on television as the terrible drama had unfolded when terrorists crashed two jet airliners into the World Trade Center. I can remember clearly the incredulity and revulsion that I had felt as the nightmarish scenes were relayed to our living rooms.

I waited in respectful silence as Frank composed himself and then began to relate his own recollections of the tragic event. His words sent a chill down my spine as he informed me that his group of firefighters, or 'ladder' as they call them in the States, was one of the first to arrive at the scene. Some of his closest friends had perished in the ensuing collapse of one of the towers.

He told me how he had woken up that morning around 7.30 and flicked on the television shortly afterwards to catch the latest news bulletin. The TV Channel was replaying the amateur video of the first plane as it hit the Center. Frank watched in disbelief, thinking that maybe they were showing a preview of some new horror flick from Hollywood, but soon realised that this was a real-life tragedy that was being reported.

He raced to the bedroom, donned his fireman's outfit and drove frantically to the scene of the devastation. He recalls that even when he saw the burning tower for the first time he still found it hard to believe that such a thing could have happened.

an unforgettable encounter

When he arrived at the scene he was told that some members of his Ladder 132 had already entered the North Tower. As he looked up to scan the building, he was horrified to see that some of the desperate workers and visitors to the floors above the inferno were now leaping from the building. He could hardly believe his eyes.

Realising that it would be almost impossible to make headway against the stampeding mob of terrified individuals now rushing from the tower, Frank did what he could to direct and assist them. When the South Tower began to collapse, he had no other option but to flee and seek shelter at the first available refuge point.

When the blinding and choking pall of dust had settled, Frank eventually returned to the devastated area to find that the towers had been reduced to debris and rubble. He spent the next few hours assisting the wounded and helping the ambulance personnel remove the bodies of those who had not survived the holocaust.

It was only when some semblance of order had been restored that he learned of the fate of seven of his workmates from Ladder 132. They had all been inside the South Tower when it collapsed. They were just some of the hundreds of New York City firemen who gave their lives in the course of their duty that fateful day.

As I listened to Frank's story unfold and saw the grief and deep sorrow etched on his face, I found it hard to hold back my own tears. When he told me that he had lost forty-five other close friends to the disaster we both fell silent, as if we had both agreed to observe a respectful period of mourning.

As the powerful impact of what he had experienced began to sink in, I wondered to myself how I would have reacted in those circumstances. I wondered if I would have had the courage to venture into the danger zone with no thought other than to help those who might need my assistance. I told Frank that I felt as if I'd met a real-life hero and how much I admired his preparedness to risk his own life to save others. When Frank then asked me if I understood why he had been so moved by Greg's sculpture, I nodded in silent acquiescence.

Later, when I rang Greg in his studio and told him about the remarkable encounter, he immediately began to wonder if there was any way that we could donate the sculpture to Ladder 132 and send it across to their Department in New York.

The following day I was able to tap into the local grapevine and ask if anyone had met this amazing firefighter from New York, and did they have any idea where he might be staying. It wasn't long before the answers were provided, and I was able to contact Frank at his hotel.

He was lost for words when we outlined our plan to him, but when he eventually found his voice he said it would give them all a wonderful lift to think that their deeds had been appreciated by people as far away as the place they called 'Down Under', and that the sculpture would have pride of place in their Fire Department.

It was only a few days later that we had the piece ready for shipping, after we had added a brief message to the work stating: 'May the American

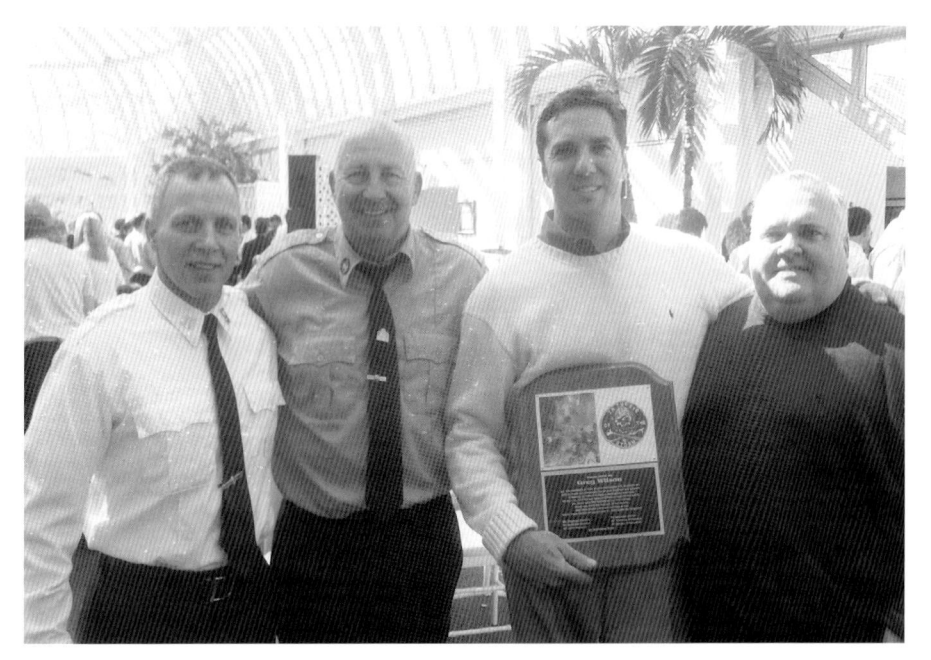

In good company: Fire-Chief John Plante (left), veteran fire fighter Frank Ancona, Greg, and Vice President of the International Association of Firefighters Kevin Gallagher. The courageous fireman presented Greg with a plaque for his art contribution to the Brooklyn fire department during a commemorative luncheon held in the Brooklyn Botanical Gardens.

an unforgettable encounter

spirit continue to shine. Best wishes from Greg Wilson and all your mates Down Under.'

When the sculpture arrived some two weeks later, Greg was contacted by the department and was invited to attend a plaque dedication ceremony in New York for the members of Ladder 132 who had lost their lives. He was told that the Fire Chief would like him to present his sculpture to the Ladder in person and attend a dinner for the members of the families who had lost their loved ones in the tragedy of September 11.

Accordingly, two months later, Greg and Josie swapped the peaceful serenity of the Hunter Valley for the frenetic pace of the Big Apple. They were greeted on their arrival by the Fire Chief of Ladder 132, John Plante, and the Vice President of the International Association of Fire Fighters, Kevin Gallagher. Both men expressed their gratitude for such a thoughtful gesture on Greg's part and told him that there would always be a special link, from that day forward, between the Ladder and the Greg Wilson Gallery.

Part of the commemorative observance included a tree planting ceremony that was held in the magnificent Brooklyn Botanical Gardens to pay tribute to each of the firefighters who had lost their lives. During a luncheon organised for 300 guests, Greg was presented with a plaque of recognition from the fire department to thank him for his thoughtfulness and his generous contribution.

During the rest of their stay in New York Greg and Josie spent most of their time in Frank's company and found it hard to say goodbye when the day came for them to return home. Their admiration for such an outstanding individual had grown considerably during their stay. The tragedy that could well have left him bitter and vengeful had instead given him a greater appreciation of the value of human life and the time that we each have left to enjoy it. They both felt privileged to be able to call such an outstanding individual their friend.

One of Greg's first assignments when he was back at work was to replace the donated sculpture with another that would commemorate their visit to America and the great spirit of friendship they had experienced. It featured the twin towers in a mirror-like finish and was entitled 'Reflections'. It carries a small replica of the Australian coat of arms. As Greg explained to Frank, the kangaroo and the emu are two animals that are unable to take a backward step (just like Frank and his heroic firefighter friends) and could also be seen as representing the ongoing alliance and friendship that both of our countries enjoy with each other.

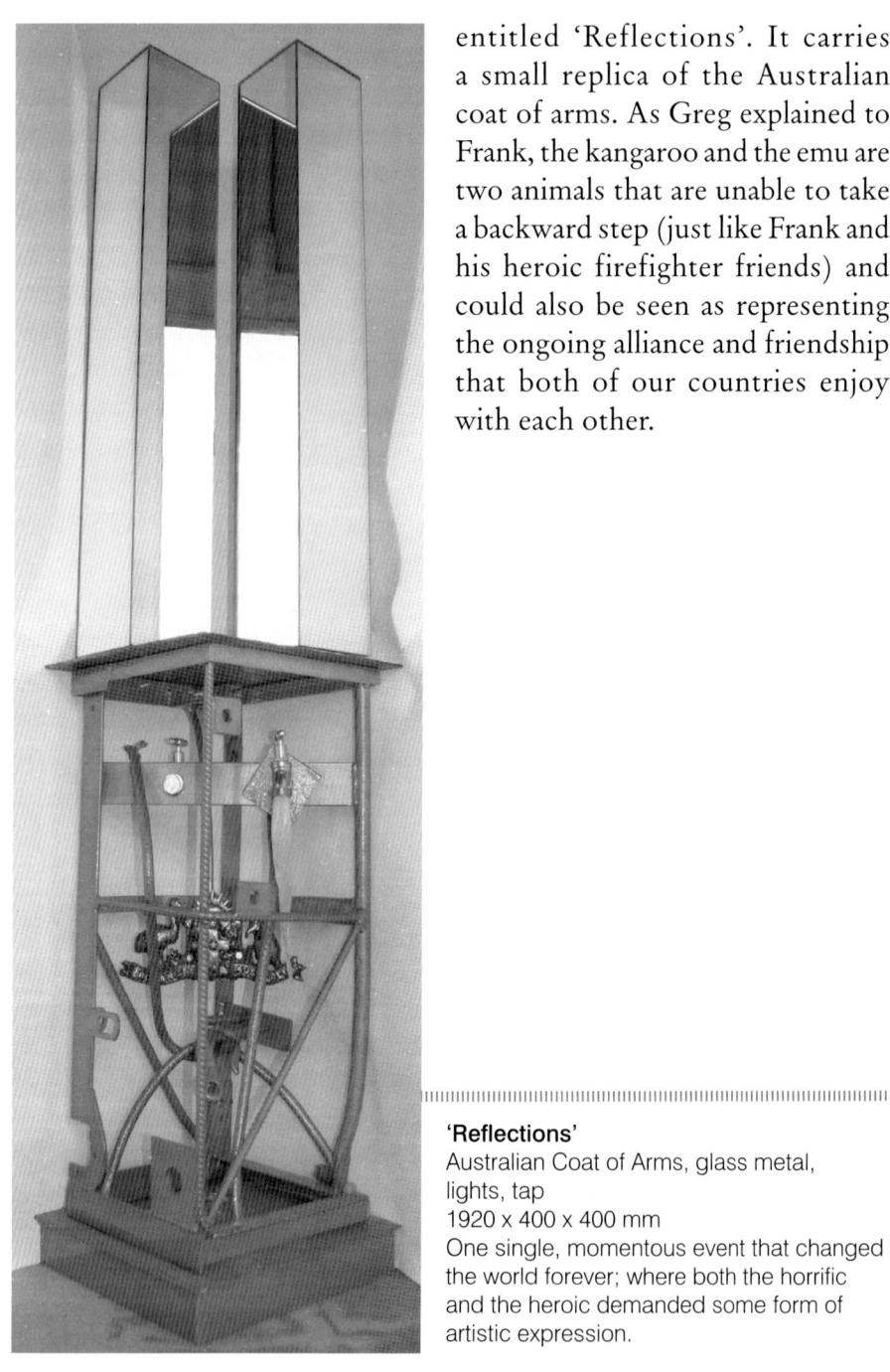

'Reflections'
Australian Coat of Arms, glass metal, lights, tap
1920 x 400 x 400 mm
One single, momentous event that changed the world forever; where both the horrific and the heroic demanded some form of artistic expression.

chapter twenty-five
sharing his inspirational story

'The grapes will be ready to pick soon,' Greg remarked to me one afternoon as he eyed the large bunches that had grown on the vines closest to his studio. I removed a small handful of the ripening green fruit, and squirted some of the juice into my mouth. The bitterness that I tasted caused me to grimace in disgust. Greg realised my stupidity and chuckled. When the acid taste finally left my mouth and I was able to speak, I asked Greg if he would like a peach from our fruit tree. After all, wine grapes certainly hadn't eased my hunger pains.

'No thanks,' he replied and he headed for his studio to continue work on 'The Seat of Wisdom,' a coloured steel chair made out of recycled metal and gemstones. He had told me about the inspiration for this particular work in an earlier discussion we had. 'Sometimes our greatest achievements come in the face of our greatest adversities,' he had stated. His recovery from the accident was hard and austere. His period of recovery was spent in a hard, cold chair, but it was in these difficult circumstances that his future as an artist had begun to crystallise. It certainly was an uplifting message that he was trying to convey through the work.

As his welder sent sparks flying into the air like a fireworks display, I marvelled at the fertility of his imagination, and paused for a moment to consider how lucky I was to witness such a talented artist creating such wonderful and fanciful works.

Desperate to get the lingering unpleasant taste of the sour grapes out of my mouth, I walked hurriedly towards a nearby tree full of fruit. I pulled a succulent peach from a branch and took a large bite. The juice flowed down my chin and dripped onto my shirt. After a short time, when I had swallowed the tasty mouthful, I walked back to Greg's studio and sat on a bench.

As he worked we discussed some of his upcoming speaking engagements. I thought how the sparks that lit up the room were almost an analogy for the way in which Greg was using his motivational talks to bring light into the lives of those with depression. He was being regularly asked to address youth groups, church groups, mental health groups and even private audiences.

His willingness to give such talks came as quite as a surprise to me in the beginning. I noticed a transformation in his bearing when it came to public speaking. A normally shy and retiring Greg Wilson talked openly about his experiences without hesitation and with confidence.

When I asked him why he felt compelled to speak to people in this fashion, he told me that as he looked back he no longer feared his past. Nearly ten years on, the mental demons that once threatened his life were now manageable. He still had his illness but he had learned to control it. More than anything else, he told me, he wanted to communicate to people that there is always hope, that it is possible to rid the mind of those demons that sometimes torment the spirit.

I paused for a moment and devoured the rest of my juicy peach.

Greg admitted that when it comes to crowds and public speaking he would much rather avoid them. However, when the topic that he was given related to mental health issues he was really passionate about his talk. He would do whatever he could to help promote better awareness in the community, even if it meant confronting his fear head-on and standing up before a large audience to tell his story.

sharing his inspirational story

Greg believed that men in particular found it hard to talk about themselves and their emotions. His message to them was straightforward, that he was a male who suffered from depression, and if he had learned to deal with it then so could other men as well.

Greg admits now that it would have made a significant difference to him if he had been able to listen to somebody who suffered from depression and be reassured by them that the battle against the disease could be won. When he had his depression there were times when he actually believed that he was the only one who suffered from the condition.

His constant awareness of depression makes it easy for Greg to recreate his fight against the disease when he speaks in public. If he can reach even one person who has been where he has been, then he figures that his own life has been worthwhile. To share what he has learned along the way and to see it ease the torment of others gives him a great deal of personal satisfaction and happiness.

Unfortunately, he comes into contact with sad cases on a disturbingly regular basis. In one month alone, Greg was given the sad news of three people killing themselves as a consequence of depression. When he hears of these cases and the circumstances that surround the victims, he is vividly reminded of his own close calls. He laments the fact that the suicides occur because the support network was either not present or was not well enough equipped to handle the crisis.

At times like this he feels an urgent need to intervene and enlighten whenever he can. He has noticed that his own experiences give added conviction to his advice, and that people who suffer from depression are more inclined to listen to a fellow sufferer!

This is why Greg has become a regular speaker at functions concerned with mental health and why he's been invited to present his story in venues all around Australia. Because depression affects all age groups he talks with quite a cross-section of the community.

During Mental Health Week he has a particularly busy schedule. Greg was invited to attend the opening of Mental Health Week 2003, at Sydney's Government House. He was asked to be a guest speaker along with Jessica Rowe, Damien Lovelock, vocalist of the band The Celibate

Rifles and Frank Sartor, the Acting Minister for Health. Greg was given a special certificate of recognition for his contribution to services in the mental health field. Greg was delighted that dedicated Cessnock mayor, John Clarence, attended the day to lend his support. .

Greg particularly enjoys speaking with senior students at high schools. He feels that this is quite a pivotal time in their lives, and it is not uncommon for depression to rear its ugly head during this phase of young people's development. In his experience, an alarming proportion of young adults become so stressed that they attempt either self-harm or suicide.

His talks to students have been so successful that Senator John Tierney and his wife Pam are keen to arrange for Greg to extend his talks to children. Greg has been asked to be a patron of Lifeline in Newcastle to help people with suicidal tendencies, to raise the profile of Mental Health issues as well as help families understand why and how a person can reach the decision to end their life.

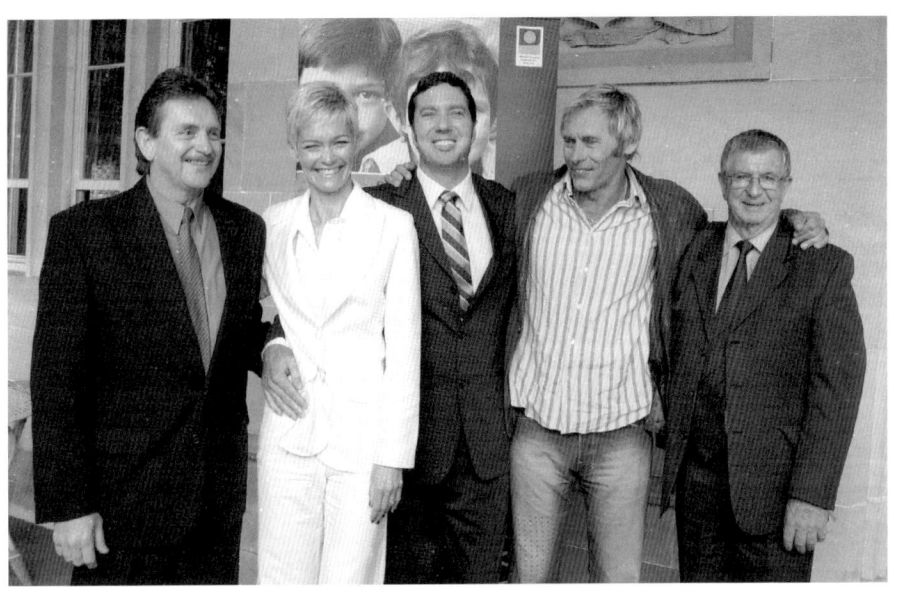

One for all and all for the mental health cause. Don Champagne (left), Jessica Rowe, Greg Wilson, Damien Lovelock and Councillor John Clarence, Mayor of Cessnock, at the opening of Mental Health Week 2003 at Sydney's Government House.

sharing his inspirational story

Pam Tierney told Greg that it was a documented fact that one Australian takes their life every four hours. Every three days somebody takes his or her own life in the Hunter Valley Region. Each day Lifeline answers about three calls relating to suicide.

Greg has also worked to raise money for beyondblue, Australia's national mental health initiative, set up by former Premier of Victoria, Jeff Kennett.

During his talks, Greg relates his own story openly and honestly. He comes across as a genuine person who just wants to make a difference to the lives of others. He tells people that he is not cured, and that he still has depression. With maintenance he has been able to control it. He understands what causes it and how to avoid it.

No topic is too sensitive when he speaks. Greg even talks about his time in the psychiatric ward with a compelling frankness and honesty. Initially, I wondered if this was such a good idea. To me it seemed an intensely private matter, and I felt he might have had serious reservations about its inclusion. Greg, however, says he feels compelled: he needs to discuss every aspect of his illness and to tell the truth! He wants people to know how desperate he felt, so that those with depression or people who may be spending time in mental institutions can listen to his words and know that he can empathise with them and understand their plight.

Greg's willingness to discuss his time in the clinic so candidly has always been a quality I have admired. He talks openly about his experience in the hospital. Never does he seem concerned about the stigma or condemnation from others that could often result from such a detailed and intimate disclosure. His only thoughts are for those living with their depression. By discussing his story honestly and frankly, he hopes it will help others, even if it means he exposes himself to personal misunderstanding and criticism. I greatly respect his courage.

As well as talking to people on the mental health issues, he spends a lot of his time working with children in art classes. During his recovery, Greg's artwork was to provide the ideal medium for giving new meaning to his life, and an ideal opportunity for him to express his innermost feelings through his paintings and sculptures. It became a tool that enabled him to work through some of the problems that he was facing.

He wanted to develop this concept further, drawing on his personal experiences of depression, so that children and teenagers could also benefit from art. Greg did not want others to undergo the suffering and the pain that he had personally endured.

So he decided to provide his own art classes for kids. They aim to provide fun for the children but they also give him an opportunity should the children communicate that they are feeling depressed, to give the participants and their families support and skills to help alleviate any detrimental feelings or thoughts. Josie, Joyce and I have helped Greg arrange these classes.

The idea of having art classes for children occurred to Greg when Josie was working as a natural medicine practitioner from their house at Church Point. One of her clients was a 12-year-old boy named Josh. He was shy, and Greg could tell that he was also quite sensitive. He didn't have much self-confidence and was being bullied at school. Greg decided that he would try and help the boy by talking with him. They went for a walk and Josh told him about his fear of being picked on, saying that he often felt nervous at school. Later, when they returned home, Greg made up a canvas for him and suggested he paint. He told Josh that whenever he felt a bit down in life he would often turn to painting to help him get through a sad time.

Josh took to the idea immediately and painted a little beach scene. Greg said it was amazing to see the transformation in his attitude. He was no longer thinking about his problems; instead, he was smiling. He was so proud of his efforts. He took the painting and went home.

His mother later rang Josie and said that Josh had not stopped talking about his time with Greg. She asked him if he would mind painting with Josh some more because she had seen such a dramatic shift in his attitude. Greg said he was really happy to oblige and painted with him regularly during the following month.

At the end of that time his mother entered one of Josh's artworks in the local art show and was absolutely delighted when he won first

sharing his inspirational story

place in his age group. The young boy was ecstatic to have collected first prize. He had never won anything before in his life. When Greg saw how happy painting had made his young protégé, and the dramatic improvement in his attitude, it became a goal of his to one day open his own art school for children.

A year later, when we moved to the Hunter, he began conducting the classes on our property and from the gallery. The classes are continuing to grow in numbers and have meant that we are presently looking for a new location. Councillor John Clarence, Mayor of Cessnock, Kavita Payall, and the staff of Cessnock Council have offered to help us find a bigger location should we ever need it in the local area. It is another example of the dedication and support we have gained through the Council. They have been wonderfully supportive, with a strong commitment to helping the children of the community.

As dusk began to spread the first of its evening shadows across the valley I stood in silence, looking over the rugged and beautiful bushland that stretched out before me. I felt immensely proud of what we had achieved in the short time we had been in the Hunter, and was looking forward to yet another first for our little group: Greg was shortly to make his maiden appearance on national television! I trusted that the beautiful sunset, with its brilliant array of yellows and purples and blues was a favourable omen.

Ben Molenaar and Ginny Fisher at Greg's art classes. It brings great joy to see children come out of themselves during art classes, and use their imagination. The canvasses come alive with their colours and their thoughts.

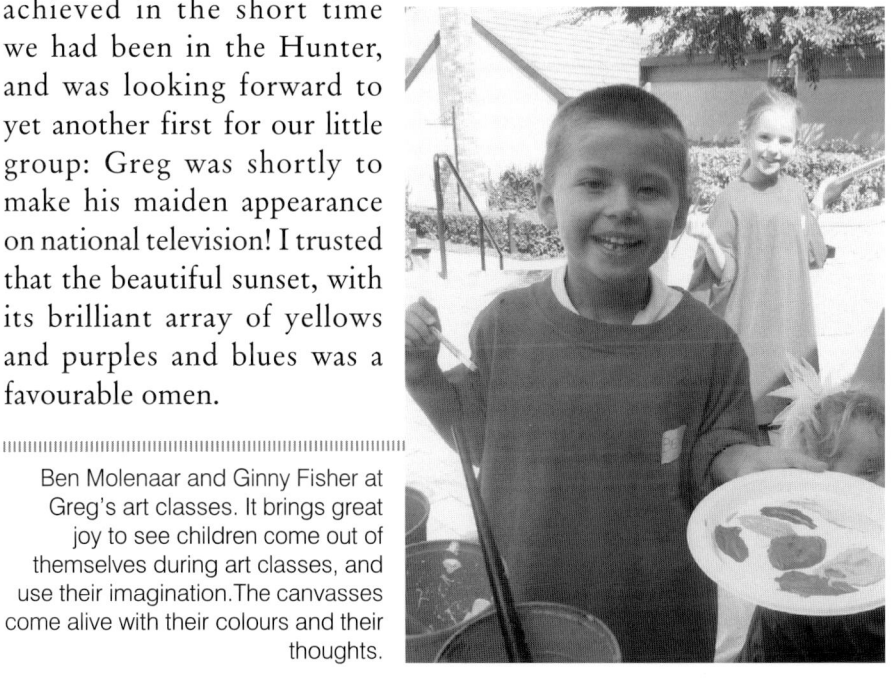

chapter twenty-six

lights, camera, action

I started to feel the excitement mounting in the pit of my stomach the moment the Channel Ten Eyewitness News van pulled up in front of the gallery. Greg had already told me that he was not going to get nervous, but intended to focus on the importance of the story and the seriousness of his message to quell any anxiety he may have felt.

The interview was to have been conducted originally at the Park Hyatt when Greg agreed to hold his exhibition there and donate proceeds from the function to the Mental Health Association of New South Wales Incorporated. Because fierce bushfires had broken out in many parts of the state during that week, however, the camera crews had all been assigned to cover the conflagrations and none was available to do Greg's interview.

Greg greeted Evan Batten, the journalist assigned to cover the story, with a wry comment that it was a case of 'second time lucky' for us, and that he hoped no bushfires would break out in the Hunter to prevent the crew from completing the story.

When the lighting technician began to turn on her special lamps inside the gallery, we were amazed at the transformation to the place. The colours of the paintings seemed exceptionally bright and almost leapt

lights, camera, action

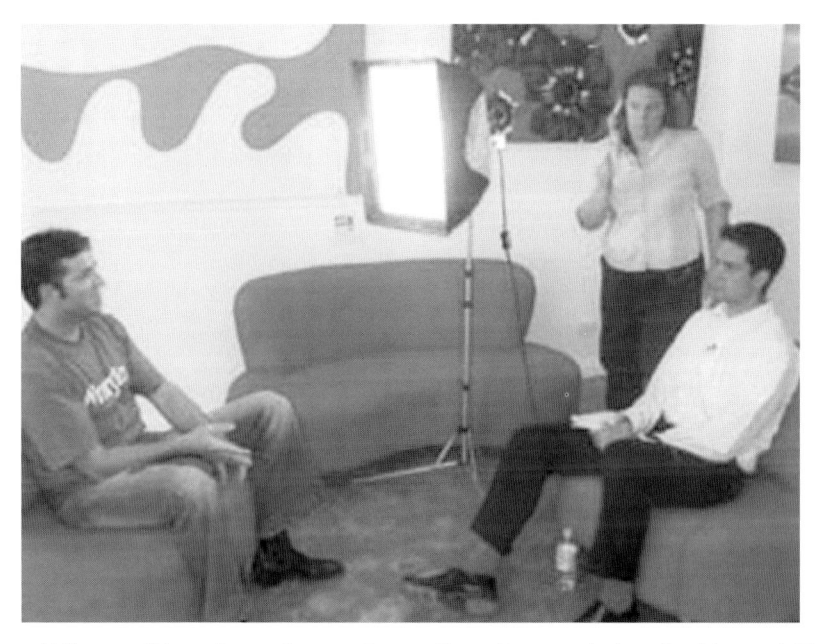

Greg Wilson talking about depression to Evan Batten during the Network Ten interview. Evan's thoughtful and caring personality made it easy for Greg to talk honestly about some of the more traumatic details of his life.

off the canvases. When the spotlight was turned onto Greg's face and he saw his image come up on the nearby monitor, he burst out laughing and said he couldn't believe that he was going to be on TV.

Evan sat Greg on one of the gallery lounges, and took up a position in front of him that was just off camera. He told Greg that since the introduction of videotape interviews were so much easier, simply because any segments that weren't satisfactory could be repeated any number of times until all concerned were happy with the result.

When Evan asked Greg to give him some idea of the message he was hoping to convey to his viewers, Greg summarised his thoughts by telling Evan that approximately one in five Australians suffer from depression; that there is always hope for those suffering from the disease, that it can be managed with the correct medication and a strong support group. Evan had obviously done his homework, and the interview progressed

my brush with depression

seamlessly with few pauses or second takes. He fed a number of pertinent questions to Greg, and it was amazing how much ground had been covered in a short time. They touched on matters relating to suicide, the symptoms of depression, recognising the disease, and its treatment.

Eventually, when there were no more questions and both Evan and Greg were happy with the outcome, the cameraman and lighting technician wrapped up their gear and packed it away in their van. We had time for a quick lunch of cut sandwiches before they headed off down our driveway on their way back to Sydney.

It was two days before the story went to air on Eyewitness News. Greg, being so deeply committed to raising the profile of mental illness and to alleviating people's depression, watched on anxiously, hoping the piece would have an impact. We all held our breath when Jessica Rowe introduced the news piece, but when Greg first appeared on the screen, we all started grinning like a row of Cheshire cats. It just seemed so funny to see him on the evening news. But then we listened intently as Evan directed the first question to Greg. We were riveted to the screen. Evan had done a great story and had certainly captured the real essence of Greg's message. I couldn't help but think what a powerful medium television was, and what a wonderful tool it could be when used to bring messages like Greg's to the world.

We were delighted with the piece. Not only because it had presented the gallery in such a favourable light, but because the interview had helped draw attention to Greg's ongoing crusade to help sufferers of depression. It had some really positive repercussions for the Mental Health Association NSW Incorporated as well. A number of people contacted the organisation through its website address which was displayed on the screen during the interview. The graph on the facing page, compiled by Gillian Church, shows the large number of enquiries that the television coverage generated.

Greg was so thrilled that his efforts produced such an outstanding response. He hoped that there were some positive results for those who contacted the organisation on the night of the interview. Deep down, he later confided to me, he even hoped that someone who had seen the

lights, camera, action

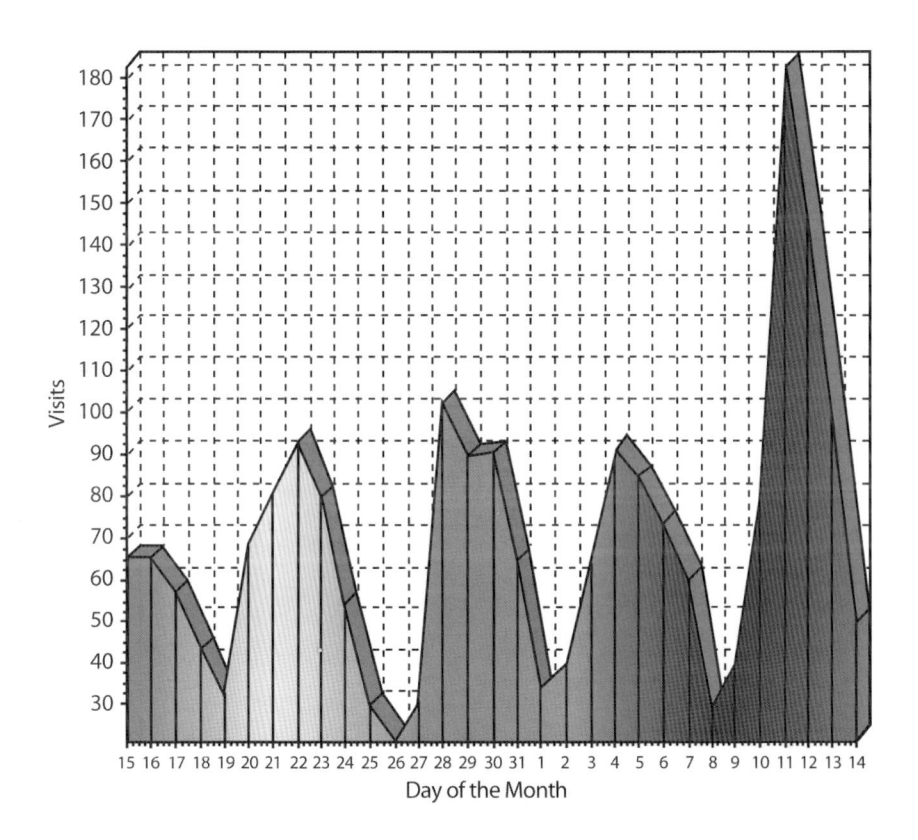

Source: Mental Health Association of NSW Inc. The spike in the graph shows a dramatic upsurge in the website hits shortly after Greg's television appearance.

programme had taken his message to heart, and that maybe, just maybe, his intervention in somebody's life had even prevented an attempted suicide.

Channel Ten's broadcast generated a lot of interest in Greg's message and work and there was a steady stream of requests for interviews on television and radio over the next few years.

ABC Television filmed a documentary on his life for the Australian Story, a half-hour programme that profiles the lives of interesting Australians. It was this show that really propelled Greg into the spotlight. The producer of the show had been contacted by Kavita Payell from the Cessnock City who believed Greg would be a excellent candidate for

my brush with depression

the show. I sent a brief biographical account of his life to the producer and waited. Not long after, he came to see us for a series of interviews. A week later they phoned us with the good news that Greg was going to be featured in the show.

The three-crew members, John, Quentin and Ross, went to extraordinary lengths to tell Greg's story. At one point during filming, the producer and cameraman climbed a tree to ensure that they could get the best angle.

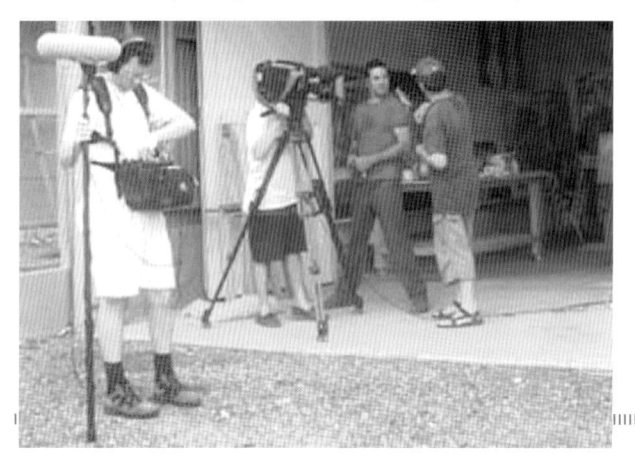

Sound recordist Ross Byrne, cameraman Quentin Davis, and producer John Millard were more like friends than film crew during the filming of the ABC documentary 'Australian Story'. They produced an enthralling narrative of the artist's remarkable odyssey that saw him eventually settle in the Hunter Valley.

Passers-by glanced at the tree in surprise, unsure of why two grown men were perched precariously in the branches above.

We were impressed with the professionalism and the dedication that the team exhibited in their efforts to convey the essence of Greg's story. Greg is delighted that the estimated audience of nearly one and a half million people got an insight into what his life had been like.

We were overwhelmed with the e-mails and phone calls we received for weeks after the show was broadcast. Even though our contact details were not listed on the programme we were inundated with enquiries about Greg and his work. One phone call would end and immediately the phone would ring again. Many people felt compelled to contact us and tell us how touching the story was. Many said they had been given new hope in their struggles with depression.

The wheel cover of my four-wheel drive carried an image of one of Greg's paintings, along with the address and telephone number of the gallery. One viewer obviously recognised the vehicle shortly after the programme went to air, and left a message under the windscreen wiper. Although we had never met face to face, I was quite touched by his note:

'Mr Cootes,

I saw the Australian Story the other night. I am a long-term sufferer of depression and the show gave me great hope. This week I stopped trying to cope on my own and sought medical assistance. I admire Greg for working through it and I admire you for giving him support.'

When I read this letter I was deeply moved. To know that Greg's story had touched so many lives and prompted others to get help gave me a personal satisfaction that I had never before experienced in my life. I felt we were contributing in a significant way to the battle against depression. If people were overcoming their inhibitions and actively seeking help, then we were definitely making a difference. It made the four of us feel quite splendid!

The interviews now follow a familiar pattern. Greg begins by discussing his artwork but inevitably draws the conversation back to his favourite topic of mental health. Greg would prefer not to be the centre of attention on these occasions, but he does it for one reason. He understands that if he continues to conduct his crusade in such a public forum, then the profile of mental health issues will certainly be elevated as well.

chapter twenty-seven

international recognition

At the beginning of 2004, our life was beautifully balanced. We were selling paintings and sculptures, making deliveries, maintaining the property, playing the odd round of golf, and entertaining the occasional guest.

One of our favourite visitors was Barbara Williams, a friend of Josie's who occasionally took a break from her extremely busy professional life to spend some time with us. She was always afforded a special welcome because we enjoyed her company so much. She would entertain us with the latest news from the 'big smoke', as we now regarded Sydney, and keep us informed of the latest political developments, happening in Canberra.

Josie and Barbara had first met in 1995, when Barbara was working as an executive assistant to the chairman of Blackmores Limited, a company that sold natural healthcare products such as vitamins, minerals, herbs, and nutrients. Josie would make regular trips to the health food supplier to pick up orders for her patients. Whenever Josie went to collect her goods she and Barbara would chat. It was not long before they were meeting outside the work place for coffee and soon they became close friends.

international recognition

Before her appointment to the position at Blackmores, Barbara had worked as a private secretary to five senior politicians, two of whom were our State Premiers, the Honourable Nick Greiner and the Honourable John Fahey. She enjoyed the pace of life at this level and the involvement with some of the country's leading decision makers. She had little hesitation, therefore, when she was asked to leave Blackmores and return to Canberra to take up a position as the senior private secretary to our Australian Prime Minister, the Honourable John Howard.

The ensuing period from 1996 to 2002 was the busiest period of Barbara's life, and her time was divided between living in Sydney and Canberra and accompanying the Prime Minister on his national and overseas engagements. Whenever she came to Sydney she always tried to include a quick visit to her friend, Josie, to catch up on all the local news. In 2002 she decided that a change of pace was in order and when asked to accept the position of secretary to the Speaker in Federal Parliament, she readily accepted the new assignment.

When Josie first introduced me to Barbara, I was intrigued as the story of her fascinating life unfolded. I listened in amazement as she recalled the times she had spent in the company of some of the most well-known and recognisable personalities on the world stage. She recounted her unexpected encounters with people like Nelson Mandela, Princess Diana, the Queen and the Duke of Edinburgh, as well as a number of American Presidents, including George Bush Senior and Bill Clinton.

She had one experience, however, that made me shudder when she recounted the details. She had been attending an official visit to Washington with the Prime Minister and was due to fly to New York on the following day. The date was 11 September in 2001. It was the day that the plane, hijacked by terrorists, was deliberately flown into the heart of the Pentagon.

The Prime Minister and his party were immediately advised that Air Force Two was waiting to transfer them to Hawaii. It was on the way to the airport that Barbara witnessed one of the most horrifying scenes that she has ever seen: the remaining tail section of the crashed airliner protruding grotesquely from the Pentagon building. Barbara described it as one of the most obscene and shocking sights of her life.

I never tired of listening to the stories that Barbara related to us, especially those that involved her extracurricular activities – these included charitable works for breast cancer. Her experience from working with people suffering from depression was another great support for Greg also, and Barbara gave freely of her time and advice to help him keep his own depression at bay.

She was extremely generous with the precious few hours of leisure time that she had, and we all grew to love her for her generosity and kind-hearted nature. They were qualities that we greatly admired. Whenever Greg was involved in fund-raising activities for the Mental Health Associations, Barbara was the first to volunteer her help if she had the time available. Not only did she help with our charitable endeavours, however, she was also responsible for organising one of the most exciting trips and exhibitions that Greg could have imagined.

We were all sitting having lunch one afternoon at our favourite eatery in the Valley, Beltree@Margen's Winery. It has a delightful little boutique restaurant that serves seasonal Mediterranean inspired cuisine and provides diners with a splendid view of the surrounding bushland from the verandah. During the course of our meal Barbara asked us about the time Greg and Josie went to New York to meet with the firemen from Frank Ancona's Ladder. They told her that they had been enthralled with the trip and had never stopped talking about the wonderful city that New York was. They also explained how impressed they had been by the bravery and courage of the firefighters on September 11, and how Frank had become such an inspiration to them both.

Greg told Barbara he enjoyed the trip so much that he had vowed to return some day if he possibly could, not only as a tourist but as a serious artist. He said that he had visited quite a number of galleries in the city and believed that he could hold his own with many of the works that he had seen on display. He acknowledged, however, that it would probably take him years and years of hard work before he could ever hope to realise such a dream.

international recognition

When Barbara almost casually observed that it might not necessarily take that long to achieve his goal, Greg's interest was instantly aroused. He asked her what she had meant by such a remark. Barbara replied by telling Greg that she knew someone who could probably give him some guidance and assistance in arranging a showing of his works in the great metropolis.

Greg was astonished and for a moment he didn't quite know how to frame his next question. He asked Barbara if she were really serious and if she really thought that there was a possibility that he could actually display his paintings to the Americans. Barbara smiled when she saw the incredulity on Greg's face, but hastened to reassure him that she had every reason to believe that an exhibition could be arranged.

She informed us that she would approach Ken Allen, the Australian Consul-General in New York. Greg and I were both stunned. We were both completely lost for words as we realised what Barbara was suggesting.

She told us that Ken had just returned to Australia for his annual holiday and that she would get in touch with him as soon as she could to run the idea past him. She would then let us know how she got on and what chance there was of achieving such an incredible objective.

Greg and I were almost falling off our chairs with excitement, still not quite believing that we were actually hearing what Barbara was telling us!

All our doubts were dispelled the following week, however, when Barbara invited us to drive to Sydney and meet with Ken at the beachside suburb of Avalon, not far from where Ken resided at Whale Beach. We were both feeling more than a little intimidated before the meeting, having heard so much of Ken's reputation, not only in his previous roles with leading Australian companies, but also as a senior diplomat. Our fears were groundless, however, and we soon felt quite at ease in the company of this impressive Australian.

Ken was only too willing to answer any questions we had about New York and when we asked him about some of the galleries and the art community he was straightforward with his reply. He informed us that

New York was a fiercely competitive market, with artists from all over the world vying for places to show their wares.

When we showed him some copies of Greg's work that we had reproduced in a large, glossy calendar, Ken studied the prints carefully and then thoughtfully stroked his chin. He told us that he really liked what he saw, and after further deliberation delivered the most amazing proposal we had ever heard. He explained that he had organised a few special exhibitions at the Consulate itself during his time in New York. They were rare events, but they had all turned out well. He continued by asking us to forward a resume of Greg's work and a profile to the Consulate. He said he wasn't prepared to promise anything at this early stage but, depending on the timing and any feedback he received from his staff in America, it was quite possible that an exhibition could be arranged.

Greg and I were in a state of sheer amazement, but we tried to control our youthful high spirits as we thanked Ken for his time and pretended that the possibility of a showing in New York was all part and parcel of a young artist's expectations … we were absolutely agog with concealed excitement.

When Ken had driven off, we could hide our elation no longer. We both turned to Barbara, grabbed her roughly in a group bear hug and squeezed her petite frame, bouncing her up and down, until she squealed in protest! Even though nothing had been confirmed, we were certain that Ken had been impressed enough with Greg's work that he would make every effort to get us to New York. It was a window of opportunity that we had never imagined in our wildest dreams.

Joyce had Greg's resume and media kit ready that afternoon, and it was on its way to New York before nightfall.

Three weeks later – a period that seemed more like three months to us – Ken contacted Barbara to let her know his decision. The Consulate had agreed to help support the young Australian artist and would be keen to promote not only his art, but his mental health crusade as well.

We were overjoyed when Barbara rang to give us the good news. Greg and I ran around the house like children, screaming with excitement. We

international recognition

both began dancing, throwing our hands in the air, and spinning around until we collapsed in a heap, totally consumed with laughter.

When Josie heard the commotion, she rushed into the lounge room to see what was wrong. When she saw the strange spectacle that greeted her and heard the news, she showed a little more restraint and simply told us to stop horsing around, that we looked quite ridiculous! Upon which Greg and I immediately resumed our childish antics.

Never before did Greg have such an incentive to throw himself into his work, and he began what he would surely acknowledge as one of the most productive periods of his career. We excitedly discussed the type of work that we thought might appeal to the sophisticated art lovers of New York, and agreed that a strong Australian theme would more readily distinguish his work from any other and provide a refreshing difference to the type of paintings one would expect to find in the Big Apple.

'Swaggie'. Oil on linen, 1010 x 760mm
'When you are touched by the spirit of Australia, you will come to know the joy of the open road, the warmth of sunshine on your face, and the freedom of the wind.'

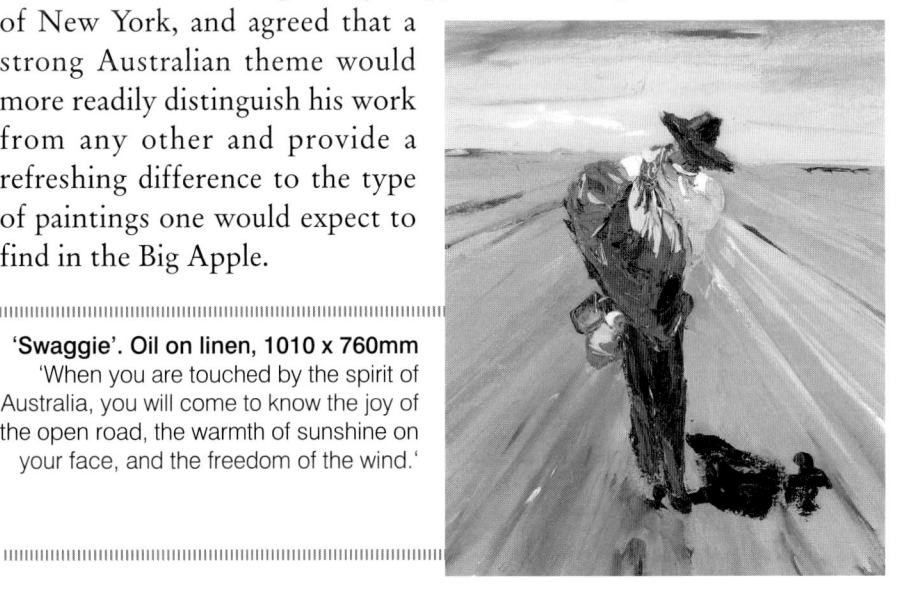

He began painting swaggies and jackaroos and the Australian outback with its strong reds and ochres, embracing the theme that the journey of life had taken Greg down many roads into many different landscapes – some harsh and inhospitable where he has felt isolated and alone, and others quite breathtaking in their beauty, where he has been simply overwhelmed by the dazzling colours and the sheer glory of creation.

Scenes from the Hunter Valley also featured in his collection. The wine region provided him with regular bursts of inspiration: the grapes ripening on the vines, reflections on the dam, early morning mists on the nearby mountains, and the welcome rains that brought new life to the valley.

After four months he selected twelve pieces from his latest works and from those on display at the gallery. We freighted the paintings out a few weeks before the exhibition was due to take place. Not long afterwards we received a glossy invitation in the mail from the Australian Consulate. It was one of the most beautiful things we had ever seen.

The Australian Consul-General,
The Honourable Ken Allen,
cordially invites you and a guest to a
unique evening with Australian Artist Greg Wilson,
showcasing work from his Hunter Valley Gallery.
Wednesday, 30 June 2004
at the Australian Consulate General.

We had to pinch ourselves to make sure we weren't dreaming!

It wasn't long before Greg and Josie had made arrangements to travel abroad. Another friend of Greg's, Dr Dianna Wheeler, also volunteered to tour with the group and lend her support. Dianna was an avid collector of Greg's work and had already acquired seven of his paintings to hang in her unit. (We often refer to her place as the second Greg Wilson gallery and have jokingly offered to leave a stack of our business cards at her front door.) Joyce and I drew the short straws and had to stay behind to keep the gallery open during the rest of the team's absence. As we wistfully waved goodbye and wished them all 'Bon Voyage', they promised to keep us fully informed of all that happened during the trip.

True to their word, they phoned us regularly over the next two weeks and gave us a detailed description of the wonderful opening night of the exhibition. Over two hundred people attended, expressing enthusiastic appreciation for the artist's work and applauding his dedication to the cause of helping people who were suffering from depression. Ken and his dedicated staff did a wonderful job putting on the show.

international recognition

Elizabeth Charles, one of Australia's outstanding 'exports', has a successful fashion outlet in York. After viewing Greg's work at the Consulate, she was so impressed that she offered to sell his work on consignment through her boutique shop in Hudson Street.

During the exhibition Greg was also lucky enough to be introduced to Jennifer Hawkins, the newly crowned Miss Universe, and the two Hunter Valley residents were able to congratulate each other on their recent achievements.

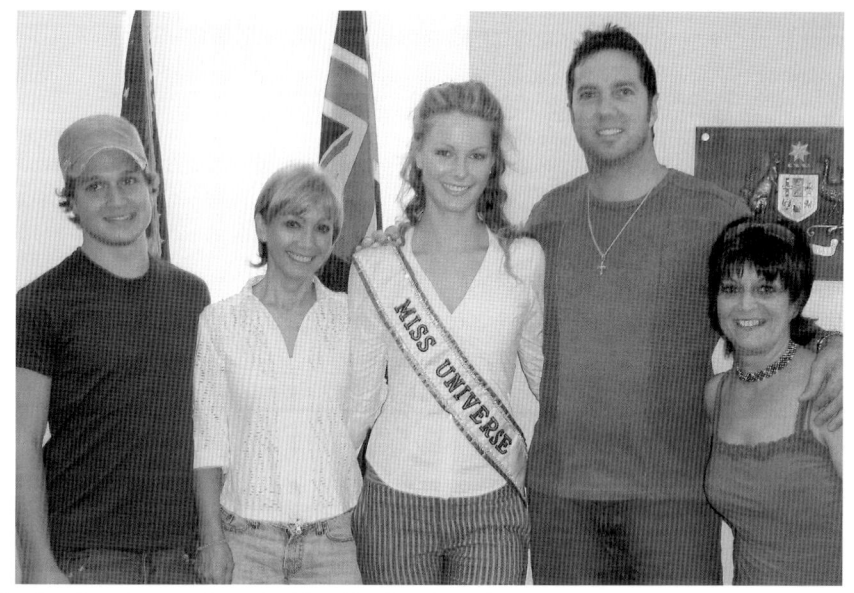

The hard work was all worthwhile. Sharing the celebrations at the Australian Consulate: Jonathon Alder (left), Barbara Williams, Miss Universe Jennifer Hawkins, Greg, and Josie.

There was another group, too, who made a special effort to attend the opening night: members of Ladder 132, the firefighters who had welcomed Greg on his previous trip. By a quirk of fate, Frank Ancona was unable to be present: he was Down Under in Australia, enjoying his annual holidays!

The next two weeks passed in a flurry of activity for Greg and Josie. Ken Allen and his wife Jill proved to be the most wonderful hosts and arranged for them to attend a dinner in Greg's honour, spend some time aboard the 'HMS Enterprise', and be introduced to some influential art critics in New York.

Greg could hardly believe the warmth and hospitality that Ken and his wife extended to the group. They were outstanding ambassadors for Australia, and Greg will be forever grateful for the tremendous support they showed him during his time with them.

Greg confided to me during one of his phone calls that the protocol and proprieties practised in diplomatic circles left him fascinated and a little bemused at times. I chuckled to myself as he described his disorientation on a number of occasions, one of which was the night that he and Josie were invited to Ken's residence for dinner. When he began making comparisons with our humble abode in the Hunter, the contrasts were quite amusing. When he asked me how many times I had been greeted at our front door by a butler; how many times I had been confronted with six separate items of cutlery laid out on a dining table; how many times I had been waited on by a uniformed maid; I warned him not to become too familiar with a lifestyle that we could hardly afford to perpetuate!

During the meal, Ken congratulated Greg on the success of the exhibition and told him that there had been some positive and encouraging feedback from those who had seen his work, especially the Australian expatriates who enjoyed seeing the familiar subjects of Greg's paintings. Overseas visitors had also been complimentary of the work and Ken had been inundated with questions from people wanting to know more about the young Australian artist. They had told Ken how much they loved the unique style of the paintings and the strong colours that were a feature of the landscapes. Ken paid him a final compliment when he echoed the words of one of our promotional campaigns back home: Everyone will want to own a Wilson!

Towards the end of the evening Ken took Greg and Josie on a guided tour of the residence. It provided a wonderful, exciting time of the visit that Greg could never have anticipated. When the group entered one of the entertainment areas of the house, Greg stopped in amazement. Hanging in one corner of the room was an unmistakable work by Arthur

international recognition

Boyd. When Ken pointed out that it was indeed an original by the great artist, Greg could barely contain his admiration, and told Ken about his regular visits to 'Bundanon'; how he regarded Arthur Boyd as his mentor and one of his greatest inspirations.

Then, in what was to become a fairy tale for Greg, Ken put forward an unexpected proposition. He asked Greg if he would like to hang his work alongside Arthur Boyd and in the Consulate. Greg was dumbfounded. Just to view one of Boyd's original works was a great joy in itself, but to be asked to display his own work alongside his mentor would for him be a dream come true. He told Ken that such an offer was one of the greatest honours he had ever been accorded.

When Greg and Josie finally said goodbye and thanked their hosts effusively for such a wonderful evening, Greg said he floated down the street, and had to pause while the enormity of Ken's offer began to sink in. He was choked with emotion as the magnitude of what had just unfolded dawned on him. Never in his wildest dreams did he imagine that his work would find its way onto the hallowed walls of the Australian Consulate in New York. Even more unbelievable, his work would be displayed alongside one of Australia's great painters, Arthur Boyd. Greg suddenly realised that all the hardships, the struggles of the past decade had finally paid off. It was the proudest moment in his career. In fact, he rated the exhibition and his time in New York among the best experiences of his life.

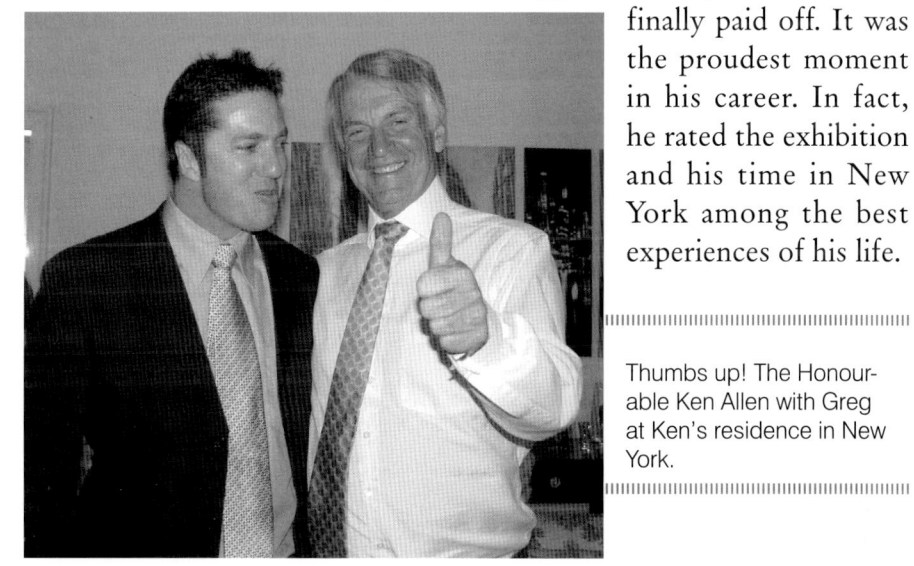

Thumbs up! The Honourable Ken Allen with Greg at Ken's residence in New York.

greg wilson — 243

chapter twenty-eight
the rainbow's end

It is one of those evenings when the Hunter Valley weaves its own special magic and favours its residents with a crystal clear night, almost demanding a reverential silence and awe. My gaze is drawn skyward to the brilliant display that greets me as I make my way to a favourite spot on a hilltop near our property.

The sky is ablaze with stars, and the full moon sheds a soft light over the vineyards and the sleeping village below me. I imagine Van Gogh sitting beside me and informing me that it was just such a scene that inspired his wonderful masterpiece, 'Starry Night'. It is one my favourite works.

It is not the first time that I have reflected on the tragic life of the great Dutch master. There are times, in fact, when I almost believe that his spirit has been reincarnated in my young artist friend. Although I sometimes chide myself for being far too presumptuous, I still consider some of the similarities quite extraordinary.

Both were gifted with an undeniable passion for their art. Both suffered from severe bouts of depression and had stints in mental hospitals. Both were jaded by city life and sought refuge in the country. Both found expression for their anguish and pain through their artwork. Van Gogh sliced off the lobe of his ear; Greg drove a nail through his hand. Vincent

the rainbow's end

aspired to be a minister and teacher; Greg teaches art to children and dedicates himself to the cause of mental health issues. Van Gogh relied heavily on the support of his brother Theo; Greg had Josie – as well as myself and Joyce – to assist him through his crises.

Tragically, Vincent ended his life in 1890, aged 37, with a self-inflicted gunshot wound to his chest. He despaired of ever being cured or of overcoming his loneliness. Greg Wilson attempted to take his own life with a deliberate overdose and almost succeeded.

It always makes me sad to think how misunderstood, lonely and desperate Van Gogh must have been in those final haunting days. It is hard to imagine that one of the world's most respected artists died feeling a failure. How terrible that he was not accorded the recognition he deserved while he was still alive. In his lifetime he had completed some fifteen hundred oil paintings and drawings, but had sold only one at the time of his death. It is an incredible contradiction that someone who had so many reasons to live wanted so desperately to die.

As I begin to make my way back down the hill towards our property, I am overcome with a sense of melancholy as I wonder how many other souls, with their own range of talents and reasons to live, have taken that final desperate step as well. Nearly one million people commit suicide each year – and that is one million too many!

I pause for a moment by the dam, where my spirits are revived by the reflection of the moon and stars on the surface. I'm gradually overcome by a reassuring wave of gratitude that washes over me. Even though there are times when Greg feels the spectre of his depression still lurking in the shadows, when even his love of painting momentarily recedes, the real crisis seems to have passed. I hope and pray that his worst days are behind him, even though the memories will forever remain as a vivid reminder of the frightening experiences we have been through together. Greg has gradually learned to cope with his illness and knows that he can always rely on our support.

I am no longer afraid of his depression. I understand that Greg is prone to recurring cycles of hope and despair. I accept it as a part of who he is and do everything possible to help if I can.

my brush with depression

There was no defining moment, no key to unlocking the door of his depression. There was the medication, there was the diet, there was the move to a more peaceful and carefree lifestyle in the country, there was his new-found strength of mind, and there was his art and the sense of meaning it gave his life. But Greg is convinced that above all else it was the support of his friends that was the most crucial element in his recovery.

Greg still has his illness, and doctors have not as yet come up with an absolute cure. However, his depression is now under control. He is delighted that life has given him another chance. He wants to continue portraying the beauty of a world that he has rediscovered.

He acknowledges, and has come to terms with the inescapable fact, that he has a mental illness through causes that are completely unknown to him. It does not mean that he hasn't been able to keep it at bay and live a happy and successful life. His progress has been truly remarkable: at age thirty-three both his reputation and the demand for his work are growing appreciably.

He has slowly conscripted a willing army of helpers to achieve his goal of bringing hope and light to the thousands of victims of depression.

His business is growing steadily both in Australia and overseas, and his works are regularly being shown to an appreciative group of patrons. Already a number of collectors possess multiple selections of his paintings and sculptures. Another interesting project on the drawing board is a proposed exhibition in London.

Don Champagne, the Manager of the Hunter Export Centre, has helped showcase his work for an expanding international market. He has invited Greg to be one of a number of Hunter Valley contributors at a special shop in downtown Shanghai. Some of his work is already on show at the Peace Building as part of the China Made Easy initiative.

Greg has also recently joined forces with Tyrrell's wines, one of Australia' oldest and most awarded wine making families. They're using his artwork to label a new selection of premium wines. Through this association we have also been fortunate enough to sample an assortment of Pauline Tyrrell's cooking. The lamb roast and the apple cake were

the rainbow's end

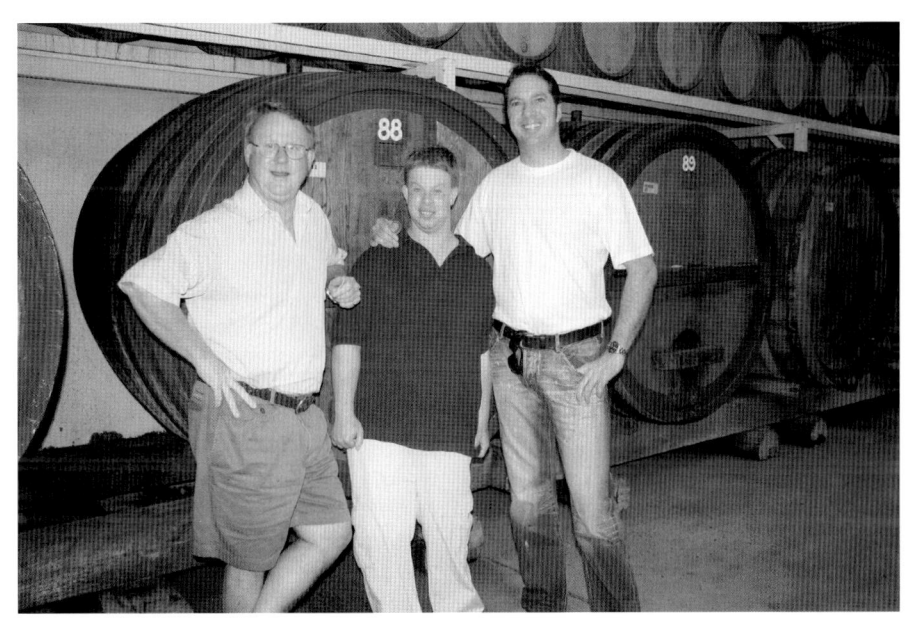

Bruce Tyrrell (left), John Tyrrell and Greg in the winery's cellar. Bruce is never too busy to take time out, and you can rely on him sharing a few stories and adding some humour to your day. We all look forward to John's new jokes – keep them coming J.T.

absolutely delicious. We have made it clear to her son John that even though we have an extremely demanding schedule, we would never be too busy to attend another dinner (hint, hint 'JT').

Greg regularly returns to the United States where there is a growing interest in his work. Arrangements have been made for the artist to return to New York to spread the word about the Hunter Valley at an Australian Tourism launch there. He's been asked to take on the role of 'Goodwill Ambassador' for the area and will be joined by other well-known Australians at the event.

Greg welcomes any and every opportunity to pass on the invaluable lessons that he has learned on his remarkable journey. He even regards the trauma and the suffering as an essential part of his ongoing progress. It has been truly a baptism by fire! However, he is convinced that he is a stronger person today because of the trials that he endured and managed to overcome. While he acknowledges the value of those hard-fought

my brush with depression

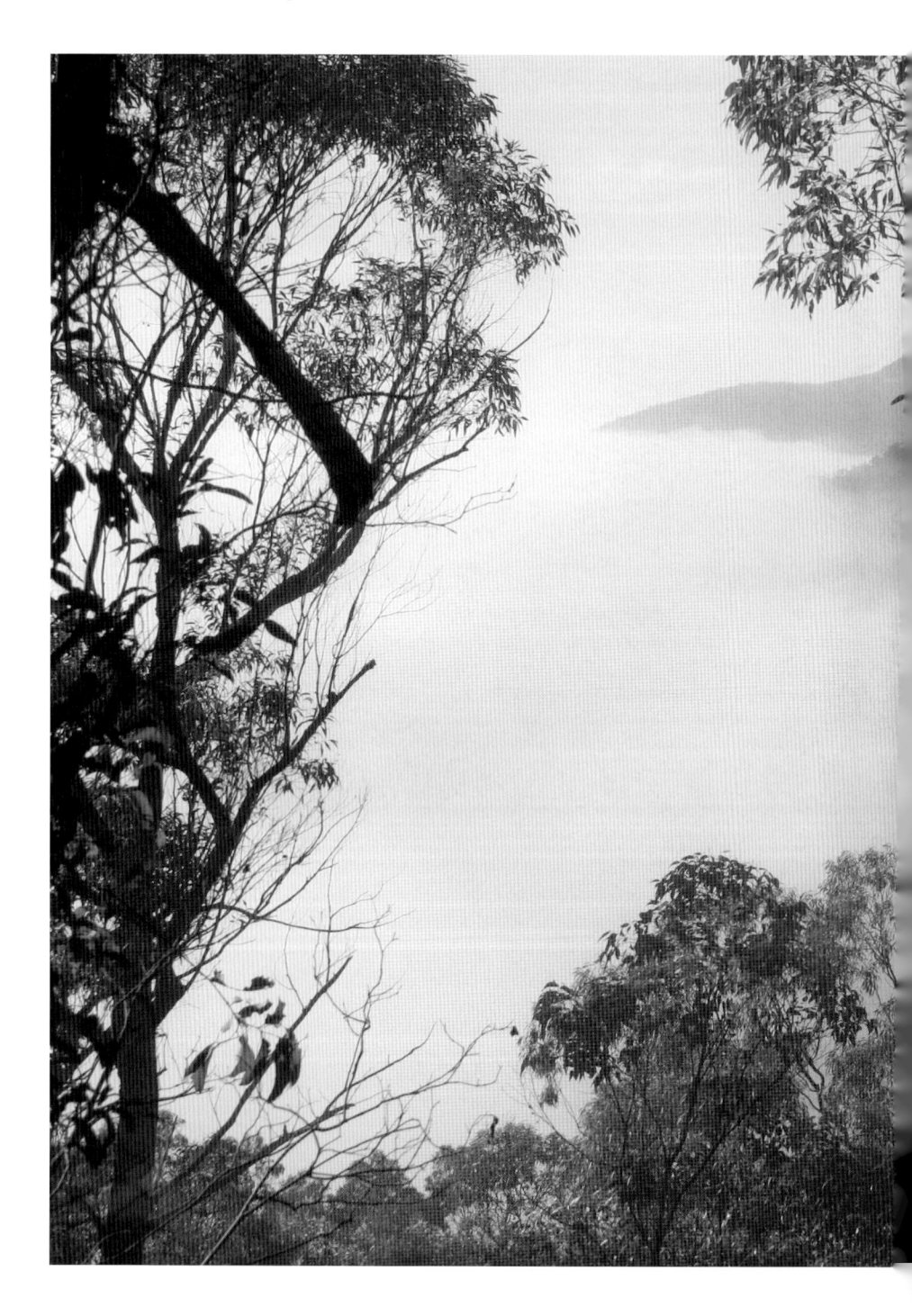

the rainbow's end

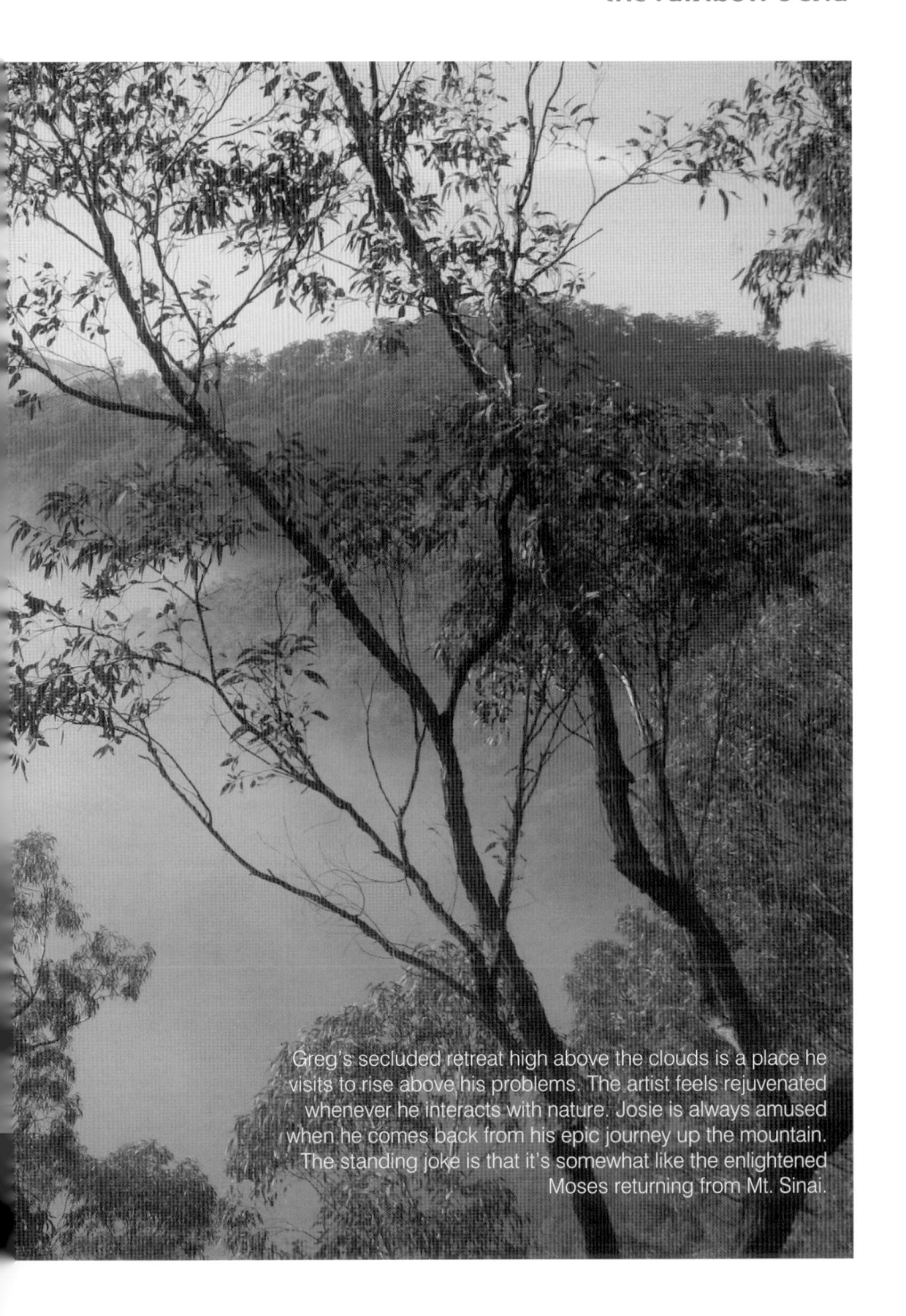

Greg's secluded retreat high above the clouds is a place he visits to rise above his problems. The artist feels rejuvenated whenever he interacts with nature. Josie is always amused when he comes back from his epic journey up the mountain. The standing joke is that it's somewhat like the enlightened Moses returning from Mt. Sinai.

battles, he is quick to affirm that a return to those times is the last thing he would want to happen!

He has come to appreciate more than ever that true success and happiness comes not from any material goods that one may accumulate, but in the presence and support of loyal and true friends. If honesty, trust and respect are the true yardsticks of wealth and accomplishment, then Greg regards himself as one of the wealthiest men in the world!

We have all shared the learning experience with Greg, and we have all savoured the wonderful outcome that our efforts have been able to achieve. To see Greg where he is today is one of the most satisfactory results that any of us could have expected.

The four of us all remain close friends living and working in the Hunter Valley, where we each have our own role in the business.

Josie works in the gallery, selling Greg's artwork and coming up with ideas to expand the business. She shows a real propensity for networking and developing new initiatives for the business. She still reaches out to as many people with depression as she can, and continues to be a tower of strength in supporting Greg.

She now has the garden that she's always so desperately wanted. With forty acres of arable soil beneath our feet it was only a matter of time before she began planting. She can often be seen raking a path, watering a flower bed, turning the soil to plant vegetables, or even pulling out the odd offending weed that threatens to steal nutrients from her nectarine, peach, orange, and lime trees. She is especially proud of her sunflowers and roses that line our driveway.

Joyce also works in the gallery, doing the accounting and acting as a sales assistant to Josie when things get busy. She keeps all facets of the operation running smoothly. Her reliability and dedication to the job means she is a big support to us all. She spends a lot of her time coming up with ways to improve the gallery. She has been arranging reproductions of Greg's work to be put on clothing, calendars, prints, and stationery items. She spends her leisure time walking amidst the serene vineyards and indulging in her passion for cooking. It's even better than she imagined in her daydreams all those years ago: 'It's French Kiss with an Australian twist.'

Greg loves his life in the Hunter Valley. He still has a great affection for animals. In fact, Greg continues to bring home the injured animals that he finds in the countryside and the property is now starting to resemble an animal shelter. We've had two birds and a turtle turn up in the last week alone! Greg was fortunate not to end up on the wrong end of a four-wheel drive bull bar just recently. He was moving three cows off a nearby road and into a paddock, concerned that a car might hit them. He almost became the victim himself.

Jess, our cockatiel, continues to sit on his shoulder and bring a lot of joy into his life. Jackson is his constant attendant both in and out of the studio. While Greg works solidly at the easel, Jackson inspects every can of paint and usually manages to collect at least a smudge from each one. We then refer to him as the dog with the coat of many colours!

Greg has never been a regular churchgoer. In fact, there have been many moments in his life when he has had distinct reservations about Divine Providence. Today, however, there is something deeply spiritual about his life. When he becomes overwhelmed with problems he and Jackson will often walk to the top of the mountain behind our home. There he sits and asks for guidance.

It was on that mountaintop that he was eventually given some of the answers that he longed to know all those years ago. Why was he singled out? Why wasn't he allowed to end it all when he was ready to give up? Greg says it was as if the answer was carried to him on the gentle breeze that brushed his face. An inner voice told Greg that he first had to learn what it was like to be the victim of depression, that he had to experience the pain and anguish that it entailed so he could understand the plight of others who were inflicted with its torments. His own battles with depression would now help others in their fight against the debilitating illness.

Certainly, his experiences have given his life a deeper sense of meaning and purpose.

With the same determination that has made him a successful painter and sculptor, Greg is sharing his inspirational story with others, hopeful that it will enable sufferers and their families and friends to understand and cope with the everyday stresses that are part and parcel of depression.

He works tirelessly to raise much-needed funds for charity, especially those associations dedicated to the treatment of mental illnesses. He has donated quite a number of paintings to these organisations for auctions and has raised tens of thousands of dollars for these worthwhile causes.

As long as there are people afflicted with depression, then he will continue to conduct his own special crusade – to try and extricate others from the horrible and destructive illness and lift them to a happier and more enriching way of life. Greg puts colour onto a canvas, but more importantly he wants to put the colour back into the lives of those who have depression.

It is a cause to which Greg is prepared to dedicate the rest of his life. He wants to convey the reassuring message that no matter what others say, no matter what difficulties we endure we can find happiness in our lives, even against the greatest odds.

He reminds us that through any journey there will be moments when we are confronted with criticism. It is important to remember that when we stand united we can overcome anything.

Perhaps his mission was most succinctly outlined during one of his observations during 'Australian Story'.

'I'm not saying that I have all the answers to overcoming depression. I am not saying do this, do that, or follow me! That's not what I am about whatsoever. All I want to say is that there is hope. Depression is not a dirty word. Now that I've reached the other side, and it's not as scary, I really owe it to people to share my story and say hey, you can do it too!'

He hopes that his story helps in some small way to enhance the lives of those afflicted with depression. His most fervent wish is that medical and psychological research will eventually lead to complete elimination of depression. Even though his purpose is to assist as many people as he

the rainbow's end

can to overcome the disease and lend his total support to mental health organisations, his dream would come true if the world were free of this mental torment.

Remarkably, the simple action of wanting to help a friend and share his message of hope with others has led me to venture into untried waters. The daunting prospect of committing to paper some of Greg's experiences and conveying his encouragement and recommendations caused me considerable misgivings! I launched myself into the project, buoyed by the simple hope that by enabling others to share such an inspirational story they might find the courage to emulate some of the principles that Greg had discovered on his epic journey.

However, I was faced with self-doubt; I feared that I wasn't good enough, and that I was wasting my time. Then, just as I had lent my support to Greg while he was developing as an artist, he gave me his full support as I attacked the formidable task of recounting the story of his eventful journey. His words and his example have taught me to have courage to follow my own path in life, even when it is intimidating and sometimes fearsome.

It's getting late, and as I approach the house I can see that Greg is still at work in the studio. He always turns out the lights when he has finished for the day. It is such a beautiful night, and the peaceful stillness that has descended on the valley causes me to smile with contentment.

What an incredible journey it has been, I think to myself. I only hope that this book conveys some of the hope and optimism that I feel as I survey the world that we now enjoy. I hope that it enables others to find that same peace in their own lives. I hope they come to believe that this demon, this ogre that we know as depression, does not always prevail as it did with the tragic figure of Van Gogh. I hope those with depression will continue their struggle with renewed vigour and determination, taking heart from the way in which my best friend overcame all the adversity that life threw at him.

As I continue to fix my gaze on the heavens, an old Hollies' ballad starts playing in my mind, and I begin to sing the beautiful lyrics beneath the starry evening sky.

'The road is long, with many a winding turn
That leads us to who knows where? Who knows where?
But I'm strong, strong enough to carry him
He ain't heavy, he's my brother … so on we go!
His welfare is of my concern, no burden is he to bear
We'll get there. For I know he would not encumber me,
He ain't heavy, he's my brother!
If I'm laden at all, I'm laden with sadness
That everyone's heart isn't filled with the gladness
Of love for one another.
It's a long, long road from which there is no return.
While we're on the way to there – why not share?
And the load doesn't weigh me down at all,
He ain't heavy – he's my brother!
He's my brother. He ain't heavy – he's my brother!

Greg interrupts my performance, as he opens our door and walks from our house.

'Are you okay standing out here in the dark?' he enquires.

'I'm fine,' I say. The song is still echoing in my ears, and I'm so moved by the words and the beautiful sentiments they express that I walk right up and embrace him!

'Hey, what's that for?' he asks.

He doesn't notice that my eyes are brimming with tears.

'That's just because I'm so darned proud of what you've achieved and what you've done. It's because I'm just so happy to be a part of our closely-knit group, our special family. I'm just over the moon that we still have each other, despite the incredible trials that we've been through … But we did it, Greg, we all did it!

I put my arm around his shoulder, and he chuckles softly as we go inside to rejoin the ladies. Tomorrow's a new day, and I just can't wait to see what's in store for us!

the rainbow's end

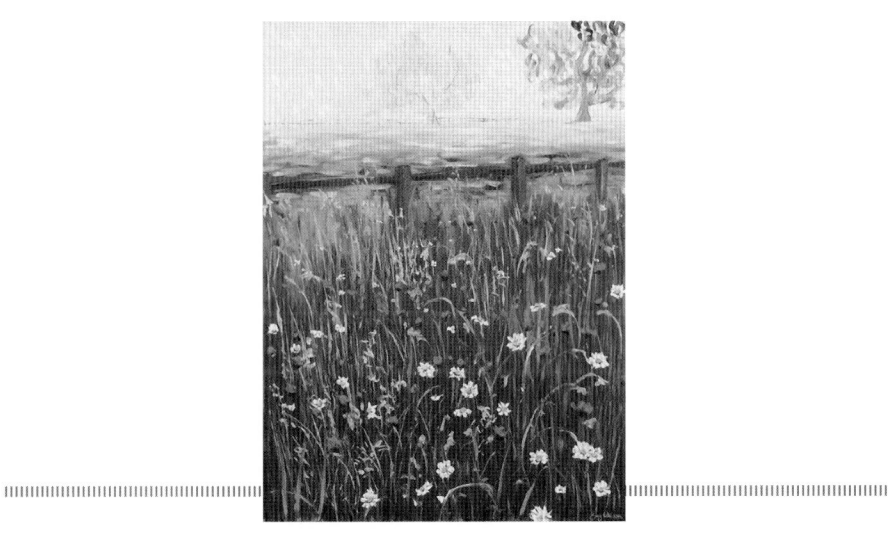

'New Day, New Beginning'
Oil on canvas, 910 X 760 mm

With each new day comes the
opportunity for new beginnings. We must never let anyone or any
situation break our spirit for it is ours to keep forever.

– Greg Wilson

appendix one

endorsements and testimonials

The ABC programme, 'Australian Story' was telecast on 26 April, 2004 under the title 'Colouring the Dark'. The TV programme guide included the following description:

'Successful international artist Greg Wilson once saw life as a series of browns and blacks. Suffering the agonies of depression from adolescence, he sought escape from its demons by speeding on powerful motorcycles and with other high-risk activities.'

The phones at the Greg Wilson Gallery in Pokolbin rang almost continuously for weeks after the show was put to air. We received over one thousand e-mails from viewers who felt compelled to express their appreciation. The following represent a small selection of those sentiments.

I watch Australian Story all the time and this is the first time that I have ever wanted to contact someone from these stories. The story that was told gave me goose bumps.

endorsements and testimonials

I will admit that I know nothing about depression and that I actually don't understand it either. I don't want to offend any of you by saying that I don't understand depression, it is just that I could not see myself thinking anyone would be better off without me so I don't have the understanding of how anyone could think that way.

The reason why I felt compelled to contact the three of you is to say two words – thank you! I know that your story was about the illness of depression, but it was also about the beauty of friendship.

I was in awe at the friendship, trust and understanding that the three of you have. You showed me what a true friendship is, standing by each other no matter what.

Today I have rung all of my closest friends just to say hello, it brought a smile to my face. I hope I wasn't intruding by sending this e-mail, I really just wanted to wish all three of you eternal happiness and every success in the world.

'Colouring the Dark' should be mandatory viewing for every adult who has never suffered depression in the form that Greg Wilson has suffered.

I have been suffering from depression since my teens, but to a point I have hidden it and continue to do so because family, friends and even health care professionals don't seem to take me seriously or to be more accurate 'don't believe in depression' – all of them have the attitude of 'just think happy thoughts and you'll be right'.

The saddest and most frustrating thing is I even find myself thinking this – I force a smile on my face and some cheer in my voice just so people think that I am normal, maybe even so I can try and feel normal. I suppose to a point, I have never been able to articulate exactly how I feel – tonight I finally heard it.

I was dumbstruck listening to Greg Wilson tell his story – his words, his feelings, his actions are almost a mirror reflection of my words, my feelings, my actions, my life.

My life at this moment is the darkest it has ever been. I feel lonelier and more helpless than I can ever recall. I can't sleep, I can't move, don't want to leave the house or even the bedroom, sometimes I can't even get out of bed at times, even simple tasks like cleaning my teeth seem pointless – even when something good happens to me I just can't find the joy in it …

I am still in the darkness, but after watching that story I now think there is hope… I find I tell no one about my illness … it is a hidden illness … Greg has helped me more than anyone will know.

Thank you.

I would just like to say THANK YOU to Greg Wilson, Josie Alder and Aaron, for giving us Greg's story. To Greg, I feel your hurt all the way, to Josie thank god there is someone like you out there to see through the Psychiatrists blur, and to Aaron everyone needs a friend like you. To Australian Story thanks for bringing such a revealing story to us. I imagine there are a lot of us trying to come to terms with depression, but with Greg's hope, I believe all of us can overcome this, as Greg has. Thanks once again the Australian Story, and keep up the good work.

A very inspiring story!

I have a wonderful 19-year-old daughter Jessica, who suffers from depression/bi-polar and like Greg's story Jessica too is learning to cope with her illness.

She is an artist, and I find that it is a creative outlet for her, but I am afraid to say at the moment she can't do it, what can I say to her, where do I turn. It's a long and difficult road.

She struggles with life at the moment and is ashamed to let people know about her illness. I wish all people with illness such as Jessica's, are empowered by talking about it.

Thankyou Greg.

----

endorsements and testimonials

As a sufferer from chronic depression since my teenage years I'd simply like to say how inspiring your story on 'Australian Story' on the ABC TV on Monday night last was to me.

Many home truths … hit home in your absolutely brilliant profile and the way you have battled this terrible condition from which so many of us suffer was an absolute inspiration to me …

Having read a sample of the many hits on the site, I realise that mine is very basic and perhaps lacking the flair and colour of those who have written to you, but as a fellow inhabitant of the Hunter Valley (I'm in Newcastle) … your story both moved and inspired me to keep on battling the black dog that is depression.

PS I would give anything to actually see an exhibition of your amazing art!

Thank you for your inspiration, am doing it the hard way, have my good days and bad days. My art has saved my life more than once. Some days it's all too hard. Trying to do the right thing by everyone.

Thank you Greg & Josie for your wonderful story. It has taken me years to acknowledge & accept my mental illness even though I'm still not out of the woods, but with people like you telling your story, I am no longer ashamed of my depression.

Greg, I am glad to hear your story. You are an inspiration to others with depression. Keep up the fight & keep educating the people. Glad to hear your dog is bringing you much peace and happiness. I know what you mean about finding beauty in everyday things.

To those with Depression – please seek professional help. You don't need to suffer with depression!

I thank you very much for the story, it has helped me to understand the feelings that I carried for many years, it brought me to the beyondblue

website and I have come to realise that I can't do this on my own.
I have reached out, thank you for bringing me my first step.

I feel that society, friends and doctors aren't getting close to helping people with mental health issues, but further away – it seems to be a problem that very few people want to address or care about.

Maybe Greg's story may open a few eyes, a few doors and a few minds that are closed to the idea that 'depression' really is a serious and painful disease.

I know that my depression will never go away, but maybe now, just maybe, I can feel there is a reason to get up in the morning, that eventually for me I will also see the other side of this dark, endless hell, just as Greg has.

Thank you ABC, Greg and your very good friends for sharing your life and putting your life and experiences into words that many of us are unable to find.

Wow …

I was totally enraptured in the Australian Story tonight. I could relate to Greg and his supportive friends. I am a recent graduate of art therapy and I was once again shown how art can be a supportive friend. Being creative in my life has been so central, it has given me my own unique voice, it has allowed me to create my own meaning of the world, without it surely I would not have coped. Greg's story has given me inspiration for my career and has given me inspiration on coping with the life I seek. When Greg said 'all he wants is peace' I heard my own voice echo. I encourage all the people who have supported Greg, to hear his story and the strong friendships and love that have supported him rekindles my faith in us, all of us.

As I watched Greg's story last night I found that I could relate to so much of what he was saying. As a city girl who has been through many bouts of depression, particularly over the past year or so, I have noticed my condition improving and my outlook on life lifting the more I escape from the city and get 'back to nature'. We are all so lucky to live in such a beautiful country and it is easy to find inspiration and motivation for life when we realise that we are meant to be part of this beautiful world too. Thank you, Greg.

I have suffered from depression, for many years, with similar experiences to Greg Wilson.

Tonight's programme assists in many ways, including … to reinforce the message that depression is not 'in my head,' that depression IS an illness and NOT my fault … and it also reinforces that message to 'well-meaning friends and family', that think you just need to 'get your act together'.

Well done Greg, great courage … I wish you more success and happy days in the future.

I would like to commend Greg on speaking out about his depression. I grew up in a family where both parents suffered depression and I never understood them until I was in my mid twenties when I experienced severe depression and again only recently. It is wonderful to hear of Greg's story how he has come through the dark periods of his life and is now 'living' life. Stories like Greg's give people with depression inspiration. I believe that you can manage depression in severe cases and in milder cases it can be overcome but only with persistence and assistance from people who love you and can support you. God bless you Greg, and also Josie and Aaron who have helped you through.

Greg, you have no idea what comfort I have drawn from your story. I suffer from Major Depressive Disorder & am currently going through the worst 'flareup/relapse/episode', that I have ever experienced before. When you spoke of your thoughts & feelings tonight and your desire to end not only your suffering, but the suffering of your family & friends, I felt like I was you or you were me that's how close to what I am going through now is to what you experienced. I know many depressed people, but none of them, by their own admission, have been to the depths of depression I am right now. I have felt so alone and I thought that no one could understand the 'pits of hell, misery & hopelessness' I am in right now. I have been in hospital recently due to being physically ill. During my illness this time I am suffering some debilitating physical problems as well. My doctor & psychiatrist tell me that the depression is so extreme this time that it is effecting areas of my brain, therefore effecting my whole body, even my immunity. I have had depression for as long as I can remember, even as a child. I have had at least four extreme 'episodes' of depression, but this one is the worst. I am 39 years & feel I have nothing more to look forward to other than more episodes of illness, each becoming worse than the next. I had dreams of being loved by someone but I feel that with this illness I would be no good to anyone. Greg I have never heard the words out of someone else's mouth that describes exactly how I feel, until your story tonight. I am heartened by your recovery to date. I know the illness is always there, but you have done the right thing & made your lifestyle & environment so that you lessen the chances substantially of a 'relapse/episode etc' ... Good luck, stay well & I will include you in my prayers tonight.

Greg's story on tonight's programme moved me to tears. I'm 18 and have lived with depression for a long time, and it was amazing to finally hear someone else voice their experiences. It's hard enough coming to terms with the diagnosis of a mental illness, but the social stigmas and misconceptions surrounding it make living with depression so much more difficult. I'm so grateful to Greg for bringing depression out of the shadows and giving hope to people who share his illness. There will always be a place for counselling and other medical treatments but I think the voice of someone like Greg, who has experienced and beaten depression, is the greatest inspiration of all. Realising that there is hope has made me determined to keep fighting.

---

endorsements and testimonials

There have been instances in my life when I've heard or seen just the right thing at the right time ... Thank you Greg Wilson ... tonight it was you.

I am just going through my third diagnosed depression, & so is my family. Listening to you talk about the way everyone who experiences depression feels was like a breath of pure air.

Everyone should hear it from the inside, because you are so right...empathy is very difficult, if not impossible unless you have been there.

We all need to inspire each other ... tonight ... you inspired me ... & made me cry ... & made me smile ... & I gave my children an extra cuddle for the day. Keep it up.

appendix two

how can you help if someone has depression?

Greg Wilson offers the following observations and advice based on his own experience.

WHAT IS DEPRESSION?

According to the *Diagnostic and Statistical Manual of Mental Disorders IV*, published by the American Psychiatric Association, to get a doctor's diagnosis of clinical depression you need to have at least five of the following symptoms, including number 1 or number 2, for at least two weeks:

1. Depressed mood (feeling low or sad)
2. Loss of interest or pleasure (in activities you normally enjoy)
3. Significant appetite or weight loss or gain
4. Insomnia or hypersomnia (sleeping too little or too much)
5. Psychomotor agitation or retardation (being restless and jittery, or alternatively, slower than usual)
6. Fatigue or loss of energy
7. Feelings of worthlessness or excessive guilt
8. Impaired thinking or concentration; indecisiveness
9. Suicidal thoughts/thoughts of death.

how can you help if someone has depression?

It's unfortunate that we sometimes use the same word for two different conditions – a low mood, and a diagnosable illness.

WHO'S AT RISK OF GETTING DEPRESSION?

Depression can affect anyone, and it is not limited to any specific background. Nor is any group immune to its effects. It disturbs many families and reaches into all socio-economic backgrounds. People with a mental illness are prone to recurring cycles of despair.

You are more likely to experience depression if you:

- Have a family history of depression;
- Are under stress;
- Are a perfectionist.

Mental illness is something that touches all of us. Most people have experienced some form of depression at some stage in their lives. It can be triggered by many causes: a relationship failure, illness, a dramatic life change, or losing a loved one. If we can 'normalise' depression and remove the stigma that is often attached then more people will feel comfortable approaching someone with depression. They will realise that it's not shameful to have depression and be less fearful about talking to others about their problems.

SYMPTOMS

One thing that I've observed from our classes is that people with depression often carry guilt. It is a very common symptom of depression, along with slowness and crying. People feel as though they can't do anything right. They feel as though everything they do is wrong. Normally they don't exhibit outward signs of guilt, but it is often an underlying element of the depression. Guilt is one of the biggest contributors to depression and it can be overpowering.

SUICIDE WARNING SIGNS

- Feelings of hopelessness or helplessness;
- An overwhelming sense of shame or guilt;

An obvious change in personality or appearance;
Irrational or strange behaviour;
Changes in eating or sleeping habits;
A severe decline in school or work performance;
A lack of interest in the future;
Written or spoken notice of plan to commit suicide;
Giving away of possessions.

WHAT CAUSES DEPRESSION?

Nobody is entirely sure what causes depression, but an imbalance in the brain chemistry is thought to be the most likely source.

It is a medical condition that is aggravated by stress.

Sometimes the causes of depression can be misunderstood. I remember one child in my classes said to me: 'People with a lot of money don't get depression.' This is not true, of course. Money can give us better opportunities, but it cannot make us a better person. No matter how much money we have it will not guarantee peace of mind. No amount of money in the world could have made me happy during my darkest times. It was not the dollar that alleviated my depression. It was my friends and a change in attitude that made the difference.

Aaron once told me a story about his visit to the local bakery. Whenever he went to collect his bread he would ask the baker how he was. He would reply, 'Terrific, Aaron, love follows me! I feel it and touch it everywhere I go. It is a beautiful day!' Rain, hail, or sunshine he would greet people in the same way. Aaron never saw him unhappy once, and his six children all grew up to be wonderful and successful people.

One of the major causes of depression that I have observed in my dealings with the children and adults is negative self-talk. The thoughts that they have about themselves are a significant factor in determining whether they feel happy or depressed.

Family situations can also be a factor: unrealistic expectations by family members; being unable to communicate with other family members; the fear of failing in the eyes of parents or siblings; and aggressiveness within the family can all cause depression. But before we go and point the finger of blame, remember that often parents are simply living the way their own parents taught them. We should remember to put our efforts into changing rather than blaming.

There are some harmful consequences for those who are reluctant to express themselves because they fear the consequences of doing so. They keep their thoughts to themselves. When they come across a problem in life, instead of voicing it they keep it in while pretending everything is all right. They are intimidated and scared of expressing themselves. Eventually a number of problems surface. Then one day the build up of tension inside is so great that their feelings cannot remain inside any longer. There is an outburst of emotion and their feelings explode. They may become physically violent or they might become quite abusive. All the feelings they have concealed come rushing out in a surge.

What I have learned through my own experience is that if we act on our feelings immediately they don't become so volatile later. I have noticed that if we continue to suppress our concerns they can rapidly develop into depression. As we've seen in my own case, sometimes a chemical imbalance might be a cause of disruptive behaviour. Depression can run in families. If we suspect a child has a chemical imbalance, we encourage the parents to contact the local doctor. Many types of chemical imbalances can be counteracted through the use of medication and support.

WHAT YOU CAN DO?

What I have seen is that when families instil in their children a sense of importance and worth, then those children are less likely to suffer depression. Having two parents doesn't mean that the chances of children getting depression are any less. Some of the most confident children that have come through the art school live in single-parent households. Some even live with relatives or a grandparent.

WHAT CAN WE DO TO MANAGE DEPRESSION?

To become skilled in any area you need plenty of practice and hard work. Beating depression is also something that takes time. It took me nearly five years before I finally broke the cycle that caused me so much pain. However, by being patient, following some simple techniques and putting them into practice, people can overcome it, or at least learn to manage it.

When we are trying to beat depression it's important that we try and put ourselves into a good frame of mind. We must be willing to change, and believe that happiness is possible for us. It is critical that we have the love and understanding of friends and family, and the love and understanding of ourselves, when we are tackling depression. If we don't have the support in these areas then mental health associations, telephone counselling services such as Lifeline, or the local doctor will try and refer us to appropriate supports in our area. Having support means we are far more likely to conquer depression.

It is equally important to identify any trigger that causes the problem. Normally, I believe it's a subconscious thought generating a negative feeling that causes depression. When we determine what that trigger is, we have to focus on changing or eliminating the particular train of thought that sets it off. We must redirect our thinking process, so the mind starts to dwell on more pleasant associations.

In order to defeat depression it is necessary to rid the mind of negative thoughts by slowly reprogramming the mind with positive thoughts. In many instances negative thoughts and poor self-esteem develop from our upbringing. The real challenge lies in breaking down some of the conditioning that is handed down from generation to generation. It's those demons – the harmful thoughts – that we hand our children that we must learn to destroy. We must teach our children to break these chains, so they avoid passing it on to their own children. Only in this way will these harmful ideas be eliminated.

I developed the following exercise to help me get rid of fear and negativity. I often use this same exercise when I am under pressure. Remember the time I was about to show my work at Paddington. My underlying fear could be traced to a single thought that had been slowly crystallising during my youth: 'I am not good enough.' What I needed to do was reprogramme that thought in my mind. An easy way I have found to do this is to superimpose a pleasant experience over the negative thought.

how can you help if someone has depression?

One of my favourite colours is blue, and one of my favourite songs is 'True Blue' by John Williamson. When I have my next unpleasant thought of 'I am not good enough', I will use this exercise by hearing the song in my mind, closing my eyes and imagining a brilliant, clear blue sky. The fear of something has now been replaced by far more positive impressions. Reprogramme the thought and it becomes less fearful. Every time we do this we can gradually break down the fear.

There are a number of additional steps that can help. To help children avoid depression we can follow some further recommendations. Teach them to be children by encouraging them to laugh, to paint, to draw, to read, to write, and to ride bikes!

Avoid TV shows and video games filled with violence that instils fear into their minds. My observation is that violence in these areas frightens kids and can make them act violently. Depression can easily follow such behaviour.

Another thing that is essential in helping children with depression is to make them feel secure in the knowledge that adults are here to help them make their own choices. It's important that we don't use them vicariously to achieve the things that we were unable to accomplish when we were their age.

We should also encourage children not to be afraid to express how they are feeling. Give them the confidence to ask for help and to communicate with others. Don't make them feel fearful or ashamed when they don't understand something. If they are having problems, we should teach them to confide in us so their problems don't escalate in their own minds. That's why Josie and I came up with a simple principle to remind us of the benefits of speaking up – and it's not something that has come easily to either of us.

We named the formula the *three R's formula: releasing, receiving and rejoicing*. The first step in the formula is releasing. If we release heavy thoughts in our mind – the harmful thoughts that go back and forth in our minds – then we free the mind. For instance, we might be having issues with somebody. If we express the thought to the person who is disturbing us, or at least express it to somebody that is close, then we will feel better and won't harbour resentment.

Fear of losing love, fear of not being accepted, fear that others know better, fear that we're not meeting other people's expectations – all of these can prevent us from releasing. Expressing themselves can be very difficult for many people, especially when they don't like to be in conflict with others.

We must learn to speak up. We must not lose our free will and freedom of choice by surrendering them to others. Who are the 'others' anyway? They are simply other human beings. Everybody is entitled to live the way they choose, as long as it is not harmful to another. Nobody has the right to destroy our dreams.

Provided we firmly believe in what we are about, we must be prepared to face criticism and even ridicule. What matters most is that we are being true to ourselves, and if we have this conviction then we are much less likely to fall prey to depression.

The second component of the formula is receiving: a natural consequence that follows on from the first. Once we have divested ourselves of our negative thoughts and feelings, we must dispose ourselves to welcome the stability and peaceful state of mind that will ensue if we allow it to come.

The third and final element of the formula is rejoicing. Once we have learned to speak up, rejoicing comes about because we are being true to ourselves and to our own ideas. We learn to love ourselves; we reach out and embrace the love that is all around us. We no longer fear and we are free to be who we really are.

We must never be afraid to follow the path to our dreams and goals. We have the power within us to achieve all our dreams.

There are some further observations I have made that should help children avoid depression. We definitely need to continue our children's education in the home, especially to reinforce the difference between right and wrong. We need to provide them with guidelines. This is surely one of the most important duties and roles of a parent!

how can you help if someone has depression?

Sometimes it's as simple as taking the time to explain why things are regarded as 'wrong', and encouraging the children not to make the same mistake again. We need to show them how their actions can sometimes have harmful or detrimental effects on others – and that such behaviour needs to be curbed. It is only by giving them a sense of moral responsibility, a sense of being an important and integral part of society that we can then expect them to undertake the responsibility that being a member of that society entails.

We must also keep in mind that no medication comes with a guarantee: we are all different, and what might work for one individual might not necessarily work for another. We mustn't be disillusioned if we don't seem to be getting the results we expected from our medication. We may need to try another kind and persevere until we find the one that is right for us. I took several types of medication before I discovered the medication that worked best for me.

To help someone overcome guilt, family and friends need to tell the person they are worthwhile and that they are important, even though the person may indicate they are not feeling receptive to any kinds of comments at all. Only by being consistent and regular in these types of comments can we chip away at their insecurities and give them a sense of worth. We should tell them at least several times a day that we love them, that they have a friend. Only in this way will we be able to build their confidence and trust, two essential qualities for people with depression.

Another thing we can do is point out the beauties of life to those with depression. We should encourage people to do things; to go for walks; go to the beach; visit the Botanical Gardens; go on a picnic; to be a part of nature and of life!

During our discussions with children and adults, I have made a simple yet powerful observation. I have noticed that *what my brain wills and believes in and is convinced it can achieve, the body will usually follow suit and fulfil*. Put simply, a wish is simply a thought. What we think is what the brain holds, and what the brain holds, the body can fulfil.

The brain is the strongest influence in these situations and can will almost anything: it can make us happy, it can keep us sad, and it can keep us depressed. The idea, then, is to keep the happy thoughts flowing and prevent the negative thoughts from prevailing.

We have seen first hand at the Greg Wilson Art School and through my talks how thoughts can influence behaviour . If children or adults have been filled with negative thoughts they become negative and far more prone to depression. If we programme a child or adult with love and hope then the opposite occurs. Children will grow up to be more positive and stronger adults who can achieve because fear or negativity can't get in the way. The thoughts children and adults have about themselves will largely determine how they lead their lives.

Here's an exercise that can encourage children to think more positively about themselves: get them to simply write down statements that promote positive thoughts, like 'I am clever', or 'I can do it'. Then get them to keep repeating this exercise until they start to believe what they are writing.

If children are saying comments that carry negative connotations about themselves, then it is up to us to discourage this behaviour. We are the ones who need to prevent destructive thoughts entering a child's mind. If we don't teach them, who will? Unless they are told otherwise they will continue to have these damaging thoughts and grow up believing they are useless.

Gently correct a child if you notice them implying that they are no good. For example, a child might believe that they are stupid. They say, 'I can't do this', or 'I am not smart'. Don't let them entertain these thoughts any longer. Tell them, 'It isn't so', say to them, 'of course you can do it', or 'I think you're really clever'. Then follow this up by giving them an example of how clever they are. 'You are so good at your drawings.' This will promote good thoughts and in turn it will generate good self-esteem.

We encourage all parents to give at least five positives to a child each day. Here are some examples: I love you! You're fantastic! You're wonderful! What a terrific job! You're amazing! Well done! I'm proud of you! Get the picture? These sorts of comments encourage good thoughts

how can you help if someone has depression?

about an individual. We must mean this when we say it, otherwise don't say it at all. Children know intuitively if we are being genuine.

We must *encourage our children's dreams*. Reinforce the point that anything is possible if the child allows it. Why? Because we have noticed in the classes that if a child is allowed to use his or her imagination and allowed to dream, and if you tell the child that anything is possible, they can will it to be. It helps generate their belief in themselves and in life. When we do it in the art school, we see some amazing results. With support, the shy retiring child who would not pick up a paintbrush is suddenly splashing colour onto a canvas and creating a little masterpiece.

Give children the permission to dare to dream. Because when they dare to dream they can make their dreams come true and all is possible. They can reach the stars. Nothing is stopping them from achieving anything. We stop ourselves from achieving because of thoughts that are left over from a past memory; often it is a harmful comment made to us in our formative years, things like: 'You won't amount to anything', for example. 'You're an idiot', 'Don't be so stupid, you can't achieve that'. When we say these words we are stopping a child from visualising and achieving their dreams. If you are a child or teenager and hear these phrases then strengthen your own resolve to believe in your dreams. Achieving is a goal that you set yourself. No one can take away your hopes and dreams unless you allow it. Don't ever let anyone break your spirit – it's yours to keep forever. Whether or not we achieve our goals depends on our state of mind. We must have belief in ourselves.

I think it is equally vital to tell people that they can achieve their dreams through effort and determination. Anything is possible but it normally has to be achieved through hard work. Doors will open but only if we reach up and turn the knob.

We mustn't give up on life when things don't work out as planned. We must keep trying and eventually we will find what is right for us. Life is a journey of many highways.

As my friend Martha says: 'Life is a journey, and the journey of life is far more valuable than the destination, because what we learn along the way will help us reach our destination.' Remember that it is up to us to decide what path we take in life and what our ultimate goal will be. Every one makes choices to determine their own destiny.

It is also important to tell our people that reaching their dreams often takes time. Tell people that life will be full of hurdles that they need to overcome. I often normalise this by talking about some of the hurdles I have had to overcome. Believe me when I say, there have been many. Tell them that making mistakes is all part of life, and that we learn from these mistakes and move forward. The word mistake is probably not the best choice of words. I prefer to use learning experiences because it doesn't carry any negative connotation.

We also teach children to *look upon life as a challenge: a chance to succeed*. In our classes we often tell children that they have a choice in life. If they want to work towards their goals they can achieve them – or they can sit back and miss out! We ask them what they would rather do. The answer is obvious. They all want to build successful lives. When life throws curves, and threatens to disrupt their dreams, children should be encouraged to look upon it as a challenge. A challenge becomes reachable, and the more determined they are to take the challenge, the higher are their chances of them succeeding.

If we can encourage our children to see life as a challenge, then they will grow up regarding life's difficulties not as insurmountable obstacles, but as rungs up the ladder of opportunity.

I use painting to encourage the children's ideas and to build their confidence. Helping children with their artwork gives me an opportunity to tell them that their ideas and efforts are good.

I believe with artwork that if the kids can do something they're proud of it builds self-esteem. If the kids are doing this at an early age they can actually take what they have learned into their adult lives. Painting can develop confidence and self-belief. It can also be a tool to help them overcome their troubles in the world. If they are feeling a bit blue and they do enjoy painting, they can use a canvas and colours to paint their worries away. It's almost like your worries flow out through your brush when you are painting.

how can you help if someone has depression?

We all need help; we all need someone to believe in us; we can't always achieve everything on our own; and we all need friends and family, or someone that understands us.

We all have a special ability, a purpose. Everyone has something to offer. It might not be as a painter or a writer, but we all have a gift deep in our souls. Sometimes it takes a shock to the system to uncover our soul's desire. In my case it took an horrific motorcycle accident to unveil my talent. I had to overcome my inner demons and fears before my desire to paint and sculpt could be unravelled. Sometimes we don't even understand what that desire is until we are forced into it. In other cases it might be more simply understood. It might only be the realisation to try something new. When we understand our purpose then life takes on a whole new meaning. It is then that we find real joy.

THINGS TO AVOID

Words such as 'cheer up', 'get your act together', 'just think happy thoughts and you will feel better' don't work. Telling people with depression they are weak-minded doesn't help, either. People with depression would get better if they knew how.

We've seen many children who are continually put down by their parents throughout their lives. Often the parents are firm and rigid. They tell their children that they will be unable to achieve their goals. Children who come from abusive backgrounds fall into this category. They grow up unable to speak their minds, fearing the consequences of the adult or parent. They hold in their feelings and thoughts because they fear the consequences of being themselves. They are not true to their own thoughts and ideas and are unable to fulfil their dreams. Their dreams are discouraged and they grow up with depression.

If they do not break the chains of their parenting they create similar situations in their own adult lives and for their own children. They grow up still fearing to speak their own mind, still fearing to dream – and so they re-create the same shortcomings.

Always remember, if we feed children positive thoughts, give them hope and challenge them to dream, then they can achieve great things.

If we give them darkness and doubt they will try and hide from such a dismal world, and they will always be fearful.

My own self-talk was self-defeating when I had depression. I was never made to feel confident so I thought that I was useless. This made me think my whole life was useless. Because I told myself that life was not worth living, I nearly made it become a reality, and attempted to take my own life.

Only when I started getting some positive feedback from those around me did my mind change. Phrases like: 'Yes you can, you are good, and you have plenty to offer the world' reversed my thinking. I began to believe that I could be something in this life. The positive thoughts given to me by you, Josie, and Joyce, helped me alter my state of mind. My fears slowly began to dissolve as I came to believe in my own ability. This change in attitude has allowed me to do things I never dreamed of being able to do. I always had the talent as an artist, but until I had the belief in that talent I could get nowhere. With a change of thoughts came a change in action. I have reached my own version of the stars by becoming an artist and by becoming someone who inspires others who have depression.

Try not to hold on to hurtful memories. Whenever I did this it only served to make me feel worse. Craving for my past only created despair. I came to the conclusion that I had to let go so that I was free to walk down new roads, so that I could make way for new and better memories. I had to learn to forgive. To forgive is to let go.

Don't let your mind think that you need something else to make you happy. Fantasy is not as good as the reality. Often we chase our fantasies, only to realise that when we have achieved them, that they're not what we thought they would be at all. We might want a new car, for example. We work tirelessly trying to earn the money to get the car. 'I need this to be happy', we tell ourselves. Finally, we get the car. We are happy for a while before the reality sets in and the fantasy is blown away. Having the car doesn't really make us any happier. Many of us move on to the next fantasy, unhappy with our present lives. The trick is to look at what we have, not at what we don't have. Be happy in the moment.

how can you help if someone has depression?

THE STIGMA OF DEPRESSION

Unfortunately for me, my need to take medication for my depression was not always regarded in an understanding manner. Some of my acquaintances actually confronted me and expressed their concerns to me personally. They felt there was a stigma attached to taking medication for mental problems, as if I had contracted some incurable disease or that I belonged in a mental institution.

Taking medication is nothing to be ashamed of. Yet you mention to someone that you are on antidepressants and they can become uncomfortable. It conjures up images in their mind that maybe you are just a little bit crazy or out of control. I have noticed that people can even become uncomfortable if you admit to having periods of depression.

Could you imagine approaching someone who had just broken a leg, and suggesting they didn't need any painkillers or a splint for the injury? Imagine taking them by the hand and telling them, 'We'll just walk it off! Time heals all wounds. You'll be all right!' Can you imagine the pain they'd experience, and how they would respond if you asked what they were crying about, what all the fuss was about? It would be inconceivable, and we would certainly be classified as either insane or sadistic! Yet these types of comments are still being used towards those who take medication for depression. Because some people can't see any physical signs of an injury they assume that those who have depression must be making it all up. Of course this is not true.

Compare depression with other conditions and you soon realise that it is somewhat unique. For instance, there is no stigma attached to the diabetic injecting insulin to control sugar levels. Nor is the chronic asthmatic ridiculed for taking an anti-inflammatory to make sure the airways remain open. The diabetic and asthmatic hardly feel bad for taking their supplements. Nor should the person with depression feel bad for taking medication to enhance the quality of his life. The medication makes me feel better, simply replacing the chemical that my brain is unable to make in adequate quantities. It simply acts on the part of the brain responsible for controlling emotion much the same way the medication an asthmatic takes works on the lungs. Just because it is an illness of the brain doesn't mean that people can't lead happy and successful lives.

    We need to shift people's perception so that they don't feel bad taking medication for depression or condemn somebody else for taking their medication. At the end of the day, it is important that we have quality of life. My life is certainly better for taking the medication, and I will continue to use all the help that medical science can offer me.

index

A
ABC Australian Story 231-3, 252, 256-63
 – response to 233
Alder, Josie 67-74 (*see throughout*)
Allen, Ken 237-8, 242
Ancona, Frank 215-20
apprenticeship 47-9, 52
art, as life-force 83-5, 100, 145, 152-3
art classes
 – for children 225-7, 274
art reviews 172
Australian Consulate, New York 237, 238, 240, 243

B
Batten, Evan 228-30
Belltree@Margen's Winery 236
beyondblue 225
Biviano, Joyce 81-5 (*see throughout*)
Blackmores Limited 234
Boyd, Arthur 151, 243
Bundanon 151, 243
bushfires 181, 228

C
carpentry 47-8
Champagne, Don 246
Channel Ten interview 228-31
Church, Gillian 165, 198, 230
Clarence, John 198, 224, 227
Cootes, Aaron 86-91 (*see throughout*)

depression
 – and children 267, 268, 269, 270-4
 (*see also art classes, for children*)
 – and suicide 224-5, 245, 265-6
 – causes of 266-7
 – effects on others 124-9
 – help, how to 267-74
 – onset of 62-6
 – patterns in 101
 – stigma of 277-8
 – triggers of 116-17, 121, 148, 229
 – understanding of 79, 115-16, 146-53, 245
destruction of paintings 93-5, 113
diet 69, 150-1

emotional isolation 41-6, 62-3
employment 52-3
 – self- 53
exhibitions
 – first, Pasadena Hotel 92-4
 – second, Global Gallery 155-63
 – third, Park Hyatt 164-6
 – fourth, Aust. Consulate, New York 240-3

F
fund-raising 252

G
Gallagher, Kevin 219
Greg Wilson Gallery 27, 194-5, 196, 197-201, 213, 250
 – as 'sanctuary' 201, 213-4
Greg Wilson Art School 272

H
Hawkins, Jennifer 241
Hunter Export Centre 246
Hunter Valley 27, 173, 184, 244, 250
Hunter Valley Gardens 173-7, 181

greg wilson — **279**

I
interior design   82-3

J
'Jackson'   28, 91, 251
'Jess'   33, 251
Johnson, Peter   38-41

K
Kennett, Jeff   225

L
Ladder 132   217, 218, 219, 241
Lifeline   117
   – Hunter Valley Region   225
   – Newcastle   224
lifestyle choices   150
Lord, Gillian   152
Lovelock, Damien   223

M
medication   79-80, 116, 118, 149, 229, 277-8
   – side-effects of   122-3
Mental Health Assoc. of NSW Inc., 164-5, 166, 198, 230
Mental Health Week 2003   223
Miletic, Robert   164, 166
mood swings   93-4,101, 113, 146
motorcycles   55-8, 70-1, 76
motivational talks   222-5, 251
   – to students   224
Mulham, David   180

N
New York firemen   216-20, 236
Norris, Dr Greg 'Becker'   79, 117

O
overseas travel   52

P
painting studio   32

parents   38
   – divorce of   51, 53
Payell, Kavita   231-2
Plante, John   219
Pokolbin   29, 181, 184, 192
primary school education   40
psychiatric treatment
   – disillusionment with   65-6, 73-4
   – hospitalisation   77-8

R
road accidents   49-50, 56-9, 76-7
   – injuries from   57, 58-61, 62-4
Rowe, Jessica   165, 197, 201, 223, 229
   – and mother's depression   198, 200-01

S
Sartor, Frank   224
sculpting studio   35
sculpture   101-2, 112
secondary school education   41-6
   – art classes   43
   – failing grades   46
   – leaving   46
   –woodwork   43
self-confidence   145, 149, 152-3
self-doubt   98-9, 119, 154, 169
self-harm   74, 119-121, 244
self-respect   151-2
self-talk   96, 148, 276
September 11, 2001   235, 236
stocktake of life   142-3
   – coming to terms   143
stonefish   44-5
substance abuse   49-50
suicidal feelings   77, 100
suicide attempts   22, 71-2, 129-33
   – effect on health   135-7
support network, importance of   116, 229, 246

index

T
TAFE 48
Tierney, John 224
Tierney, Pam 224
Tyrrell's Wines 246-7

V
van Gogh 244-5
  – self-harm 244
  – suicide 245
vineyards 29, 173, 178-9, 194, 221

W
Walker, Janice 165
Westmore, Dr Bruce 79, 115-16
Wheeler, Dr Dianna 240
Williams, Barbara 234-8
Williamson, Paul 45
Wilson, Lynda 38, 70
Wilson, Robyn 38, 66, 67, 70
World Trade Center 216-17, 235
worthlessness, feelings of 65, 94-9, 134

First published in Australia in 2005 by:
Pennon Publishing
59 Fletcher Street
Essendon Vic 3041
www.pennon.com.au

Text copyright © Aaron Cootes and Greg Wilson
All rights reserved. No part of this book may be reproduced, stored in a retrieval system, or transmitted in any form or by any means electronic, mechanical or otherwise, without the prior written permission of the publisher.

Every effort has been made to ensure that this book is free from error or omissions. However, the publisher, the author and their respective employees or agents, do not accept responsibility for injury, loss or damage occasioned to any person acting or refraining from action as a result of material in this book whether or not such injury, loss or damage is in any way due to any negligent act or omission, breach of duty or default on the part of the publisher, the author, or their respective employees or agents.

The National Library of Australia
Cataloguing-in-Publication entry:

Cootes, Aaron.
    My brush with depression.

    ISBN 1 877029 91 2 (cased edition)
    ISBN 1 877029 96 3 (paperback edition)

1. Wilson, Greg (Gregory Robert), 1970-. 2. Painters -
    Australia - Biography. 3. Depression, Mental - Australia.
    I. Title.

    759.94

Designed by Allan Cornwell
Printed in China through Bookbuilders

Photography:
Ian Hamilton – Limelight Films
Richard Gates photography

Where to find the Greg Wilson Gallery:
Shop 13, Hunter Valley Gardens Village, Broke Road, Pokolbin, N.S.W. 2320
www.gregwilsongallery.com
Phone: 61 2 4998 6772

Disclaimer: The diagnosis of mental health disorders requires trained medical professionals. The information in this publication is to be used for educational purposes only. It should not be used as a substitute for seeking professional care in the diagnosis and treatment of mental health disorders.

Some names have been changed in this story to protect people's privacy.